Fatigue in Sport and Exercise

Fatigue is an important concern for athletes at all levels, recreational sport and exercise participants, athletic coaches, personal trainers, and fitness professionals. The study of fatigue is also important for students of the sport, exercise, and health sciences, as it enables a deeper understanding of fundamental physical function and the limitations behind human performance.

There remains considerable debate about the definition of fatigue, what causes it, its impact during different forms of sport and exercise, and the multitude of factors that can influence the nature and severity of fatigue. The vast body of literature in these areas can make it challenging to understand what we know and what we still need to understand about fatigue in sport and exercise.

The second edition of this book presents a fully revised and updated overview of the contemporary research evidence into sport and exercise fatigue. The book examines the latest thinking into how we conceptualise fatigue, as well as how we measure it. The fundamental science of fatigue is introduced, focussing predominantly on physiological aspects of energy depletion, metabolic acidosis, environmental challenges, electrolytes and minerals, and the perception of fatigue as it relates to mental fatigue and the central regulation of sport and exercise performance. Each chapter includes real case studies from sport and exercise, as well as useful features to aid learning and understanding such as definitions of key terms, guides to further reading, and discussion questions. *Fatigue in Sport and Exercise*, Second Edition is an invaluable companion for any degree-level course in sport and exercise science, fitness and training, or strength and conditioning.

Shaun Phillips, PhD is Senior Lecturer in Sport and Exercise Physiology at the University of Edinburgh, Scotland, with 15 years of experience teaching undergraduate and postgraduate sport and exercise science, strength and conditioning, and physical activity for health students. His research interests focus on fatigue and human performance, and high-intensity interval exercise as a population health tool. Alongside his academic expertise, Shaun has provided research and consultancy services for elite and professional sport and health organisations, including the FIA Young Driver Excellence Academy and Rally Star programmes, Heart of Midlothian Football Club, The Scottish Institute of Sport, the Scottish Female Hockey Team, and the National Health Service.

Fatigue in Sport and Exercise

Second Edition

Shaun Phillips

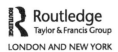

Routledge
Taylor & Francis Group

LONDON AND NEW YORK

Designed cover image: Getty images

Second edition published 2024
by Routledge
4 Park Square, Milton Park, Abingdon, Oxon, OX14 4RN

and by Routledge
605 Third Avenue, New York, NY 10158

Routledge is an imprint of the Taylor & Francis Group, an informa business

First edition published by Routledge 2015

ISBN: 978-1-032-35267-1 (hbk)
ISBN: 978-1-032-35265-7 (pbk)
ISBN: 978-1-003-32613-7 (ebk)

DOI: 10.4324/9781003326137

Typeset in Galliard
by codeMantra

Contents

Figures

Tables

Preface

Since the beginning of sport and exercise science as a standalone discipline, many questions about the function of the human body during sport and exercise have been posed and a great deal have been answered with a good degree of certainty. However, there is one question that, despite our vast increases in knowledge, research output, and technological innovations, remains to be answered conclusively: why do we fatigue during sport and exercise?

You would be forgiven for thinking that such a question would be relatively easy to answer. Most exercisers and sportspeople will have experienced some of the signs and symptoms of fatigue such as breathlessness, muscle soreness/ burning, heavy, tired limbs, and a feeling that the exercise is too difficult to continue with. Why don't we just trace the root causes of these signs and symptoms, and surely, we'll then discover the cause of fatigue? That's what fatigue researchers have been doing for over a century, and rather than lead us to a clear cause of fatigue, this work has served to show us the incredible complexity and sensitivity behind what appear on the surface to be fairly rudimentary physical and mental sensations. Whereas early fatigue research attempted to lay the cause of fatigue at the feet of only a very few possible causes, we now know that the number of variables that can influence fatigue processes during sport and exercise, along with the intricate and integrated functioning of the human body, is partly responsible for this complexity. This means that the reasons behind why we fatigue during sport and exercise are more keenly debated now then they probably have ever been.

The study of fatigue is important and useful for students of the sport, exercise, and health sciences. Not only does it provide greater insight into how and why performance (athletic, clinical exercise, physical activity, etc.) can be limited and therefore improved, but it also provides an excellent framework for better understanding fundamental discipline-specific knowledge (whether this be physiology, psychology, biomechanics, or others). Unfortunately, the teaching of fatigue is often overlooked or limited to a superficial overview of the "classical" theories. These theories often are outdated, significantly challenged by contemporary research, or simply wrong. I believe that one of the reasons sport and exercise fatigue is not more substantially taught is that the body of literature is so large and diverse that it is difficult to condense into an appropriate form. This was the inspiration behind this book: to address in one volume some of the key hypotheses and current thinking behind how and why humans fatigue during sport and exercise.

The aim of the book is two-fold: (1) to bring together current thinking on some of the key hypotheses behind fatigue in sport and exercise in order to help students understand and appreciate this fascinating area of investigation, and (2) to encourage students to widen their thinking and challenge their existing beliefs behind what causes fatigue in sport and exercise. Some ideas regarding the how and why of sport and exercise fatigue have entered general consciousness (at the expense of other equally valid ideas) despite significant evidence against them. Both the well-known and the not so well-known ideas will be discussed critically and fairly. I have no agenda behind this book other than to inspire a greater level of teaching and understanding of an important topic.

To devote as much space as possible to the topic at hand, the book is focussed exclusively on sport and exercise fatigue and will not include detailed discussions of common biochemical or physiological principles. The reader should consult any of the excellent existing undergraduate texts in exercise physiology to support their reading as required. The book focusses on prevalent hypotheses of sport and exercise fatigue that have generated significant research interest, along with contemporary ideas that are shedding new light on the topic. This approach allows old concepts to be clarified and corrected where necessary and new thinking to be showcased.

The book focusses predominantly on fatigue from a physiological perspective. The reader should consider that other factors not exclusive to physiology can also play a prevalent role in the fatigue process. Interested readers can contact me for further discussion of any information included in the book, or indeed of any information not included. The topics discussed in the book are intricate and often subject to intense debate. To fully appreciate this, the reader is encouraged to use the chapters as a foundation for further study by accessing some of the references cited in each chapter.

One final important point: do not read this book expecting that come the end you will know precisely what causes fatigue in an exercising human. You will not! This is not a failure of the book or of your engagement with it but is instead an accurate reflection of the state of knowledge in this field. I offer an insight into a fascinating, frustrating, and ever-changing topic of sport and exercise science research. I hope your time with this book is informative, intriguing, challenging, and enjoyable.

Shaun Phillips

Section 1

What is fatigue?

1 Conceptualising, measuring, and researching fatigue in sport and exercise

PART 1: CONCEPTUALISING FATIGUE

The study of fatigue in humans has been a source of interest for over a century, since the early work of Mosso[1] and Hill.[2] Despite huge forward strides in technology that provide us with a much clearer and in-depth perspective of the function of the body, many of the observations made by these early pioneers still provide the foundation on which we study fatigue today:

> The first (phenomena characterising fatigue) is the diminution of the muscle force. The second is fatigue as a sensation. That is to say, we have a physical fact which can be measured and compared and a psychic fact that eludes measurement.[1]
>
> With young athletic people one may be sure that they really have gone 'all-out', moderately certain of not killing them, and practically certain that their stoppage is due to oxygen want and to lactic acid in their muscles. Quantitatively the phenomena of exhaustion may be widely different; qualitatively they are the same, in our athlete, in your normal man, in your dyspnoeic patient.[2]
>
> (The limit of exercise) has often been associated with the heart alone, but the facts as a whole indicate that the sum of the changes taking place throughout the body brings about the final cessation of effort.[3]
>
> Fatigue of brain reduces the strength of the muscles.[1]
>
> Strength is kept in bounds by the inability of the higher centres to activate the muscles to the full.[4]
>
> It is not will, not the nerves, but it is the muscle that finds itself worn out after the intense work of the brain.[1]

It is outside the scope of this book to provide a detailed history of all aspects of fatigue research. However, before progressing, it is important to appreciate the historical nature of research into human fatigue.

DOI: 10.4324/9781003326137-2

1.1   Defining fatigue

Given its long history, it could be assumed that an unambiguous, universally accepted definition of fatigue has been developed, which all researchers and students of fatigue can use as a benchmark for understanding and applying knowledge. Unfortunately, this is far from true. The long history of research has only served to extend the number of available 'definitions' of fatigue (a non-exhaustive sample of these is in Table 1.1).

The definitions in Table 1.1 highlight one of the main issues in sport and exercise fatigue research: the inability to agree on a single definition of fatigue. This inability clouds the scientific investigation of fatigue, as there is no single meter on which to gauge and compare study results.[5] Why are there so many definitions of fatigue? This is likely due to three main reasons. Firstly, fatigue has wide applications across almost all forms of sport, exercise, physical activity, occupational performance, and many clinical and health conditions. Investigating fatigue in any one of these areas requires fatigue to be defined as it applies to that area (this has been termed in the literature 'fragmentation of fatigue' into discipline-specific niches such as clinical medicine, occupational health research, psychology, and physiology).[6] This fragmentation/compartmentalisation will have two primary effects: (1) it will inevitably make the definition of fatigue exclusory of (almost) all other areas, and (2) it will require fatigue researchers in those other areas to develop their own niche fatigue definitions. Et voila-you have almost as many fatigue definitions as there are fatigue applications! Secondly, fatigue can arise due to changes/impairments in the function of any of the processes involved in muscle contraction, from supraspinal initiation of the motor command through to the actual contractile processes themselves (Figure 1.1). This fact makes it very difficult to home in

Table 1.1 Different definitions of fatigue found in the scientific literature on fatigue in sport and exercise. These varied definitions emphasise the degree of variability in the quantification and interpretation of fatigue, even between those studying the topic

1   The moment when a participant is unable to maintain the required muscle contraction or performed workload.
2   Extreme tiredness after exertion; reduction in efficiency of a muscle, organ, etc. after prolonged activity.
3   The failure to maintain the required or expected force.
4   Fatigue produced by failure to generate output from the motor cortex.
5   A loss of maximal force-generating capacity.
6   A reversible state of force depression, including a lower rate of rise of force and a slower relaxation.
7   Any exercise-induced reduction in the ability of a muscle to generate force or power; it has peripheral and central causes.
8   Failure to continue working at a given exercise intensity.
9   Any exercise-induced reduction in the ability to exert muscle force or power, regardless of whether or not the task can be sustained.
10   A progressive reduction in voluntary activation of muscle during exercise.

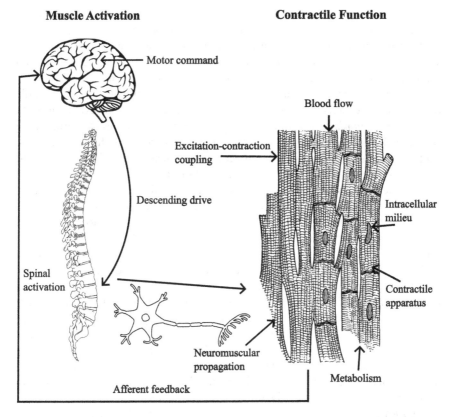

Figure 1.1 An overview of the physiological processes that can contribute to fatigue in sport and exercise. These include central (muscle activation) and peripheral (contractile function) processes, but the important point here is that any and all processes involved in voluntary muscle contraction are potential locations of fatigue. Re-drawn from Enoka RM. Neuromechanics of Human Movement. 5th ed. Champaign, IL: Human Kinetics; 2015:333.

on the specific site(s) of fatigue in different contexts. To assist in this, much research has attempted to isolate specific components of the functional chain of muscle contraction and study fatigue in this manner. For example, a muscle physiologist may focus exclusively on the peripheral excitation-contraction coupling process. The problem with this is that the body does not function in an isolated manner, so studying it in this way will at best give an incomplete understanding of fatigue and at worst give wrong insights. Thirdly, there are a huge range of factors that can influence how fatigue manifests in a given situation. Some of these factors will be discussed in Section 2, but examples include: exercise intensity, exercise duration, active muscle mass, type of sport/exercise, training status, diet, muscle fibre type, presence/absence of competition, environmental conditions, and health status. What is more, many of these factors can interact with and influence one another. Perhaps now you are beginning to see why "*it is easier to experience fatigue than to study it.*"[7]

Another source of confusion is that researchers often use the terms 'fatigue' and 'exhaustion' interchangeably. A person who is no longer able to maintain a given power output during a time to exhaustion test will often be classified as having reached 'exhaustion'. However, they may still be fully capable of continuing exercise at a lower intensity. The definition of exhaustion: "*a total loss of strength; to consume or use up the whole of*"[8] implies that attaining a state of exhaustion results in a complete inability to continue functioning, not simply an inability to continue at the current intensity. Therefore, fatigue and exhaustion are different constructs that should not be conflated. This becomes more difficult when there are examples in the scientific literature of researchers using different criteria to define and discuss the concept of exhaustion.[5,9] It is important to remember that in this book, fatigue is the focus, not exhaustion.

Look again at the definitions of fatigue in Table 1.1. In particular, focus on definitions 2, 4, and 9. Do you think these definitions adequately define and describe the complex, multifaceted phenomenon of fatigue? For example, definition 2 specifically refers to a "*reduction in efficiency of a muscle, organ etc after prolonged activity*" – should we interpret this to mean that there is no such thing as (A) fatigue during an activity (the definition specifically states after activity), and (B) during or after short-duration activity? Ask an 800-metre runner what they think of that! Definition 4 states fatigue is due to "*failure to generate output from the motor cortex*". This definition appears to discount the potential influence of other central factors and peripheral factors in the development of fatigue (Part 2 of this chapter). Definition 9 defines fatigue as occurring "*whether or not the task can be sustained*". Does this definition clarify or cloud the differences between fatigue and exhaustion discussed above? As you can see, not only might the multitude of fatigue definitions cause misunderstanding, but also the available definitions are open to debate regarding their veracity for actually defining sport and exercise fatigue in all of its poten-

> **Key point 1.1**
>
> *The term 'fatigue' has many definitions, and this makes the consistent interpretation and comparison of research findings into fatigue difficult.*

tial manifestations. Clearly, it would be useful if a single, 'unified' definition of fatigue could be achieved. However, care is needed here, as "*to prematurely arrive at a definition (of fatigue) that is only accepted because no better one exists may only confirm our own biases and misrepresent the reality of fatigue*".[5]

1.2   Conceptualising fatigue

Historically, fatigue has been broadly categorised into two 'types': peripheral fatigue and central fatigue. While recent research has proposed a fundamental shift in the way that fatigue in sport and exercise is conceptualised, it is still appropriate to provide an overview of the terms peripheral fatigue and central fatigue. To accompany this overview, Table 1.2 describes the key peripheral and central sites that may contribute to fatigue.

Table 1.2 Possible sites involved in the development of peripheral and central sport and exercise-induced fatigue. Adapted from Ament and Verkerke[9]

I. Peripheral fatigue

A. Exercise-related changes in the internal environment

1 Accumulation of lactate and H^+. H^+ is partly buffered, increasing carbon dioxide production from bicarbonate.
2 Accumulation of heat, leading to increased sweat secretion. The loss of water may lead to dehydration.

B. Exercise-related changes within muscle fibres

1 Accumulation of P_i in the sarcoplasm, decreasing contractile force due to cross-bridge inhibition.
2 Accumulation of H^+ in the sarcoplasm, decreasing contractile force due to cross-bridge inhibition. Accumulation of H^+ may also depress Ca^{2+} re-uptake in the sarcoplasmic reticulum.
3 Accumulation of sarcoplasmic Mg^{2+}. Mg^{2+} counteracts Ca^{2+} release from the sarcoplasmic reticulum.
4 Inhibition of Ca^{2+} release from the sarcoplasmic reticulum by accumulation of P_i (see point 1). Ca^{2+} release is inhibited by precipitation of calcium phosphate in the sarcoplasmic reticulum and phosphorylation of Ca^{2+} release channels.
5 Decline of glycogen stores and (in extreme cases) decline of blood glucose levels.
6 Decreased conduction velocity of action potentials along the sarcolemma, probably as a result of biochemical changes in and around the muscle fibres. This has no known immediate effect on muscle force production.
7 Increased efflux of K^+ from muscle. Increased K^+ in the lumen of the t-tubuli may block the tubular action potential and lessen force due to a depression of excitation-contraction coupling.

II. Central fatigue

1 The conduction of axonal action potentials may become blocked at axonal branching sites, leading to a loss of muscle fibre activation.
2 Motor neuronal drive may be influenced by reflex effects from muscle afferents.
3 Stimulation of type III and IV nerves decreasing motor neuron firing rate and inhibiting motor cortex output.
4 The excitability of cells within the cerebral motor cortex may change during the course of maintained motor tasks, as suggested by measurements using transcranial magnetic stimulation.
5 Synaptic effects of serotoninergic neurons may become enhanced, causing increased tiredness and fatigue. This may occur from increased brain influx of the serotonin precursor tryptophan, via exercise-induced decreases in the blood concentration of BCAAs.
6 Exercise-induced release of cytokines; IL-6 induces sensations of fatigue and IL-1 induces sickness behaviour.

BCAA's = branched-chain amino acids; Ca^{2+} = calcium; H^+ = hydrogen; IL = interleukin; K^+ = potassium; Mg^{2+} = magnesium; P_i = inorganic phosphate.

1.2.1   *Peripheral fatigue*

Peripheral fatigue refers to fatigue caused by a process or processes distal to the neuromuscular junction.[9] The concept of peripheral fatigue originates from the early work of A.V. Hill and colleagues in the 1920s.[10–13] This work led to the conclusion that immediately before termination of exercise, the oxygen (O_2) requirements of the exercising muscles exceed the capacity of the heart to supply that O_2 thus developing an anaerobic state within the working muscles and consequently causing lactic acid accumulation. Because of this change in the intramuscular environment, continued contraction becomes impossible and the muscle reaches a state of failure. Hill interpreted these findings to mean that lactic acid is only produced in the body under anaerobic conditions, and that fatigue is caused by increased intramuscular lactic acid concentration.[14] Coupled with study findings that appeared to demonstrate improved exercise performance when O_2 was inhaled,[15] Hill and colleagues concluded that the primary limiting factor to exercise tolerance was the heart's capacity to pump blood to the active muscles. This theory, termed the cardiovascular/anaerobic/catastrophic model of human exercise performance ('catastrophic' due to the predicted failure of homeostatic cardiac function), became the dominant theory within exercise science teaching and research.[14] A schematic of the theory is in Figure 1.2.

There are significant issues with the cardiovascular/anaerobic/catastrophic model of exercise performance. Firstly, consider the way in which many of the studies underpinning this model were conducted, namely with Hill himself acting as researcher and as a participant. Clearly, this is not the most objective or reliable research approach. Hill's background as a muscle physiologist may also have influenced his focus on the muscle as the loci of fatigue and pre-empted his interpretation of his findings,[14] although this is somewhat speculative. Third, Hill and colleagues stated that maximal cardiac output is attained due to the development of myocardial ischemia. Simply put, the heart cannot pump any more blood as it can no longer consume O_2 at a greater rate. However, the development of sophisticated monitoring equipment has allowed us to confirm that while a ceiling of cardiac output is attained during maximal intensity exercise, a healthy human heart does not develop ischemia even during maximal exercise.[16] Fourth, the model clearly shows that the attainment of a 'maximal' cardiac output limits blood flow to the working muscles, causing an 'anaerobiosis' that prevents oxidative removal of lactic acid. This results in lactic acid accumulation within the muscle that directly interferes with the contractile ability of the muscle fibres, causing muscle fatigue. The role of lactic acid in sport and exercise-induced fatigue will be discussed in detail in Chapter 3. It is sufficient to say at this stage that there is an increasing body of evidence which seriously challenges the concept that lactic acid is the cause of altered contractile function in exercising skeletal muscle.[17–19] Furthermore, there is a lack of evidence to demonstrate that muscles actually become anaerobic during sport and exercise or that O_2 consumption or cardiac output consistently reaches a maximal point (defined by a plateau in values with

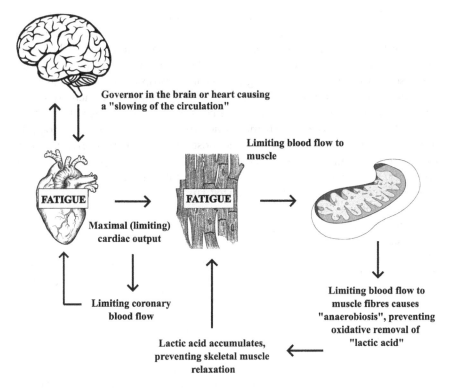

Figure 1.2 A schematic of the cardiovascular/anaerobic/catastrophic model of exercise performance. This theory became, and arguably remains, the dominant
paradigm on which the vast majority of exercise physiology teaching and research is conducted. Re-drawn from Noakes T. Front Physiol. 2012;3:1–13.

increasing intensity), which would be a requirement for their implication in
fatigue during maximal sport and exercise.[14] Fifth, Hill's model suggests that
the development of fatigue in the periphery would result in the brain recruit-
ing additional muscle fibres in an attempt to help out those fatiguing fibres
and thereby maintain exercise intensity, with this response continuing until
all available muscle fibres had been maximally recruited. Only at this point
would 'fatigue' begin to develop. However, this prediction is contradictory to
other aspects of the model, as continued recruitment of muscle would exacerbate the metabolic crisis (i.e. developing anaerobiosis) that the model predicts
causes exercise termination.[20] We now know that regardless of the duration
or intensity, fatigue develops before full recruitment of all available muscle
fibres. Approximately 35%–50% of muscle mass is recruited during prolonged
sport and exercise,[21] rising to only ~60% during maximal sport and exercise.[22]
Finally, refer again to the schematic of the model in Figure 1.1. Near the top
left of the figure is a picture of the brain with the phrase "*governor in the brain
or the heart causing a 'slowing' of the circulation*". Hill and colleagues proposed

myocardial ischemia as the cause of attainment of the 'exercise limiting' maximal cardiac output. If myocardial ischemia was allowed to develop and persist during intense sport and exercise, this would pose a clear threat to the integrity of the cardiac tissue, and hence the athlete. Hill and colleagues explained the absence of this life-threatening condition by proposing the existence of a governor, located in either the brain or heart, which reduces activity of the heart at the onset of myocardial ischemia, thereby protecting it from damage.[11] However, we have already mentioned that myocardial ischemia does not occur in a healthy heart during even the most severe sport and exercise. Therefore, different components of this model of fatigue do not appear to marry up. However, the theory remained, and arguably still stands, as the most quoted explanation of sport and exercise-induced fatigue.

Further issues occur when the model is tested against some of the definitions of fatigue highlighted in Table 1.1. Many individuals, from recreational exercisers to elite athletes, will identify with a progressive inability to maintain a given running speed or cycling cadence despite best efforts, a form of fatigue defined in example 8 in Table 1.1. Many have also perceived the reluctance of their muscles to provide them with a maximal effort when required to break away from the pack in the middle of a race, as defined in example 5 in Table 1.1. These are both definitions of fatigue where the athlete is more than capable of continuing exercise, just at a slightly lower intensity. Indeed, so are fatigue definitions 2, 3, 6, 7, 9, and 10. These definitions of fatigue, that have been subjectively experienced and experimentally demonstrated, cannot exist based on Hill's catastrophe model of fatigue. This is because the model states that fatigue is indeed a catastrophic, 'all or nothing' event that results in complete failure of the working muscles to continue producing force. However, with extremely rare exceptions, catastrophic muscle or organ failure does not occur at exhaustion in healthy individuals during any form of sport and exercise.[23] In this vein, the model also does not account for the observation that athletes begin exercise of different durations at different paces: a harder initial pace for shorter duration events, and a reduced initial pace for longer events (Section 6.4.3), and that they are generally able to exercise at a higher intensity during competition compared to training. This suggests two things: that physiological mechanisms are not solely responsible for the regulation of intensity (if they were, the athlete would surely maximise their physiological capability regardless of the duration of exercise), and that humans display an anticipatory aspect of sport and exercise regulation, possibly related to factors, including perception of task effort and motivation.[14] Clearly, this aspect of sport and exercise regulation cannot be attributed purely to peripheral components, i.e. the skeletal muscles (see the 'To Think About' example at the end of the chapter).

> **Key point 1.2**
>
> *Peripheral fatigue is the term for fatigue caused by factors that reside outside of the central nervous system, distal to the neuromuscular junction.*

Indeed, if sport and exercise is limited purely by attainment of a maximal cardiac output, as Hill suggested, then psychological aspects such as motivation, focus, and confidence have no role to play in sport and exercise performance. This is clearly

Key point 1.3

The cardiovascular/anaerobic/catastrophic model of sport and exercise performance does not satisfactorily explain many of the definitions of fatigue stated in this chapter, or many of the real-world observations and sensations when a person experiences 'fatigue'.

not the case. It therefore appears that the long-standing model of 'catastrophic' exercise-induced fatigue does not hold all the answers and is likely too simplistic to adequately explain the complex phenomena of human fatigue (Table 1.2).

1.2.2 Central fatigue

Central fatigue refers to fatigue caused by a process or processes proximal to the neuromuscular junction. Specifically, this refers to locations within the brain, spinal nerves, and motor neurons. Just as there are multiple definitions for fatigue, there are several definitions of central fatigue, although these definitions have similarities:

A negative central influence that exists despite the subject's full motivation.

A force generated by voluntary muscular effort that is less than that produced by electrical stimulation.

A subset of fatigue associated with specific alterations in central nervous system function that cannot reasonably be explained by dysfunction within the muscle itself.

The loss of contractile force or power caused by processes proximal to the neuromuscular junction.[24]

Some of these definitions are questionable. For example, assessing whether someone has the 'full motivation' to perform is difficult. However, the definitions are all similar in that they provide only vague definitions of central fatigue, with no specific information about locations or mechanisms of impairment.

On an examination of what takes place in fatigue, two series of phenomena demand our attention. The first is the diminution of the muscle force. The second is fatigue as a sensation.[1]

There appear, however, to be two types of fatigue, one arising entirely within the central nervous system, the other in which fatigue of the muscles themselves is superadded to that of the nervous system.[3]

The two quotes above were made in 1915 and 1931, respectively, indicating that awareness of the potential for both peripheral and central fatigue processes has existed for at least a century. However, the idea of a 'central' component to the fatigue process did not immediately become popular from a research perspective, perhaps because it was superseded by the work of Hill and others about a decade later that focused on the periphery as the loci of fatigue (Section 2.1).[14]

In fact, comparatively little research effort was spent on the role of the CNS in fatigue until the last few decades.[24] This seems strange, considering for how long the possibility of a central component of fatigue has been known. It is also interesting to note that the second quote above, which acknowledges both a central and peripheral fatigue, was added into the Bainbridge text at the request of A.V. Hill, the 'father' of the peripheral catastrophe fatigue model.[14] However, the central component quickly vanished from the teaching of sport and exercise fatigue, as the perceived importance of peripheral fatigue became more engrained.[14]

Central fatigue as a hypothesis may not have gained traction due to the publication of research findings that appeared to support the theory of peripheral muscle fatigue (Section 2.1). However, it may also have been due to limitations in the ability to measure central fatigue because of a lack of objective, clearly defined measurement tools (this is discussed further in the next section of the chapter). In fact, difficulties with trying to accurately test central fatigue theories remain to the present day (Chapter 6), although technological advances are making this more feasible (Part 2 of this chapter; Chapter 6).[25,26] A common research approach for studying central fatigue is the comparison of maximal voluntary contraction (MVC) force with the force generated by direct electrical stimulation (ES) of the muscle itself (Section 3.1). Studies applying this technique have reported a parallel reduction in MVC and electrically stimulated (i.e. non-CNS-mediated) force during repeated muscle contractions, leading to the suggestion that central processes do not play a role in muscle fatigue.[27,28] However, as Davis and Bailey[24] summarise, this may not be the case for the following reasons:

- Maintaining a maximal CNS 'drive' is difficult and even unpleasant and requires a well-familiarised and motivated participant.
- Even if a participant is well motivated, it is not always possible to maintain maximal CNS drive to some muscles.
- It is more difficult to maximally recruit all motor units during repeated maximal concentric contractions compared with eccentric contractions. Therefore, the reported impact of central fatigue on exercise performance may be influenced by the specific protocols used in different studies.

These issues help to highlight some of the problems associated with measuring central fatigue. However, objectivity in central fatigue measurement tools is important, as it helps to remove some of the potential subjectivity involved in the assessment of a persons' 'willingness' to continue exercise. The difficulties with objectively measuring central fatigue may be part of the reason why the presence of central fatigue is sometimes only accepted when experimental findings do not support any peripheral causes for fatigue,[24] making central fatigue almost a 'condition of exclusion'. Furthermore, quantification of the presence of central fatigue, for example by observation of reduced MVC force, does not offer insights into the causes of central fatigue (potential causes are discussed in Chapter 6).

> **Key point 1.4**
>
> *Central fatigue is the term for fatigue caused by factors that reside within the central nervous system (brain, spinal cord, and motor neurons).*

1.2.3 Peripheral and central fatigue: summary

Sections 1.2.1 and 1.2.2 have introduced the two overriding theories of fatigue in sport and exercise. It may already be apparent that both theories have limitations in terms of the research that has investigated them and in their ability to explain sport and exercise fatigue. In fact, the ability of either theory to independently, consistently, and effectively explain fatigue in all sport and exercise scenarios is highly questionable. This inability may in part be because peripheral and central fatigue are simply umbrella terms used to classify multiple specific processes that are thought to contribute to fatigue. As will be mentioned throughout the book, the body responds to sport and exercise in an integrated fashion. Therefore, it is likely that peripheral and central fatigue processes overlap and influence one another. This integrated response to fatigue may have been one of the drivers behind recent recommendations from fatigue researchers that we re-conceptualise fatigue itself, moving away from 'peripheral' and 'central' to viewing fatigue in a more holistic sense. Let's have a look at this in more detail.

> **Key point 1.5**
>
> *Considering central and peripheral processes as separate contributors to fatigue is inappropriate. The body functions in an integrated fashion, meaning that central and peripheral fatigue processes likely overlap and influence one another.*

1.2.4 Fatigue as a symptom

In 2016, the journal Medicine and Science in Sports and Exercise published a series of articles on many aspects of fatigue. One of these articles, by esteemed fatigue researchers Roger Enoka and Jacques Duchateau, proposed a new model for the conceptualisation of fatigue in sport and exercise.[6] The proposal was driven in large part as an attempt to overcome some of the known challenges with studying fatigue (see Part 1 of this chapter). As Enoka and Duchateau[6] point out, the fragmentation of fatigue has led to the absence of a universal definition of fatigue and the development of questionable experimental models to study it, which in turn has limited our ability to evaluate the functional impact of fatigue on human performance. The 'new' model attempts to provide a unified definition of fatigue, a taxonomy encompassing the range of conditions associated with fatigue, and a general experimental approach for evaluating the effect of fatigue on performance.[6] Let's begin by having a look at the proposed unified definition of fatigue and the associated taxonomy.

Within the model proposed by Enoka and Duchateau,[6] fatigue is no longer modified by adjectives that indicate the hypothesised 'locations' of fatigue (e.g. central fatigue, peripheral fatigue, physical fatigue). Instead, fatigue is defined as "*a disabling symptom in which physical and cognitive function is limited by interactions between performance fatigability and perceived fatigability*".[6] The word 'symptom' is an interesting one. If you look in a dictionary, you will see symptom defined as "*any feeling of illness or physical or mental change that is caused by a particular disease*". You would probably agree that fatigue manifests as physical and/or mental changes but caused by a particular disease? Surely this would not be relevant to sport and exercise fatigue, as neither sport nor exercise are diseases?! Well, pull that dictionary out again and look up 'disease': "*A disorder of … function…especially one that produces specific symptoms…and is not simply a direct result of physical injury*". Can sport and exercise cause disordered function? Yes, it can, even if only temporary. Can that sport/exercise-induced disordered function produce specific symptoms? Yes, it can. Does this sport/exercise-induced disordered function and associated symptoms have to be due to physical injury? No. It seems, therefore, that sport/exercise can be thought of as a disease! Or, perhaps more appropriately, something that can place the body in a state of dis-ease (not at ease), which is exactly what sport and exercise is: a (positive) stressor that disrupts the homeostasis of body systems. An obvious benefit of a single definition like this is that it should make the fatigue literature more coherent, as everyone would be framing their work within the same definition.

If we accept the definition of fatigue as it is stated in the previous paragraph, then the next step is to have a look at the proposed taxonomy of fatigue (presented in Figure 1.3). This

> **Key point 1.6**
>
> *An alternative model of fatigue defines fatigue as a disabling symptom whereby physical and cognitive function is limited by interactions between performance fatigability and perceived fatigability. This definition removes the need to modify fatigue with adjectives such a peripheral, central, and supraspinal.*

taxonomy, adapted from the work of Kluger *et al.*[29] on fatigue in neurologic illnesses, proposes that fatigue as a symptom of disease (or dis-ease) manifests via the interactive contributions of two attributes: perceived fatigability and performance fatigability. Enoka and Duchateau[6] define perceived fatigability as "*changes in the sensations that regulate the integrity of the performer*", and performance fatigability as "*the decline in an objective measure of performance over a discrete period*". While it could be tempting to view perceived and performance fatigability and their associated modulating factors as distinct entities, this separation is precisely what the model is trying to move away from. Look more carefully at Figure 1.3 and you will see that some of the moderating factors of perceived fatigability can also directly influence performance fatigability (e.g. blood glucose, core temperature, metabolites), and vice versa. Therefore, it is important to remember that the contributions of perceived and performance fatigability to the development of fatigue are *interactive*.

The proposed unified definition of fatigue and the associated taxonomy also have a significant impact on how fatigue is investigated in research. Firstly, if fatigue is accepted to be a symptom, then it can only be measured via self-report (see Part 2 of this chapter). As Enoka and Duchateau[6] discuss, common measures of fatigue such as time to complete a task and decline in power output are components of performance fatigability (Figure 1.3) but do not provide a measure of the intensity of fatigue as a symptom. To gather this information requires participants to provide responses to standardised questions. Doing so will allow quantification of the sensation of fatigue as a trait (e.g. average amount of fatigue in the preceding 7 days) or a state (level of fatigue at a specific instant in time) property.

Key point 1.7

Within the new model of fatigue, the presence and severity of fatigue can only be measured via self-report methods.

As you have probably already surmised, if we are to change how we define and therefore measure fatigue, fundamental changes to the design of fatigue research projects are also required. Historically, as touched on above, fatigue research has sought to quantify the degree of impairment in a specific outcome measure(s) during a specific sport/exercise task, usually under the guise of studying 'central fatigue', 'peripheral fatigue', 'supraspinal fatigue', etc. In contrast, the method proposed by Enoka and Duchateau[6] involves three steps: (1) choose a criterion measure of performance that is influenced by fatigue; (2) identify a laboratory test that is a good predictor of that criterion measure of performance; and (3) carry out research to understand the relative impact of the appropriate modulating factors (see Figure 1.3) on performance limitations on the criterion test. This approach would also involve self-report measurement of fatigue severity. It is important to note that this approach should not involve measuring all of the proposed modulating factors in Figure 1.3, but selecting in an evidence-based manner

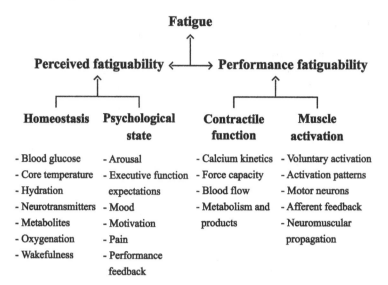

Figure 1.3 The proposed taxonomy of fatigue where fatigue is defined as a self-reported disabling symptom that develops via the interactive effects of two overarching attributes: perceived fatigability and performance fatigability. Each of these attributes has two domains that are themselves dependent on a number of modulating factors. The severity of fatigue experienced by the individual is dependent on the change in the two attributes. Re-drawn from Enoka RM, Duchateau J. Med Sci Sports Exerc. 2016;48(11):2228–2238.

those factors that are most likely to contribute to fatigue in the chosen criterion test. This approach to fatigue research may also necessitate the development of appropriately robust laboratory measures of the desired criterion performance before specific mechanistic fatigue research can be conducted.[6] However, this more standardised approach to fatigue research may enable (1) more coherent and comparable research findings, and (2) better translation of fatigue research to practice. That being said, there are challenges in this approach, primary amongst them being how to ensure accurate and truthful self-reporting of fatigue severity (particularly when working with elite/competitive performers, who may have a vested interest in downplaying the impact of fatigue on their

Key point 1.8

Within the new model, fatigue research would follow these steps: (1) choose a criterion measure of performance that is influenced by fatigue; (2) identify a laboratory test that is a good predictor of that criterion measure of performance; and (3) carry out research to understand the relative impact of the appropriate modulating factors on performance limitations on the criterion test.

performance).[6] At the time of writing, it is unclear to what extent this 'new' method of researching fatigue has been adopted. However, I encourage you to read the Enoka and Duchateau[6] paper to fully appreciate the messages it contains.

PART 2: MEASURING FATIGUE

To better understand sport and exercise fatigue research, it is important to appreciate how fatigue can be measured and assessed. The following is a brief introduction to some of the common methods of measuring fatigue. The section is split into discussion of direct and indirect methods of fatigue measurement and also includes potential tools for the quantification of fatigue as a self-reported symptom, in line with the discussion in Section 2.4. This structure most accurately reflects the way that fatigue has and still continues to be measured in research while acknowledging how this measurement may change in the future.

1.3 Direct methods of fatigue measurement

1.3.1 *Maximal voluntary force generation/ electrical stimulation*

Accurate measurement of the force-generating capacity of muscle is crucial for the reliable assessment of muscle fatigue.[30] Maximal voluntary force production (via MVC assessment) is often used for this purpose. Participants are instructed to exert what they believe to be their maximum force in a concentric, eccentric, or isometric contraction against a piece of apparatus that can measure the force produced. Strong verbal encouragement is provided to assist the participant in reaching a true maximal contraction. There are numerous examples in the literature of the use of MVC force as an indication of fatigue. For example, Nybo and Nielsen[31] investigated the influence of hyperthermia on fatigue following exercise to exhaustion at 60% $\dot{V}O_2$max in temperatures of 40°C and 18°C. Following exercise, participants undertook a 2-minute MVC of the knee extensor muscles with force output continually monitored. While force decreased over the 2 minutes in both trials, the drop was significantly greater in the hot trial, indicating a negative effect of hyperthermia on force production and, hence, greater central fatigue. However, there are concerns with the use of MVC for assessing fatigue. Force production can be limited by the voluntary effort/motivation of the participant. Not even strong encouragement and feedback may be sufficient to enable someone to achieve a true maximal contraction.[30] Furthermore, MVC can be limited by factors present within the CNS or in the periphery.

How, therefore, were Nybo and Nielsen[31] able to conclude that reduced force in the hot exercise trial was due to greater levels of central fatigue? The answer is they also utilised a technique called ES. Here, an electrical stimulus is externally applied to the motor neuron of the muscle, or directly to the muscle itself, which causes it to contract. This is usually done in short, repeated bursts, or twitches, to prevent overstimulation of the muscle that can attenuate force production and lead to an incorrect interpretation of muscle fatigue.[32] The important concept behind ES is that it removes the CNS from the equation as the ES to contract the muscle is externally and directly applied. Therefore, potential limitations to muscle contraction present in the CNS can be discounted, and the ability of the muscle itself to contract is isolated. Voluntary contractile ability can be interpreted using the simple formula:

MVC/MVC + ES

where MVC is the MVC force and ES is the force generated by direct ES, superimposed onto the MVC (and referred to as total muscle force). Solving this equation provides the voluntary activation percentage, which is the percentage of the total muscle force that can be achieved by a voluntary contraction. As the right side of the equation includes the muscle force produced by isolated, non-CNS-mediated contractile force, the voluntary activation percentage provides an estimate of the degree of central activation present in any given muscle contraction.

1.3.2   *High-frequency and low-frequency fatigue*

High frequency fatigue (HFF) is characterised by attenuated force production at high frequencies of muscle stimulation. High-frequency force production is quite well preserved in most situations, except for those involving processes that directly impair the ability of the cross-bridges to generate force (this would attenuate force equally across all stimulation frequencies).[33] This preservation stems at least in part by the fact that most voluntary muscle contractions (including those in sport and exercise) can be maintained with motor neuron discharge rates of approximately 30 Hz,[33] yet firing rates can increase to >100 Hz (although force development essentially plateaus with firing rates >50 Hz).[33,34] Therefore, there may be a buffer range of high discharge frequencies that can be utilised by motor neurons to maintain force production. However, motor neuron discharge rates will depend on the muscle fibre/group and the nature of the muscle contraction.

Low frequency fatigue (LFF) is characterised by a proportionally greater loss of force during low frequency compared with high-frequency muscle stimulation.[35] This form of fatigue can take hours or even days to dissipate and may play a key role in the decline in muscle force production.[35] LFF is typically interpreted by measuring torque responses to different frequencies of ES and examining changes in the ratio of force production at a given frequency (usually 20 Hz) to that at a standardised frequency (usually 50 or 80 Hz). Decreases in this ratio are interpreted as LFF. LFF may increase the requirement for greater CNS activation to elicit a given muscle force.[35] Consequently, this could cause an increase in effort perception for a given force production, potentially contributing to the development of central fatigue.

LFF has been reported during high-intensity and submaximal exercise[36] and therefore has the potential to be used as a fatigue measure during a variety of exercise scenarios. The use of ES to quantify LFF may be subject to limitations, including preferential recruitment of fast-twitch motor units near the sites of ES, potentially overestimating fatigue due to the greater fatigability of fast twitch units,[37] varied recruitment thresholds of motor neuron axons so that different motor units may be recruited by ES in different trials,[38] and the inability of ES to accurately account for the influence of muscle damage on LFF, as ES only stimulates a fraction of the muscle mass and damage is not uniform throughout a muscle.[39] However, Martin *et al.*[40] reported that LFF can be accurately assessed by ES via large surface electrodes (termed transcutaneous stimulation). Assessment of LFF is of course limited in its applicability by the requirement to use laboratory-based ES on a small amount of muscle mass during exercise that is not representative of most sporting situations.

> **Key point 1.9**
>
> *Many of the techniques commonly used to measure fatigue during sport and exercise are limited in their ability to measure fatigue during real-world sport-specific activities.*

1.4   Indirect methods of fatigue measurement

1.4.1   Endurance time ('time to exhaustion')

Many research studies have used an endurance test, commonly known as a time to exhaustion test, to assess and/or quantify fatigue, particularly the influence of an intervention on fatigue development. Use of these tests is partly based on the assumption that there is a relationship between the force-generating capacity of muscles and the time to exhaustion.[30] However, this assumed relationship has been demonstrated to vary considerably, at least during repeated isometric contractions.[41] Also, gross time to exhaustion tests (e.g. a cycle to exhaustion at 80% $\dot{V}O_2$max) exhibits large coefficients of variation (up to ~35%),[42] suggesting that time to exhaustion tests should not be the only measure used to determine the influence of a treatment on performance/fatigue.[43] Conversely, research has shown that treadmill-based time to exhaustion tests are inherently reliable when time to exhaustion is transformed using statistical modelling based on the speed-duration relationship.[44] However, the runs in the Hinckson and Hopkins[44] study only lasted between ~2 and 8 minutes. Most other research into the reliability of time to exhaustion tests has used longer duration exercise, which may be less reliable than shorter exercise due to the multitude of factors that can influence a person's decision of whether or not to continue, such as motivation and boredom. In addition, the variability in time to exhaustion of the shorter runs before statistical modelling (9%–16%) was still quite large. It is this variability that may be the major issue with use of time to exhaustion tests. Alghannam *et al.*[45] reported reliable time to exhaustion during two treadmill runs at 70% $\dot{V}O_2$max separated by 3 weeks. However, the mean difference in run time between the first and second run was 5 minutes. If a time to exhaustion test with a 'natural' 5 minute difference between successive tests was used to assess the effect of an intervention on fatigue, or the moderating effect of fatigue on athletic performance, then the genuine impact of the intervention/fatigue would need to manifest as a change in time to exhaustion of greater than 5 minutes (perhaps substantially greater) for it to stand out above the inherent 'noise' of the time to exhaustion test itself. This issue is reinforced by Succi *et al.*[46], who reported that the reliability of cycling time to exhaustion is affected by the intensity of the cycle, is modestly reliable, and may not be sensitive enough to detect real change. Time to exhaustion tests in fatigue research should be used with care and consideration of their ability to detect what the authors wish to observe, and if they are used, steps should be taken to minimise the variability in outcome between subsequent tests. Finally, if working with athletic populations in research or practice, the relevance of a time to exhaustion test to athletic performance should be carefully considered.

1.4.2   Electromyography

Electromyography (EMG) is the analysis of the electrical activity of muscle tissue. The two common forms of EMG are surface EMG (non-invasive) and needle EMG (invasive). For ethical reasons, surface EMG is most prevalent in the sport and exercise literature. Here, surface electrodes are attached to specific locations on the muscle (Figure 1.4). These electrodes detect the electrical signal transmitted through the superficial muscle tissue, allowing the amplitude of the electrical activity to be determined. The amplitude of the signal is related to the number and size of action potentials (electrical signals transmitted down motor neurons into the muscle). Changes in the frequency of these action potentials or in the number of muscle fibres activated can be detected; however, EMG cannot distinguish between these two occurrences.[27]

EMG amplitude falls progressively during repeated maximal isometric contractions, likely due to a reduction in the activity of motor units and, hence, a reduction in muscle force production.[40] However, this does not automatically mean that EMG is a good indicator of muscle fatigue, as the cause and effect relationship between EMG amplitude and fatigue is still under debate. During repeated or sustained submaximal contractions, a rise in EMG activity is seen in the presence of a reduction in muscle force production (i.e. muscle electrical activity is increasing yet force is reducing). This is probably due to the progressive requirement for more muscle fibre recruitment as contractions progress and existing muscle fibres begin to fatigue.[27] However, during repeated submaximal contractions, there is a large inter-participant variability

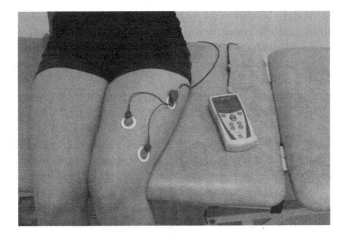

Figure 1.4 Surface electromyography of the quadriceps muscles.

in EMG response. Furthermore, EMG principally records the neural component of muscle contraction; if causes of reduced muscle force production were occurring inside the muscle, independent of neural input, EMG would not detect this.[27] Finally, EMG data is most valid during isometric contractions, as changes in muscle length alter the relationship between EMG and neuromuscular activation.[27] While acceptable EMG data can be derived from carefully controlled dynamic contractions, for example in a laboratory setting, capturing valid EMG data during muscle contractions representative of normal sport and exercise situations remains a significant challenge.

More recent research has harnessed technological improvements in an attempt to make EMG analysis a more practical tool for assessing neuromuscular function during sport and exercise. A sock-type wearable EMG device has been developed to measure EMG activity of the lower leg,[47] along with other forms of wearable and Bluetooth-connected EMG sensors.[48,49] However, these devices still have issues, such as the inability to view/analyse data in real-time and limitations on the number of EMG analysis channels and sampling frequency. A wearable EMG patch that allows real-time monitoring has been developed,[50] but the worth of these new avenues of EMG analysis in real-world sport and exercise applications is not yet clear. The overall consensus is that more work needs to be done to better standardise the EMG protocols and analysis procedures used to analyse neuromuscular function in different sport and exercise contexts.[51,52]

1.4.3 *Muscle biopsies*

In a muscle biopsy, a small piece of muscle tissue is removed from an intact human muscle for examination. In sport and exercise research, the needle biopsy is most common. Here, local anaesthetic is applied to the area after which a needle is inserted into the muscle (commonly the vastus lateralis of the quadriceps). Muscle biopsies can quantify muscle fibre composition, muscle energy content, and the concentration and activity of a multitude of enzymes involved in energy production that can provide an insight into the functional capacity of the muscle and changes in this capacity following an intervention such as a training period.

A potential limitation is that a biopsy sample may not be representative of the entire muscle from which it is drawn. In this situation, results extrapolated from a biopsy sample to the full muscle would be inaccurate. In addition, if repeated biopsy samples are required, variations in the sampling site may affect the validity and/or reliability of the data. However, the main concern with the use of muscle biopsies in fatigue research is whether the measurements made on the muscle sample are actually indicative of fatigue. For example, muscle biopsies are often taken to assess the rate and extent of muscle glycogen degradation during and after sport and exercise, with differences in the rate of degradation and end-exercise concentration often cited as a causative mechanism of fatigue. However, a closer analysis of the literature appears to indicate that carbohydrate ingestion during sport and exercise may not attenuate muscle glycogen depletion[53] (discussed further in Chapter 2). Of course, one of the primary limitations of the muscle biopsy technique is gaining the necessary ethical approval and, perhaps even more of a challenge, informed consent to conduct the procedure.

1.4.4   Blood sampling

Blood sampling is a staple tool in sport and exercise research. Methods of sampling vary, from simple fingertip or earlobe capillary sampling to arterial and venous sampling and cannulation. The frequency and method of blood sampling will depend on the aims of the research, the aims of the sampling (what blood variables will be measured and what they will be used for), and ethical and consensual restrictions. Common measurements include blood glucose and lactate concentrations and basic haematological variables, which can be accurately measured using capillary blood sampling with very small volumes of blood. Other measurements include the concentration of blood-borne substances such as hormones, free fatty acids, antioxidants, and intramuscular substances such as creatine kinase and myoglobin that can enter the blood.

Blood sampling conducted by a trained person in an appropriate environment, and adhering to appropriate codes of conduct and safety, carries minimal risk to the participant or the person taking the sample. However, as with muscle biopsies, the fatigue researcher needs to consider how representative, and therefore useful, their blood-borne analyses are in helping to quantify or explain fatigue. A classic example is the testing of blood lactate. Observation of high blood lactate concentrations at the point of fatigue led to the often-repeated conclusion that high blood lactate concentrations *cause* fatigue. However, ample evidence now exists to debate, or even refute, this claim (Chapter 3). Similarly, blood lactate concentration has been, and frequently still is, taken as a surrogate measure of intramuscular lactate concentration and, therefore, a measure of the biochemical status of the muscle. However, blood lactate concentration is not a valid measure of muscle lactate concentration during sport and exercise as it only reflects activities undertaken a few minutes prior to sampling, and the balance between lactate movement into and out of the blood.[54,55] This will be discussed further in Chapter 3, and blood-based indicators of fatigue will be discussed throughout Section 2 of the book.

> **Key point 1.10**
>
> *Blood sampling and, in particular, muscle biopsies require strong justifications before ethical approval will be granted to use these techniques in sport and exercise research.*

1.4.5 Magnetic resonance imaging

One of the challenges in understanding the complex function of the body during sport and exercise, and therefore determining fatigue mechanisms, is being able to 'see' exactly what is happening in various body systems and tissues while sport or exercise is taking place, or in the post-exercise period. Without this ability, determining the exact mechanisms of fatigue will remain a process of indirect deductions and educated guesses.

The development of magnetic resonance imaging (MRI) techniques in medical and health settings has opened a new window into the workings of the body during sport and exercise. An MRI machine produces a strong magnetic field around a person. This magnetic field acts on protons within the body. Protons are very sensitive to magnetisation and get 'pulled' in the direction of the magnet, where they essentially 'line-up' in the direction of the magnetic field. A radio frequency pulse is then directed to the part of the body to be examined. This pulse causes the protons to spin at a particular frequency and in a particular direction. When the pulse is turned off, the protons return to their natural alignment within the magnetic field and release the energy absorbed from the radio frequency pulse. This energy is detected and converted into an image, allowing the body part in question to be 'seen'.

MRI has been applied in sport and exercise research to investigate the energetics and intracellular environment of intact skeletal muscle,[56-58] skeletal muscle fibre orientation and architecture,[59] and the cardiac responses to exercise.[60] In addition, functional MRI (*f*MRI) has been employed to investigate the activity of brain regions in response to specific stimuli that are associated with performance during sport and exercise, such as carbohydrate mouth rinses.[61] The use of MRI has the potential to significantly improve our understanding of the processes involved in enhancing, and limiting, performance from a metabolic, anatomical, functional, and regulatory perspective. Unfortunately, there are obvious limitations to the application of MRI technology, not least the prohibitive cost of purchasing the equipment and the require-ment for trained practitioners to run it. In addition, techniques such as *f*MRI are still limited in their application to sport and exercise as they require a participant to lie still within the machine in order to provide accurate results. This rules out using *f*MRI to investigate most real-time or real-world sport-ing activities.

1.4.6   *Transcranial magnetic stimulation*

Transcranial magnetic stimulation is another non-invasive medical technique that is being increasingly used in sport and exercise research. Transcranial mag-netic stimulation involves placing an electromagnetic coil in contact with the head. The coil emits short electromagnetic pulses that pass through the skull and cause small electrical currents to penetrate a few inches into the brain. These currents cause activity of neurons in the areas of the brain to which they are directed. This stimulated brain activity results in an action; for example, if transcranial magnetic stimulation is used on the primary motor cortex, muscle activity is produced (this is referred to as a motor-evoked potential). These motor-evoked potentials can be used to examine the ability of the motor cor-tex to activate skeletal muscles. For example, research investigating the use of carbohydrate mouth rinses (which are thought to influence central drive to muscles) used transcranial magnetic stimulation to demonstrate significant increases in motor-evoked potentials when carbohydrate mouth rinses were used.[62] This is another example of how technology can provide fascinating new insights into the complexity behind our responses to exercise (interested readers are directed to a recent (at the time of writing) narrative review in the area[63]). Unfortunately, much like MRI techniques, the requirement for expensive equipment and well-trained practitioners limits the employment of transcranial magnetic stimulation in the study of sport and exercise fatigue.

1.5   Measuring fatigue via self-report

Numerous rating scales have been developed which attempt to quantify an individual's psychological, perceptual, and motivational responses to sport and exercise. This is a hugely complex task, and specific scales have been produced that measure varied aspects such as sensation of effort, motivation, pain, enjoy-ment, concentration, attention, lethargy, and many more. It is impractical to highlight all these scales (a 2016 review paper counted 24 self-report scales for fatigue alone!).[64] To provide an overview of this aspect of fatigue assessment, discussion will focus on some of the most commonly used scales.

1.5.1   *Ratings of perceived exertion*

The most commonly used perceptual scale is the Borg Rating of Perceived Exertion (RPE) Scale (also referred to as the Borg 6–20 scale). Developed in

1970 by Gunnar Borg,[65] the scale provides a quantifiable representation of an individual's level of exertion during sport and exercise. The scale is generally used to provide a holistic measure of exertion (the participant is free to use any and all physical and psychological 'cues' to determine their level of exertion). As a result, perceived exertion during sport and exercise is classed as having peripheral, respiratory-metabolic, or non-specific origins.[66] The seemingly arbitrary 6–20 range of the original Borg scale was developed due to the observed correlation between heart rate and RPE ratings, such that the given score on the scale can be multiplied by 10 and provide a close approximation of the exercising person's heart rate (e.g. an RPE of 12 approximates a heart rate of 120 bpm). However, this calculation is at best an approximation due to the multitude of factors that can influence both the heart rate response to and perceived exertion during exercise.

Many studies have demonstrated that the RPE scale can be used to accurately establish intensity during sport and exercise.[67-69] The scale is fairly simple to use provided appropriate instructions are given, however its use in young children is inappropriate or limited due to inabilities to cognitively rate perceived exertion (0–3 years of age) or provide a cohesive RPE score (4–7 years of age). Little is known about the validity of using the RPE scale in older children and adolescents.[70]

It is important to look a little deeper at what information is actually being provided when a person gives their 'rating of perceived exertion'. This is highlighted by the fact that the origins of how we sense and then 'perceive' exertion during sport and exercise are still not fully understood.[71,72] Furthermore, interventions can alter the relationship between intensity (usually measured by heart rate) and RPE, such as the use of music,[73] altered sensory perception strategies,[74] and provision of accurate and inaccurate feedback regarding intensity and the remaining duration of the activity (Chapter 6).[75.] Furthermore, while RPE scales may seem simple to administer, it is crucial that careful attention be paid to how the user of the scale conceptualises perceived exertion and how this is communicated to the person who is providing their perceived exertion measure. Failure to do this weakens the validity of RPE measurement. These issues are discussed well by Halperin and Emanuel,[76] but to briefly summarise:

- There are many different definitions of perceived exertion in the literature. Similar to fatigue itself, multiple definitions of the same thing are best avoided.
- Different terms are used/applied. For example, when discussing RPE terms such as fatigue, discomfort, heaviness, effort (as opposed to exertion) are sometimes used. While some of these terms may be more or less related to the concept of perceived exertion, they are different constructs and attempts to measure them using an RPE scale are inappropriate.
- Different RPE scales are used, and different instructions are given to participants (both within and between RPE scales).

- In some research, participants have been requested to provide an RPE measure for different body parts (e.g. RPE for the quadriceps during cycling). Based on existing definitions of perceived exertion, such an approach is questionable.

Halperin and Emanuel[76] recommend that to improve the validity of perceptual measurements during sport and exercise:

- The specific construct(s) to be measured (exertion, fatigue, discomfort, etc.) are carefully considered and an appropriate measurement scale is selected.
- Researchers report which scale was used, along with the instructions and anchoring procedures employed.
- Modification of validated scales is avoided wherever possible.
- An explicit question is added to measurement scales, which participants answer. This will remind participants what they are being asked to rate.

1.5.2   Brunel Mood Scale

The Brunel Mood Scale (BRUMS) was developed as a time-efficient assessment of mood state in adolescents and adults.[77] The scale consists of 24 items of mood descriptors (angry, unhappy, energetic, etc.), as well as six subscales (anger, confusion, depression, fatigue, tension, vigour), each containing four mood descriptors. Participants indicate to what extent they are experiencing the moods described using a Likert scale (0 = not at all to 4 = extremely). The standard approach is to use the scale to evaluate how a person is feeling at that moment, although other time periods have been used in the literature. The BRUMS is based on another mood state assessment tool called the Profile of Mood States (POMS). While the POMS has been shown to have good sensitivity with regard to performance prediction and the impact of environmental conditions in sporting situations,[78,79] it is a 65-item scale that takes many minutes to complete. Typical BRUMS completion time is 1–2 minutes, which although much quicker than the POMS would still limit the application of the BRUMS in certain sport and exercise situations. The BRUMS scale has been used extensively in a wide range of sport and exercise contexts.[80–83] Due to its high volume of use, normative data are now available for use of the BRUMS with male and female athletes and non-athletes.[84]

Key point 1.11

Use of self-report scales must be carried out with a good understanding of the underlying construct being measured, clear reporting of which measurement scale was used, without modifying validated scales, and ensuring participants are given clear and consistent instructions on use of the scale.

As mentioned above, the BRUMS contains subscales focussing on specific mood sub-descriptors. As a result, a lot of the research using the BRUMS only report one or more of these specific subscales, depending on which aspects of mood are most relevant to the specific research project. One of the subscales is fatigue, and this one is often reported in fatigue research. It would be valid to debate whether fatigue in sport and exercise is/can/should be conceptualised as a mood, and therefore whether the BRUMS is a valid measure of fatigue in these contexts. However, as we saw in Part 1, it has been challenging to develop a unified definition of fatigue as applied to sport and exercise, and recent attempts to do this place fatigue as a self-reported symptom. Perhaps then, this view of fatigue makes the BRUMS more relevant as a fatigue measure than it has been in the past.

1.5.3 Rating of fatigue scale

The rating of fatigue (ROF) scale was developed by Micklewright *et al.*[85] in an attempt to overcome known deficiencies with other fatigue self-report measures. These deficiencies include using rating scales that were actually designed for specific clinical populations and are therefore not generalisable, and scales that have multiple items and are therefore impractical in many sport and exercise situations.[85] The ROF scale is a single-item scale designed to be useable regardless of the context or population, and to enable measurement of fatigue distinct from perceptions of exertion.[85] The scale ranges from 0 ('not fatigued at all') to 10 ('total fatigue and exhaustion – nothing left'), with associated images to help interpret the numerical values and qualitative descriptors.

In their original publication, Micklewright *et al.*[85] established that the ROF scale has good face validity, convergent validity with a variety of physiological and activity measures during exercise, recovery, and daily living, and discriminant validity with RPE. As a result, Micklewright *et al.*[85] suggest the scale has a variety of applications across sport, exercise, health, and clinical research. Some research examples include measurement of the intensity of fatigue during sustained physical activity,[86] perceived fatigue following a tennis match,[87] and perceived fatigue during rehabilitation exercise in stroke patients[88] and during resistance training in older men.[89]

> **Key point 1.12**
>
> *Researchers must consider whether the measurements they intend to make will actually provide relevant information about the fatigue process before deciding whether or not to employ them.*

The ROF is designed to measure fatigue as a singular perception that is independent of any modifications or sub-characterisations.[85] Therefore, from a theoretical perspective, the scale aligns closely to the conceptualisation of fatigue outlined by Enoka and Duchateau[6] (Section 1.2.4).

1.6   Summary

- Human fatigue has been researched for over a century, and many of the findings and questions stimulated by this early research are still relevant today.
- Fatigue research is hampered by multiple definitions of fatigue, the myriad locations and processes that could be involved in fatigue, and the multitude of influencing factors that can modify the fatigue process.
- The two most prevalent fatigue theories are peripheral and central fatigue. Peripheral fatigue was originally modelled by Hill and colleagues in the 1920s, while the concept of a central component to fatigue was also being discussed around this time.
- Peripheral fatigue is characterised by processes occurring outside of the CNS, distal to the neuromuscular junction.
- Absence of a consistent link between any single physiological variable and the development of fatigue during sport and exercise, and contemporary refuting of many components of the peripheral fatigue model, suggests additional explanations for sport and exercise-induced fatigue are required.
- Central fatigue is the term for fatigue that resides within the CNS.
- A central component to fatigue has been speculated for over a century, but comparatively little research effort was spent investigating this suggestion until the last few decades. As a result, central fatigue is sometimes only accepted when experimental findings do not support any peripheral causes for fatigue.
- Both peripheral and central fatigue theories have limitations in terms of the research that has investigated them, their ability to explain sport and exercise fatigue, and the ability of either to independently, consistently, and effectively explain fatigue.
- Peripheral and central fatigue are umbrella terms used to classify multiple specific processes that are thought to contribute to fatigue.
- Peripheral and central fatigue should not be considered as opposing theories that have no common ground or influence over one another.
- A recent proposal suggested that fatigue should in fact be conceptualised as a disabling symptom which limits physical and cognitive function due to the interactions between performance and perceived fatigability.
- Under this proposal, fatigue has a unified definition free of modifying adjectives (peripheral, central, supraspinal, etc.), a taxonomy encompassing the range of conditions associated with fatigue, and a general approach for experimentally investigating fatigue.
- This new conceptualisation of fatigue may overcome some of the historical challenges of researching fatigue and enable research in the area to become more coherent.
- Two primary direct methods of fatigue measurement are the quantification of voluntary and electrically stimulated muscle force production and

the assessment of high and LFF. Both methods are laboratory-based and require carefully controlled procedures to produce accurate results.
- Indirect methods of fatigue measurement include time to exhaustion tests, EMG, muscle biopsies, blood sampling, MRI, and transcranial magnetic stimulation.
- A host of self-report fatigue measures exist. Care should be taken when using these tools, to ensure that the appropriate construct is being measured, the self-report tool is being used as it was designed and validated to be used, and that participants fully understand how to use the tool.
- All fatigue measurements have positives and negatives associated with their ability to shed light on fatigue development during sport and exercise. Use of any should be carefully considered based on the theoretical underpinnings of fatigue employed in the research project, the specific research design, availability of equipment, ethical and consensual restrictions, and the informed decision by the researcher of which methods will provide the most relevant and useful information.

To think about...

In 2005, the great Ethiopian distance runner, Kenenisa Bekele, set a new world record for the 10,000 metres of 26 minutes 17 seconds (which was subsequently lowered to 26 minutes 11 seconds by Joshua Cheptegei in 2020). During that race, Bekele ran the first 9,000 metres at an average pace of 2 minutes 38 seconds per kilometre. However, he ran the final kilometre in 2 minutes 32 seconds, 6 seconds faster than his average speed for the first 90% of a world-record setting race! This is by no means a 'fluke' performance; in fact, it is commonplace in endurance sports to see a significant increase in intensity near the end of a race, regardless of how hard the athlete was pushing throughout the event.

As you read the coming chapters of this book, keep this scenario in your mind. As we discuss each theory of fatigue, ask yourself: does that theory help to explain what Kenenisa Bekele did in his world record run? After all, if a theory does not explain what we see in the real world, perhaps it's time to have a re-think....

Test yourself

Answer the following questions to the best of your ability. This will reinforce the key knowledge that you require before progressing with the rest of the book. Try to understand the information gained from answering these questions before you progress with the book.

1 Write a short paragraph highlighting why the study of fatigue is complex and subject to so much debate and indecision.
2 Briefly describe the two most prevalent fatigue theories.
3 What are the key contemporary research findings that cast doubt on the veracity of the peripheral catastrophe model of exercise performance?
4 Outline how the alternative way of conceptualising fatigue proposed by Enoka and Duchateau[6] (A) is different to previous conceptualisations of fatigue and (B) may improve upon those previous conceptualisations.
5 What are the main direct, indirect, and self-report methods of sport and exercise-induced fatigue measurement?

References

1 Mosso A. *Fatigue*. London: Allen and Unwin Ltd; 1915.
2 Hill A. *Muscular Activity*. Baltimore, MD: Williams and Wilkins; 1926.
3 Bainbridge F. *The Physiology of Muscular Exercise*. New York: Longmans, Green and Company; 1931.
4 Merton P, Pampiglione G. Strength and fatigue. *Nature*. 1950;4221:166.
5 Marino FE, Gard M, Drinkwater EJ. The limits to exercise performance and the future of fatigue research. *Br J Sports Med*. 2011;45(1):65–67.
6 Enoka RM, Duchateau J. Translating fatigue to human performance. *Med Sci Sports Exerc*. 2016;48(11):2228–2238.
7 Joyner MJ. Fatigue: Where did we come from and how did we get here? *Med Sci Sports Exerc*. 2016;48(11):2224–2227.
8 Moore B. *The Australian Concise Oxford Dictionary*. Fourth ed. South Melbourne: Oxford University Press; 2004.
9 Ament W, Verkerke GJ. Exercise and fatigue. *Sports Med*. 2009;39(5):389–422.
10 Hill A, Lupton H. Muscular exercise, lactic acid, and the supply and utilization of oxygen. *QJ Med*. 1923;135–171(16).
11 Hill A, Long C, Lupton H. Muscular exercise, lactic acid and the supply and utilisation of oxygen: parts I-III. *Proc Royal Soc*. 1924;96:438–475.
12 Hill A, Long C, Lupton H. Muscular exercise, lactic acid and the supply and utilisation of oxygen: parts IV-VI. *Proc Royal Soc*. 1924;97:84–138.
13 Hill A, Long C, Lupton H. Muscular exercise, lactic acid and the supply and utilisation of oxygen: parts VII-VIII. *Proc Royal Soc*. 1924;97:155–176.
14 Noakes T. Fatigue is a brain-derived emotion that regulates the exercise behaviour to ensure the protection of whole-body homeostasis. *Front Physiol*. 2012;3: 1–13.
15 Hill L, Flack M. The influence of oxygen inhalations on muscular work. *J Physiol*. 1910;5:347–372.
16 Raskoff W, Goldman S, Cohn K. The "athletic heart." Prevalence and physiological significance of left ventricular enlargement in distance runners. *J Am Med Assoc*. 1976;236:158–162.
17 Bandschapp O, Soule C, Iaizzo P. Lactic acid restores skeletal muscle force in an in vitro fatigue model: are voltage-gated chloride channels involved? *Am J Physiol*. 2012;302:C1019–1025.

18 Kristensen M, Albertsen J, Rentsch M, Juel C. Lactate and force production in skeletal muscle. *J Physiol.* 2005;562:521–526.

19 Nielsen O, de Paoli F, Overgaard K. Protective effects of lactic acid on force production in rat skeletal muscle. *J Physiol.* 2001;536:161–166.

20 St Clair Gibson A, Noakes T. Evidence for complex systems integration and dynamic neural regulation of skeletal muscle recruitment during exercise in humans. *Br J Sports Med.* 2004;38:797–806.

21 Amann M, Eldridge M, Lovering A, Stickland M, Pegelow D, Dempsey J. Arterial oxygenation influences central motor output and exercise performance via effects on peripheral locomotor muscle fatigue in humans. *J Physiol.* 2006;575:937–952.

22 Albertus Y. *Critical Analysis of Techniques for Normalising Electromyographic Data.* Cape Town, South Africa: University of Cape Town; 2008.

23 Noakes T, St Clair Gibson A. Logical limitations to the "catastrophe" models of fatigue during exercise in humans. *Br J Sports Med.* 2004;38:648–649.

24 Davis J, Bailey S. Possible mechanisms of central nervous system fatigue during exercise. *Med Sci Sports Exerc.* 1997;29(1):45–57.

25 Graham T, Rush J, MacLean DA. Skeletal muscle amino acid metabolism and ammonia production during exercise. In: Hargreaves M (Ed) *Exercise Metabolism.* Champaign, IL: Human Kinetics; 1995:131–175.

26 Gandevia SC, Allen GM, Butler JE, Taylor JL. Supraspinal factors in human muscle fatigue: evidence for suboptimal output from the motor cortex. *J Physiol.* 1996;490(Pt 2):529–536.

27. Bigland-Ritchie B, Thomas C, Rice C, Howarth J, Woods J. Muscle temperature, contractile speed, and motor neuron firing rates during human voluntary contractions. *J Appl Physiol.* 1992;73:2457–2461.

28 Enoka RM, Stuart DG. Neurobiology of muscle fatigue. *J Appl Physiol (1985).* 1992;72(5):1631–1648.

29 Kluger BM, Krupp LB, Enoka RM. Fatigue and fatigability in neurologic illnesses: proposal for a unified taxonomy. *Neurology.* 2013;80(4):409–416.

30 Vollestad NK. Measurement of human muscle fatigue. *J Neurosci Methods.* 1997;74(2):219–227.

31 Nybo L, Nielsen B. Hyperthermia and central fatigue during prolonged exercise in humans. *J Appl Physiol (1985).* 2001;91(3):1055–1060.

32 Jones DA. High-and low-frequency fatigue revisited. *Acta Physiol Scand.* 1996;156(3):265–270.

33 Place N, Yamada T, Bruton JD, Westerblad H. Muscle fatigue: from observations in humans to underlying mechanisms studied in intact single muscle fibres. *Eur J Appl Physiol.* 2010;110(1):1–15.

34 Duchateau J, Baudry S. Maximal discharge rate of motor units determines the maximal rate of force development during ballistic contractions in human. *Front Hum Neurosci.* 2014;8:234.

35 Keeton RB, Binder-Macleod SA. Low-frequency fatigue. *Phys Ther.* 2006;86(8):1146–1150.

36 Edwards RH, Hill DK, Jones DA, Merton PA. Fatigue of long duration in human skeletal muscle after exercise. *J Physiol.* 1977;272(3):769–778.

37 Trimble MH, Enoka RM. Mechanisms underlying the training effects associated with neuromuscular electrical stimulation. *Phys Ther.* 1991;71(4):273–280; discussion 280–272.

38 Gandevia SC. Spinal and supraspinal factors in human muscle fatigue. *Physiol Rev.* 2001;81(4):1725–1789.

39 Warren GL, Lowe DA, Armstrong RB. Measurement tools used in the study of eccentric contraction-induced injury. *Sports Med.* 1999;27(1):43–59.

40 Martin V, Millet GY, Martin A, Deley G, Lattier G. Assessment of low-frequency fatigue with two methods of electrical stimulation. *J Appl Physiol (1985).* 2004;97(5):1923–1929.

41 Vollestad N, Sejersted O, Bahr R, Woods J, Bigland-Ritchie B. Motor drive and metabolic responses during repeated submaximal contractions in man. *J Appl Physiol.* 1988;64(4):1421–1427.

42 Schabort EJ, Hawley JA, Hopkins WG, Mujika I, Noakes TD. A new reliable laboratory test of endurance performance for road cyclists. *Med Sci Sports Exerc.* 1998;30(12):1744–1750.

43 McLellan TM, Cheung SS, Jacobs I. Variability of time to exhaustion during submaximal exercise. *Can J Appl Physiol.* 1995;20(1):39–51.

44 Hinckson EA, Hopkins WG. Reliability of time to exhaustion analyzed with critical-power and log-log modeling. *Med Sci Sports Exerc.* 2005;37(4):696–701.

45 Alghannam AF, Jedrzejewski D, Tweddle M, Gribble H, Bilzon JL, Betts JA. Reliability of time to exhaustion treadmill running as a measure of human endurance capacity. *Int J Sports Med.* 2016;37(3):219–223.

46 Succi P, Dinyer T, Byrd M, Soucie E, Voskuil C, Bergstrom H. Test-retest reliability of critical power, critical heart rate, time to exhaustion, and average heart rate during cycle ergometry. *J Exerc Physiol.* 2021;24(2):33–51.

47 Isezaki T, Kadone H, Niijima A, et al. Sock-type wearable sensor for estimating lower leg muscle activity using distal EMG signals. *Sensors (Basel).* 2019;19(8):1–18.

48 Xi X, Tang M, Luo Z. Feature-level fusion of surface electromyography for activity monitoring. *Sensors (Basel).* 2018;18(2):1–14.

49 Chang KM, Liu SH, Wu XH. A wireless sEMG recording system and its application to muscle fatigue detection. *Sensors (Basel).* 2012;12(1):489–499.

50 Liu SH, Lin CB, Chen Y, Chen W, Huang TS, Hsu CY. An EMG patch for the real-time monitoring of muscle-fatigue conditions during exercise. *Sensors (Basel).* 2019;19(14):1–15.

51 Rampichini S, Vieira TM, Castiglioni P, Merati G. Complexity analysis of surface electromyography for assessing the myoelectric manifestation of muscle fatigue: a review. *Entropy (Basel).* 2020;22(5):1–31.

52 Ertl P, Kruse A, Tilp M. Detecting fatigue thresholds from electromyographic signals: a systematic review on approaches and methodologies. *J Electromyogr Kinesiol.* 2016;30:216–230.

53 Karelis AD, Smith JW, Passe DH, Peronnet F. Carbohydrate administration and exercise performance: what are the potential mechanisms involved? *Sports Med.* 2010;40(9):747–763.

54 Bangsbo J, Norregaard L, Thorso F. Activity profile of competition soccer. *Can J Sport Sci.* 1991;16(2):110–116.

55 Krustrup P, Mohr M, Steensberg A, Bencke J, Kjaer M, Bangsbo J. Muscle and blood metabolites during a soccer game: implications for sprint performance. *Med Sci Sports Exerc.* 2006;38(6):1165–1174.

56 Krssak M, Petersen KF, Bergeron R, et al. Intramuscular glycogen and intramyocellular lipid utilization during prolonged exercise and recovery in man: a 13C

and 1H nuclear magnetic resonance spectroscopy study. *J Clin Endocrinol Metab.* 2000;85(2):748–754.

57 Larson-Meyer DE, Smith SR, Heilbronn LK, et al. Muscle-associated triglyceride measured by computed tomography and magnetic resonance spectroscopy. *Obesity (Silver Spring).* 2006;14(1):73–87.

58 Vanhatalo A, Fulford J, DiMenna FJ, Jones AM. Influence of hyperoxia on muscle metabolic responses and the power-duration relationship during severe-intensity exercise in humans: a 31P magnetic resonance spectroscopy study. *Exp Physiol.* 2010;95(4):528–540.

59 Sinha U, Sinha S, Hodgson JA, Edgerton RV. Human soleus muscle architecture at different ankle joint angles from magnetic resonance diffusion tensor imaging. *J Appl Physiol (1985).* 2011;110(3):807–819.

60 Wilson M, O'Hanlon R, Prasad S, et al. Biological markers of cardiac damage are not related to measures of cardiac systolic and diastolic function using cardiovascular magnetic resonance and echocardiography after an acute bout of prolonged endurance exercise. *Br J Sports Med.* 2011;45(10):780–784.

61 Chambers ES, Bridge MW, Jones DA. Carbohydrate sensing in the human mouth: effects on exercise performance and brain activity. *J Physiol.* 2009;587(Pt 8):1779–1794.

62 Gant N, Stinear CM, Byblow WD. Carbohydrate in the mouth immediately facilitates motor output. *Brain Res.* 2010;1350:151–158.

63 Moscatelli F, Messina A, Valenzano A, et al. Transcranial magnetic stimulation as a tool to investigate motor cortex excitability in sport. *Brain Sci.* 2021;11(4):1–12.

64 Gawron VJ. Overview of self-reported measures of fatigue. *Int J Aviat Psychol.* 2016;26(3–4):120–131.

65 Borg G. Perceived exertion as an indicator of somatic stress. *Scand J Rehabil Med.* 1970;2(2):92–98.

66 Robertson R. Development of the perceived exertion knowledgebase: an interdisciplinary process. *Int J Sport Psychol.* 2001;32:189–196.

67 Dunbar CC, Robertson RJ, Baun R, et al. The validity of regulating exercise intensity by ratings of perceived exertion. *Med Sci Sports Exerc.* 1992;24(1):94–99.

68 Eston RG, Williams JG. Reliability of ratings of perceived effort regulation of exercise intensity. *Br J Sports Med.* 1988;22(4):153–155.

69 Marriott HE, Lamb KL. The use of ratings of perceived exertion for regulating exercise levels in rowing ergometry. *Eur J Appl Physiol Occup Physiol.* 1996;72(3):267–271.

70 Kasai D, Parfitt G, Tarca B, Eston R, Tsiros MD. the use of ratings of perceived exertion in children and adolescents: a scoping review. *Sports Med.* 2021;51(1):33–50.

71 Marcora S. Perception of effort during exercise is independent of afferent feedback from skeletal muscles, heart, and lungs. *J Appl Physiol (1985).* 2009;106(6):2060–2062.

72 Smirmaul Bde P. Sense of effort and other unpleasant sensations during exercise: clarifying concepts and mechanisms. *Br J Sports Med.* 2012;46(5):308–311.

73 Potteiger JA, Schroeder JM, Goff KL. Influence of music on ratings of perceived exertion during 20 minutes of moderate intensity exercise. *Percept Mot Skills.* 2000;91(3 Pt 1):848–854.

74 White VB, Potteiger JA. Comparison of passive sensory stimulations on RPE during moderate intensity exercise. *Percept Mot Skills.* 1996;82(3 Pt 1):819–825.

75 Eston R, Stansfield R, Westoby P, Parfitt G. Effect of deception and expected exercise duration on psychological and physiological variables during treadmill running and cycling. *Psychophysiology.* 2012;49(4):462–469.

76 Halperin I, Emanuel A. Rating of perceived effort: methodological concerns and future directions. *Sports Med.* 2020;50(4):679–687.

77 Terry PC, Lane AM, Lane HJ, Keohane L. Development and validation of a mood measure for adolescents. *J Sports Sci.* 1999;17(11):861–872.

78 Beedie CJ, Terry PC, Lane AM. Profile of mood states and athletic performance: two meta-analyses. *J Appl Sport Psychol.* 2000;12:49–68.

79 Lane AM, Terry PC, Stevens MJ, Barney S, Dinsdale SL. Mood responses to athletic performance in extreme environments. *J Sports Sci.* 2004;22(10):886–897; discussion 897.

80 Bortolotti H, Altimari LR, Vitor-Costa M, Cyrino ES. Performance during a 20-km cycling time-trial after caffeine ingestion. *J Int Soc Sports Nutr.* 2014;11:45.

81 Bigliassi M, Leon-Dominguez U, Buzzachera CF, Barreto-Silva V, Altimari LR. How does music aid 5 km of running? *J Strength Cond Res.* 2015;29(2):305–314.

82 Marques M, Alves E, Henrique N, Franchini E. Positive affective and enjoyment responses to four high-intensity interval exercise protocols. *Percept Mot Skills.* 2020;127(4):742–765.

83 Lam HKN, Middleton H, Phillips SM. The effect of self-selected music on endurance running capacity and performance in a mentally fatigued state. *J Hum Sport Exerc.* 2021;4(17):894–908.

84 Terry PC, Parsons-Smith RL. Mood profiling for sustainable mental health among athletes. *Sustainability.* 2021;13(6116):1–21.

85 Micklewright D, St Clair Gibson A, Gladwell V, Al Salman A. Development and validity of the rating-of-fatigue scale. *Sports Med.* 2017;47(11):2375–2393.

86 Greenhouse-Tucknott A, Butterworth JB, Wrightson JG, Harrison NA, Dekerle J. Effect of the subjective intensity of fatigue and interoception on perceptual regulation and performance during sustained physical activity. *PLoS One.* 2022;17(1):e0262303.

87 Amatori S, Gobbi E, Moriondo G, et al. Effects of a tennis match on perceived fatigue, jump and sprint performances on recreational players. *Open Sport Sci J.* 2020;13:54–59.

88 Cleland BT, Galick M, Huckstep A, Lenhart L, Madhavan S. Feasibility and safety of transcranial direct current stimulation in an outpatient rehabilitation setting after stroke. *Brain Sci.* 2020;10(10):1–12.

89 Dello Iacono A, Martone D, Hayes L. Acute mechanical, physiological and perceptual responses in older men to traditional-set or different cluster-set configuration resistance training protocols. *Eur J Appl Physiol.* 2020;120(10):2311–2323.

Section 2

What causes (and what does not cause) fatigue?

2 Energy depletion

2.1 Energy metabolism during sport and exercise

It is beyond the scope of this book to provide a detailed overview of energy metabolism. Many excellent undergraduate physiology textbooks discuss this topic in detail, and the reader is recommended to consult such a text as required to support this chapter. However, a brief summary of the importance of adenosine triphosphate (ATP) in human energy metabolism is worthwhile.

ATP is the most important source of chemical energy in the body (Figure 2.1). ATP has three components: adenine, ribose, and three phosphates. High-energy bonds attach the three phosphate molecules to each other. The energy in these bonds is released when ATP is broken down in a hydrolysis reaction, and this energy is used by the cell for various functions such as muscle contraction:

$$\text{ATP} + \text{H}_2\text{O} \underset{}{\overset{ATPase}{\rightleftharpoons}} \text{ADP} + \text{P}_i + \text{H}^+ + \text{energy} \tag{2.1}$$

where H_2O is water, ADP is adenosine diphosphate, P_i is inorganic phosphate, H^+ is hydrogen, and ATPase is the name for a class of enzymes that catalyse ATP hydrolysis to allow it to contribute to its myriad functions, including muscle contraction. Only a small amount of ATP is stored in the body at any time; enough to fuel approximately 2 seconds of maximal intensity muscle contraction (only a little ATP is stored as (A) it is quite a big molecule but has a low energy density, meaning it would be inefficient to store ATP, and (B) storing it in worthwhile amounts would cause significant osmotic pressure problems). Muscle energy turnover can increase 300-fold during explosive muscle contractions, so mechanisms of ATP replenishment are critical to maintenance of muscle performance. This is where food energy comes in. While food energy cannot be used to replenish ATP *directly*, it can do so through three primary metabolic pathways/systems: the phosphocreatine (PCr) system, glycolysis, and the aerobic pathway. In glycolysis, glucose (from the blood or from glycogen stored in muscle) is metabolised to resynthesise ATP in a series of chemical reactions. In the aerobic pathway, glucose and fatty acids are metabolised

DOI: 10.4324/9781003326137-4

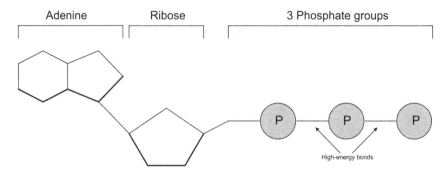

Figure 2.1 Adenosine triphosphate, the most important source of chemical energy in the body. Highlighted are the high-energy bonds between the three phosphate groups. These bonds are broken in a hydrolysis reaction, and the energy released is used for a multitude of processes, including muscle contraction.

to replenish ATP in two enzymatic systems called the Krebs cycle and the electron transport chain. The PCr pathway does not use stored glucose or fat; instead, it metabolises PCr (Section 2.2.2), a

Key point 2.1

ATP is the body's primary source of useable energy. Food energy cannot be used directly to fuel sport and exercise; however, it is required to continually replenish ATP stores.

compound present in skeletal muscle. The breakdown and resynthesis of ATP is a perpetual cycle, even at rest. Of course, during sport and exercise when energy requirements are greater, ATP turnover is also greater. Therefore, logic dictates that the availability of food energy is critical to ensuring a sufficient supply of ATP for continued sport and exercise performance.

2.2   Energy metabolism and fatigue during sport and exercise

2.2.1   *ATP depletion*

As mentioned above, the small endogenous ATP stores must be replenished continuously to avoid ATP depletion (termed the 'energy crisis' hypothesis of sport and exercise fatigue). If ATP stores were to be depleted, then the skeletal muscle would enter a state of rigor, a permanently contracted state, where the muscles are unable to relax.[1] This is a crucial statement. If sport and exercise fatigue is caused by critical depletion of ATP, then sport/exercise should be terminated due to the muscles entering rigor. However, sport and exercise-induced muscle rigor has never been documented in a human.[1]

Due to the greater rate of ATP turnover at higher intensities, it is logical to think that ATP depletion would be greater during high-intensity sport and exercise. However, repeated 6 second maximal cycle sprints can be achieved without substantial ATP depletion.[2] In fact, significant ATP depletion is not observed at the point of fatigue during progressive exercise to exhaustion (such as would be completed in a VO_2max test), high-intensity short duration sport/exercise,[3] or prolonged moderate-intensity sport/exercise.[3,4] Studies conducted on whole muscles or muscle homogenates (muscle tissues that have been mechanically 'broken up' to release their internal structures and substances) show that intramuscular ATP concentrations do not fall below about 60% of resting levels even during intense sport and exercise.[5]

It therefore appears that critical ATP depletion is not a viable direct cause of sport and exercise fatigue. Part of this reason is due to the incredibly elegant mechanisms the body utilises to tightly couple ATP hydrolysis to ATP demand (for more information on

Key point 2.2

In exercising humans, intramuscular ATP concentrations do not fall below about 60% of resting levels, regardless of the intensity or duration of sport and exercise. However, the ATP concentration of single fibres can drop to very low levels.

this, interested readers are directed to Hargreaves and Spriet[6]). Not only do these mechanisms ensure that ATP is replenished at an appropriate rate, but changes may also occur in very fatigued muscle fibres (for example, a reduction in calcium release) that reduce ATP consumption[7]; another way of preventing potentially catastrophic levels of ATP depletion.

Despite the absence of significant ATP depletion at the whole-muscle level, ATP levels in individual muscle fibres can fall to as low as 20% of resting values following maximal sport and exercise,[8] particularly in type II muscle fibres. Localised ATP depletion may also occur at crucial stages of the excitation-contraction coupling process (the process that enables muscle fibres to contract).[9] ATP depletion in just a small percentage of muscle fibres may prevent those fibres from contributing to muscle contraction and, thereby, result in fatigue of the whole muscle.[8] Given the conflicting observations regarding ATP depletion at the whole muscle and individual fibre levels, the exact influence of ATP depletion on sport and exercise fatigue is still open to debate. However, an important message to take from this discussion is that ATP depletion is far from an accepted cause of sport and exercise-induced fatigue and in fact is strongly argued against in some of the literature.

2.2.2 PCr depletion

PCr is a phosphorylated creatine molecule that is particularly important in resynthesising ATP during explosive, high-intensity sport and exercise. ATP resynthesis from PCr is driven by the reaction between PCr and ADP, catalysed by the enzyme creatine kinase:

$$PCr + ADP + H^+ \xleftrightarrow{\text{\textit{creatine kinase}}} ATP + Cr$$

where H^+ is hydrogen and Cr is free creatine. Intramuscular PCr stores equate to approximately 80 $mmol.kg^{-1}$ dry mass. In theory, this is sufficient for approximately 10 seconds of maximal work before PCr stores become depleted. However, as our energy systems work synergistically, PCr stores will not fully deplete during a single maximal effort (see Section 2.2.2.1). The recovery of PCr is biphasic. Under ideal conditions, ~50% of PCr stores are replenished in the first 30 seconds of recovery, followed by a slow component of recovery where full replenishment can take up to 8–10 minutes. However, during the slow component of recovery (and particularly in the later stages of the slow component), relatively small increases in PCr occur, meaning that PCr can continue contributing to further high-intensity efforts after relatively short recovery periods (perhaps as short as 30 seconds, although this will depend on multiple factors that we won't get into here). To discuss the potential role of PCr depletion in sport and exercise fatigue, it is useful to look at different types of activity (Chapter 8 discusses in detail the influence of different exercise demands on fatigue processes).

2.2.2.1   Maximal sport and exercise

A common protocol for assessing maximal sprint performance is a single cycle or running sprint lasting between 5 and 30 seconds. Studies of this nature have determined that PCr content drops to about 35%–55% of resting levels and contributes approximately 50% of the ATP produced during a 6 second sprint,[2] with the remainder supplied by glycolysis, aerobic metabolism, and ATP hydrolysis (Figure 2.2). As the sprint duration increases to 20 seconds, PCr content drops to about 27% of resting levels,[10] and to about 20% at the end of a 30-second sprint.[11] The significant reduction in muscle PCr content with increasing sprint duration, and the documented positive relationship between recovery of muscle PCr and muscle power output,[12] suggests that single-sprint performance is influenced by PCr availability.[13] Of course, the majority of people are able to complete a single sprint lasting 5–30 seconds without stopping. Despite this, some form of fatigue is still occurring, as the power output/movement speed at

Key point 2.3

Phosphocreatine is not exhausted during single sprints lasting 5–30 seconds, and the rate of PCr depletion and replenishment is not the sole cause of fatigue during short duration maximal sport and exercise.

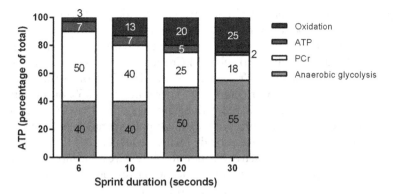

Figure 2.2 Relative energy system contribution to ATP resynthesis, as a percentage of total energy contribution, during sprints of different durations. It is important to remember that this is the contribution of energy systems to *single* sprints. The energy system contribution to repeated sprints at each duration would change progressively. Re-drawn from Billaut F, Bishop D. *Sports Med.* 2009;39(4):257–278.

the end of the sprint will be less than it was earlier in the bout. The reduction in power output may be partially due to PCr depletion and an associated reduction in the contribution of PCr to ATP resynthesis (Figure 2.2), which would reduce the rate of ATP resynthesis and necessitate a reduction in power output to prevent critical reductions in ATP concentration. However, PCr depletion is probably not the sole cause as PCr is not fully depleted in a single sprint of this length. Other possible explanations will be discussed in Chapter 8.

2.2.2.2 *Intermittent sport and exercise*

Intermittent sport and exercise refers to short periods of maximal activity (usually 5–30 seconds long) interspersed with recovery periods, or the variable intensity activity typical of many team games such as football. There is limited data on the metabolic responses to intermittent sport and exercise; however, it is known that ATP provision during intermittent sport and exercise is maintained through the coordinated contribution of the different energy systems.[13] As intermittent sport and exercise progresses, the relative contribution of the energy systems will change based on the previous efforts, and the duration and intensity of the recovery periods.[13] While aerobic and anaerobic energy provision is active during intermittent sport and exercise, the exact contribution of each is still under debate and is likely dependent on the type and intensity of exercise performed (discussed further in Chapter 8), and the individual athlete.

Significant positive relationships have been reported between the ability to resynthesise PCr and the recovery of power output during repeated cycle sprinting.[14,15] Similarly, occlusion of limb blood flow in recovery from intense activity, which prevents the resynthesis of PCr, prevents the recovery of power output in a subsequent bout.[16,17] These studies provide good evidence that performance during laboratory intermittent exercise is at least partly dependent on PCr contribution. However, it is important to reinforce the phrase *partly dependent*. Studies that have correlated PCr recovery and repeated sprint performance have shown that PCr recovery shares 45%–71% of its variance with that of the recovery of power output.[14,15] Therefore, 29%–55% of the variance in power output recovery is shared with parameters other than PCr recovery.

Studies investigating the effect of creatine supplementation on intermittent sport and exercise performance provide further evidence that the influence of PCr on fatigue during this activity is not absolute. Creatine supplementation is thought to improve performance by increasing resting PCr concentration, increasing the rate of PCr resynthesis, and buffering of intramuscular H^+.[18,19] Some research indicates that creatine supplementation increases PCr stores and improves performance during laboratory repeated sprint protocols of 6- and 30-second duration.[20,21] Conversely, other studies have found no effect, or variable effects, of creatine supplementation on laboratory and field-based repeated sprinting,[22–25] despite some instances of increased muscle creatine and/or PCr content. These differences in findings, which may be due to differences in sprint protocol and potential placebo effects in some studies, cloud understanding of the role of PCr on intermittent sport and exercise fatigue.

The potential role of PCr in fatigue diminishes as exercise duration increases. This is expected, given the shift towards predominantly aerobic ATP resynthesis with longer duration activity. However, PCr may still play a role in fatigue during long-duration sport/exercise that includes short-duration high-intensity work, such as team games. As discussed above, PCr contributes approximately half the ATP in a 6 second sprint and is predominantly resynthesised via aerobic metabolism. During team

> **Key point 2.4**
>
> *Phosphocreatine plays a role in muscle fatigue during single and repeated sprints. The influence of PCr on fatigue diminishes as sport and exercise duration increases, but it may still play a role in long-duration activity that involves bouts of short duration, high-intensity work.*

games, sprint durations of 2–3 seconds with recovery durations of two minutes have been reported.[26,27] Gaitanos *et al.*[2] stated that 30 seconds was sufficient recovery time for continued contribution of PCr to sprinting. Based on the finding that up to 85% of team game time is spent in low-intensity activity,[27,28] it would seem that despite the inherently random pattern of work and recovery, there is ample opportunity for resynthesis of PCr during team games (Section 8.2.2.1.1). However, single or multiple sprints with short recovery durations take place during team games.[27,29] Therefore, while PCr depletion may not cause exercise termination, it cannot be discounted that it may cause a transient loss of muscle force production during this type of activity (Section 8.2.2.1.1).

2.2.3 Glycogen depletion

Carbohydrate, in the form of muscle and liver glycogen and blood glucose, is the primary fuel during sport and exercise. The contribution of carbohydrate to exercising energy metabolism becomes greater with increasing intensity. Carbohydrate is metabolised in glycolysis (anaerobic) and the Krebs cycle (aerobic). Therefore, it is a fuel that can be metabolised to generate ATP across a wide range of sport and exercise demands.

A large amount of research has investigated various aspects of carbohydrate metabolism, far more than can be included in this book. Therefore, discussion will focus on the historical research that first demonstrated the potential link between carbohydrate and sport/exercise performance, subsequent work that reinforced the perception that glycogen depletion causes fatigue, and more recent perceptions of the role of carbohydrate in sport and exercise fatigue.

2.2.3.1 Brief historical perspective

Study into the links between carbohydrate and exercise performance began as far back as the 1920s.[30,31] It was not until the introduction of the muscle biopsy technique in the late 1960s that the study of carbohydrate manipulation became more focussed. Two classic studies[32,33] demonstrated that:

1 Prolonged submaximal exercise can deplete muscle glycogen.
2 Following exhaustive exercise, a high-carbohydrate diet can restore muscle glycogen to higher levels than before exercise (supercompensation).
3 The effect of exercise on the muscle glycogen concentration of inactive muscle is negligible, provided blood glucose levels remain fairly stable.
4 Muscle glycogen is the primary fuel source during prolonged moderate- to high-intensity exercise, and muscle glycogen content at the onset of exercise can determine the duration for which exercise can continue (Figure 2.3).

Following this early biopsy work, a wealth of research investigated carbohydrate and sport and exercise performance from the perspective of manipulating dietary carbohydrate intake and providing carbohydrate supplements before and during sport and exercise. The overall findings of this research further reinforced the importance of carbohydrate on sport and exercise performance, and the acceptance of key theories behind how carbohydrate exerts its performance-enhancing effects. Some of these theories have over the years, and almost via a word-of-mouth acceptance, become staples for how athletes, coaches, sports science students, and even academics explain the influence of carbohydrate on sport and exercise performance. To state that carbohydrate does not play a role in fatigue would be indefensible given the wealth of research to the contrary. However, despite the link between muscle glycogen content and exercise performance being made over 50 years ago, the fact is that we

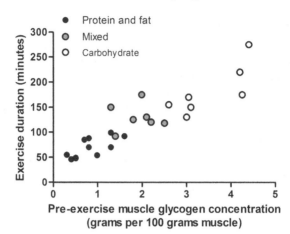

Figure 2.3 Exercise duration at a set intensity on a cycle ergometer following ingestion of one of three different diets (high protein and fat, mixed macronutrient, high carbohydrate). The progressive increase in exercise time with increasing dietary carbohydrate content demonstrates that the ability to continue exercising depends in part on pre-exercise muscle glycogen concentration. Data from Bergström J, Hermansen L, Hultman E, Saltin B. Acta Physiol Scand. 1967;71(2):140–150.

still do not conclusively know why muscle force is depressed (i.e. fatigue develops) when muscle glycogen levels are low. It is important to look closely at the older research and the more contemporary studies with a critical eye, as doing so may change our opinion of what ef-

Key point 2.5

The importance of carbohydrate as a muscle fuel has been known for many decades. However, more recent research is providing knowledge on an expanding number of potential roles of carbohydrate in the regulation of sport and exercise performance.

fect carbohydrate actually has on sport and exercise performance and fatigue, and how it exerts that effect.

2.2.3.2   *Potential carbohydrate-related causes of fatigue during sport and exercise*

One of the most commonly cited reasons for impaired sport and exercise performance, particularly of a long duration, is depletion of muscle glycogen concentration leading to an inability to resynthesise ATP at the required rate. This theory has been reported and re-stated so many times that it has taken on the status of fact. Of course, the logic behind it makes sense: glycogen is an important fuel source during sport and exercise – we only have a limited amount of it stored in our body – when it runs out, we can no longer maintain the same intensity – the end result: fatigue. Problem solved. Unfortunately not. The next sections will take potential carbohydrate-related fatigue mechanisms and provide a contemporary viewpoint of whether the literature supports, refutes, or is equivocal on the veracity of each mechanism.

2.2.3.2.1 GLYCOGEN DEPLETION REDUCES ATP RESYNTHESIS

As shown in Figure 2.3, the link between carbohydrate availability and exercise duration was made several decades ago. We also know that development of fatigue during prolonged sport and exercise often coincides with low muscle glycogen content. However, remember the discussion at the beginning of this chapter about ATP resynthesis during sport and exercise (Section 2.2.1). We discussed that if ATP is depleted during sport and exercise (if ATP use far exceeds the rate of ATP resynthesis), then the muscle will enter a state of rigor: something that has never been documented in an exercising human. In line with this, there is little evidence to support the idea that low muscle glycogen concentrations lead to a reduced ATP supply. In contrast, there is evidence to show that fatigue occurs during prolonged sport and exercise when muscle glycogen concentration is low, but ATP concentration is not significantly different to that measured at rest (Figure 2.4).[34–37] This data therefore suggests that reduced ATP resynthesis due to muscle glycogen depletion is not a direct cause of fatigue during prolonged sport and exercise.

However, the observation of high muscle ATP concentrations at fatigue does not rule out the possibility that glycogen depletion reduces ATP concentrations in localised areas of the muscle cell. Contrary to general perceptions, glycogen is not uniformly distributed in a muscle but rather is localised in clusters. The three primary glycogen clusters are subsarcolemmal glycogen (located just under the sarcolemma, or muscle fibre membrane), intermyofibrillar glycogen (located between myofibrils), and intramyofibrillar glycogen (located within the myofibrils).[38] The largest glycogen cluster is the intermyofibrillar one (approximately 75% of total glycogen stores), but the exact distributions are dependent on factors such as muscle fibre type, training status, fibre use, and the type of activity performed.[38] Depletion of specific glycogen clusters may negatively influence ATP concentrations in such a way that would not be detected by measuring 'whole-muscle' ATP concentration. Unfortunately, we don't currently know much about the exact effects of these distinct muscle glycogen depots on ATP resynthesis.[39] However, it seems that exercising muscle should be viewed as a compartmentalised structure where glycogen depots are used to support localised ATP resynthesis in response to specific demands placed on the muscle.[39,40] Therefore, localised muscle glycogen depletion could impact specific aspects of excitation-contraction coupling and contractile function.[39] The differential impact of specific muscle glycogen depots on sport and exercise performance is supported by evidence showing

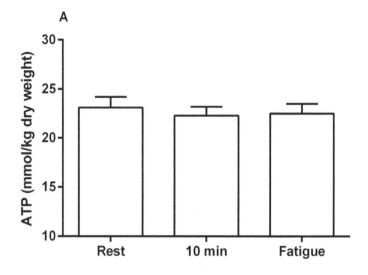

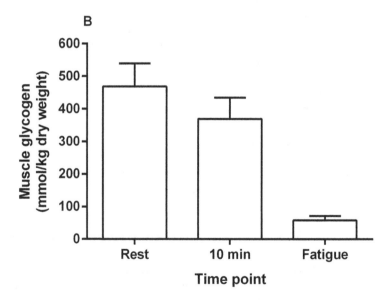

Figure 2.4 Muscle ATP concentration at rest and various stages of prolonged cycling exercise (A) and muscle glycogen concentration at the same points during the same exercise (B). It is clear to see that muscle glycogen concentration is low at fatigue, yet muscle ATP concentration does not change significantly from that at rest. Therefore, muscle ATP concentration is 'defended' even in the presence of low muscle glycogen. This does not support the contention that low muscle glycogen concentrations cause fatigue due to an inability to resynthesise ATP at the required rate. Data in these graphs were created by the author.

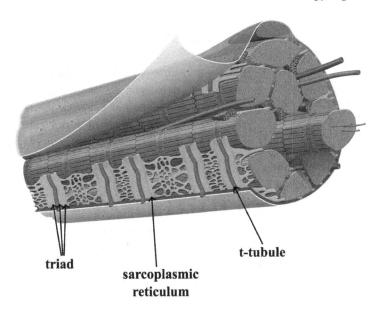

t-tubule

triad

**sarcoplasmic
reticulum**

Figure 2.5 Schematic of a muscle sarcomere and surrounding membranes. Identified
are the t-tubules, the sarcoplasmic reticulum, and the location of a t-tubule
and terminal cisternae of the sarcoplasmic reticulum that forms a triad. Re-
drawn from Thibodeau KT, Patton GA. *Anatomy and Physiology.* 4th ed.
Elsevier – Health Sciences Division.

that changes in intramyofibrillar glycogen concentration have been linked with
changes in exercise tolerance and muscle function during exercise.[38,41]

Localised ATP depletion has been linked with fatigue via alterations in calcium release from the sarcoplasmic reticulum. The intramyofibrillar glycogen
cluster is preferentially depleted during most forms of sport and exercise.[42] Most
intramyofibrillar glycogen is stored close to the triads (a t-tubule surrounded on
both sides by an enlarged area of the sarcoplasmic reticulum, termed terminal
cisternae; Figure 2.5).[42]
This glycogen cluster
is thought to gener-
ate ATP for the triads
so that they are able to
perform their important
role in the excitation-
contraction coupling
process,[38,42] namely the
release of calcium from
the sarcoplasmic reticu-
lum (which plays a cru-
cial role in formation

Key point 2.6

*A popular theory is that muscle glycogen deple-
tion leads to an inability to replenish ATP at
the required rate, and hence the development of
fatigue. However, there is little evidence to support this hypothesis. In fact, most research shows
little change in whole-muscle ATP concentration with muscle glycogen depletion.*

of actin-myosin cross-bridges and development of muscle force). Depletion of intramyofibrillar glycogen may cause localised ATP depletion at the triads, impairing this important step in the excitation-contraction coupling process. This is supported by research that

> **Key point 2.7**
>
> *Localised muscle glycogen depletion may reduce ATP resynthesis at specific locations in the excitation-contraction coupling machinery, which could lead to impaired muscle function. This would support an energy deficiency hypothesis of muscle glycogen depletion on fatigue.*

shows impaired sarcoplasmic reticulum function and calcium kinetics following sport and exercise, and an association between muscle glycogen depletion and this impaired function (further discussed in Chapter 5).[42-45] These findings appear to support a metabolic energy deficiency theory of muscle glycogen depletion that manifests as localised ATP depletion at critical steps in the excitation-contraction coupling process, primarily sarcoplasmic reticulum calcium release, despite global ATP concentration remaining constant. However, more research is required to confirm or refute the suggestion, as some studies have not found a link between reduced muscle glycogen concentration and altered calcium kinetics. Therefore, a non-metabolic role of muscle glycogen in excitation-contraction coupling cannot be discounted (Section 5.6.1).

2.2.3.2.2   GLYCOGEN DEPLETION CAUSES HYPOGLYCAEMIA, WHICH LEADS TO
            FATIGUE

The pattern of use of the four primary fuel sources (muscle glycogen, muscle triglycerides, blood glucose, free fatty acids) during sport and exercise will depend on many factors, including the exercise mode, intensity, duration, the training status, metabolic makeup, and pre-exercise fuel status of the athlete, and environmental conditions, particularly ambient temperature. However, the general pattern of use during moderate-intensity sport and exercise is summarised in Figure 2.6. Intramuscular fuel sources (glycogen and triglycerides) are predominant for approximately the first 90 minutes. If activity continues for longer than this, blood-borne fuels (glucose and free fatty acids) become more important due largely to muscle glycogen depletion. Blood glucose levels during sport and exercise are maintained by the breakdown of liver glycogen (there are other non-carbohydrate sources of glucose, such as amino acids and the glycerol portion of triglycerides, but generally these sources are utilised minimally and will not be discussed here). An increased use of blood glucose as a metabolic fuel will tax the finite liver glycogen stores, potentially leading to a situation where the liver can no longer maintain blood glucose levels within their optimum range and hypoglycaemia can develop (hypoglycaemia is defined as a blood glucose concentration < 4 mmol.L^{-1}).

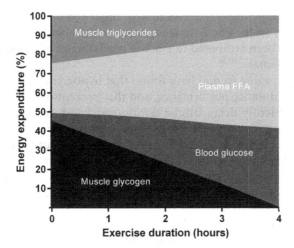

Figure 2.6 Contribution of the four primary energy sources to energy expenditure during moderate-intensity sport and exercise of increasing duration. Note that in the earlier stages (approximately 0–1 ½ hours), intramuscular fuel sources are the primary energy suppliers. If activity continues for longer, blood-borne fuel sources become predominant. The exact profile of fuel use will depend on factors such as exercise mode and intensity, training status, pre-exercise fuel status, and environmental conditions.

During prolonged sport and exercise, blood glucose is an important fuel for working muscles and the central nervous system (CNS). Brain glucose stores are limited; therefore, the uptake of blood glucose is crucial for the brain. Once blood glucose concentration drops below a critical level (approximately 3.6 mmol.L^{-1}), brain glucose uptake begins to decline.[46,47] Therefore, hypoglycaemia may contribute to fatigue in prolonged sport and exercise by limiting fuel supply to the brain. However, significant brain glycogen depletion also occurs in the absence of hypoglycaemia, suggesting a role for exercise-specific brain neural activity on brain glycogen depletion.[47]

Muscle force production is also greater after prolonged sport and exercise when blood glucose levels are maintained, with this greater force production related to better neuromuscular drive.[48] Experiments conducted in rats demonstrated that electrically stimulated muscle force production in hypoglycaemia was not different to that in euglycaemia, despite hypoglycaemic rats reaching exhaustion much earlier in the exercise bout.[37] This indicates that low muscle glycogen and hypoglycaemia did not affect the contractile ability of the muscle itself. By electrically stimulating the muscles, therefore bypassing the CNS, the authors concluded that depletion of muscle glycogen and hypoglycaemia contribute to fatigue, but that this fatigue is likely to be 'central' rather than 'peripheral'. However, hypoglycaemia may also contribute to fatigue by impairing fuel availability to the working muscles. As we have already discussed, during prolonged sport and exercise, blood glucose becomes a progressively more important fuel source. Improved prolonged submaximal exercise capacity with carbohydrate ingestion in the absence of muscle glycogen sparing has been attributed to a better maintenance of blood glucose and muscle glucose uptake.[49,50]

Interestingly, some studies have found that hypoglycaemia does not negatively affect endurance performance, and that prevention of hypoglycaemia does not consistently delay fatigue during sport and exercise.[51] Exercising in a hypoglycaemic state may not reduce muscle carbohydrate oxidation compared with euglycaemia, and maintenance of euglycaemia can produce a highly variable effect on endurance capacity, with some participants performing similarly whether hypoglycaemic or euglycaemic.[52] It appears that there is an inter-individual response to hypoglycaemia, with some people displaying symptoms such as nausea, confusion, and dizziness, but others showing no outward signs. This makes a consensus on the influence of hypoglycaemia on fatigue difficult. Currently it appears that hypoglycaemia is not a consistent cause of fatigue during sport and exercise[53] but may still be a potential cause in specific situations perhaps related to the intensity and duration of activity, and the nature of any carbohydrate ingestion strategy.

> **Key point 2.8**
>
> *While there is evidence that hypoglycaemia may contribute to fatigue via central and peripheral mechanisms during prolonged sport and exercise, this is not consistently observed and the inter-individual response to hypoglycaemia appears to be highly variable.*

2.2.3.2.3 WHAT DO CARBOHYDRATE SUPPLEMENTATION STUDIES TELL US ABOUT THE ROLE OF CARBOHYDRATE IN FATIGUE?

It is generally accepted that carbohydrate supplementation can delay the onset, and/or reduce the impact, of fatigue during sport and exercise. However, the exact mechanism(s) behind this ability are unknown. A classical theory is that carbohydrate supplementation spares muscle glycogen, as the body preferentially utilises the carbohydrate entering the systemic circulation from the supplement. Muscle glycogen sparing would then provide a readily available energy store for later in the bout, enabling sport/exercise to continue for longer. Studies have reported a sparing of muscle glycogen with carbohydrate supplementation during various exercise protocols.[54-57] However, when viewed as a whole, the literature does not conclusively support sparing of muscle glycogen with carbohydrate supplementation, at least during moderate-intensity sport/exercise.[53] In fact, back in 1986 a study showed that participants could continue cycling for an extra hour when they consumed carbohydrate during exercise, but their muscle glycogen use was almost identical to when they exercised without consuming carbohydrate.[49] The authors attributed the increased exercise duration to prevention of hypoglycaemia and associated continuation of muscle carbohydrate uptake and oxidation. However, as discussed in Section 2.2.3.2.2, there is debate about the exact importance of hypoglycaemia to fatigue. Also, it is interesting to note that in studies demonstrating an association between improved endurance capacity and maintenance of muscle carbohydrate oxidation rates with carbohydrate supplementation, fatigue still occurred despite those high oxidation rates. This raises the question of whether maintenance of plasma glucose and/ or carbohydrate oxidation rates is actually a mechanism for delaying fatigue.[53] The influence of carbohydrate supplementation on sarcoplasmic reticulum function and calcium kinetics during exercise is also equivocal. Clearly, it is difficult to get a straight answer regarding carbohydrate supplementation and exercise performance! This may be further hampered by recent more critical views of the carbohydrate supplementation literature. This critique will not be presented in detail, and interested readers are referred to a key paper for more information.[58] However, in light of the aims of this book, it is relevant to highlight. The fundamental critique of the carbohydrate supplementation literature is three-fold:

1 A number of prominent authors have close financial and professional ties to large sports supplement manufacturers, suggesting a conflict of interest between research findings and an industry worth hundreds of millions of pounds.
2 The aforementioned links between research and industry is a factor in why there are hardly any published studies showing a negative or no impact of carbohydrate supplementation on sport and exercise performance.
3 The quality of the research designs used.

Issues one and two are outside the remit of this book, and the reader is invited to draw their own conclusions after reviewing the evidence. However, the issue of research quality is worth discussing.

The proposed issues with carbohydrate supplementation research designs are in Table 2.1. Small sample sizes are a general feature of sport and exercise research, particularly when compared to clinical or medical fields. There are many probable reasons for this. For example, a specific subset of

Key point 2.9

A common perception is that carbohydrate supplementation delays fatigue by sparing muscle glycogen stores. However, the consensus from the literature is that carbohydrate supplementation does not in fact spare muscle glycogen during moderate-intensity sport and exercise, at least at the whole-muscle level.

Table 2.1 Some of the methodological and design criticisms of research into carbohydrate supplementation and exercise performance

1 Small sample sizes limit generalisability of findings.	Small sample size in research means that the study findings cannot be applied beyond people with the characteristics of the study sample. This is a fair criticism of research in general, but it should be noted that most sport and exercise research, particularly physiology research using interventions, is usually done with much smaller sample sizes than, for example, clinical research.
2 Exercise tests used are not externally valid to sports performance.	Many studies use time to exhaustion tests, which are not valid to real-world sports performance where the goal is usually to complete a set distance in the shortest possible time.
3 Differences in study approach.	Much of the research uses different protocols, environmental conditions, work intensities, carbohydrate interventions, and outcome measures. Therefore, comparing studies proves difficult.
4 Lack of solution blinding.	Some studies do not blind the investigators or participants to the interventions being assigned. Therefore, both an investigator expectancy and participant placebo effect cannot be discounted in these studies.
5 Measurements made not valid to fatigue.	Some of the measurements made in the research have questionable validity to fatigue. For example, muscle glycogen sparing has not been clearly correlated with improved performance or delaying of fatigue, and VO_2max has been shown to be a poor predictor of sports performance in a homogenous sample.
6 Pre-testing nutritional manipulation	Many studies put participants on a fast for the night before and on the morning of the study. These fasts usually lasted for 8–16 hours and would notably reduce liver and muscle glycogen stores which could improve the likelihood of a carbohydrate supplement having a positive effect on performance.

Source: Adapted from Cohen[58]

people are often required for a study (i.e. males aged 18–25 who have been active football players for at least 2 years). Such specific inclusion criteria are set not to be picky (the researchers' life would be much easier if they could recruit anyone to their study!) but because it will make the data more valid (a single gender removes possible gender differences in responses/outcome measures; a narrow age range reduces performance variability; a specific subject demographic makes the data more applicable to the target population). Recruitment practices are also somewhat different in sport and exercise research, where people from a small initial population are often asked to take part in a tough, time-consuming study with no financial or personal gain, compared with clinical or medical research where there is often access to a much larger population and the research may be carried out across multiple locations/organisations to maximise recruitment. Small sample size is a critique that can be aimed at most sport and exercise research but is defensible.

The use of non-specific or unreliable exercise tests, and measurements that have questionable links to fatigue, is a limitation of specific research studies and it would not be appropriate to speculate on why the researchers chose to use the tests and measures that they did. The use of appropriate blinding techniques is very important to counter both the researcher expectancy and participant placebo effects, and lack of blinding must be seen as a fundamental limitation. Differences in study approach (exercise protocol, environmental conditions, carbohydrate supplementation regime, etc.), while obviously rationalised as part of the research, is unfortunate as it makes reaching a consensus about the effects of carbohydrate supplementation difficult.

One of the biggest issues associated with carbohydrate supplementation research is the use of a fasting period prior to exercise. Usually, this is done to standardise participants' liver and muscle glycogen levels across trials, thereby removing differences in energy levels between participants as a possible confounding factor in the data. However, fasting will reduce muscle and liver glycogen concentrations. Therefore, participants will begin exercise with suboptimal glycogen stores, which is likely to enhance the effect of supplementing carbohydrate during exercise. Conducting a fast is uncommon for athletes prior to training or competition, and asking research participants to fast reduces the external validity of the data. It could also be argued that fasting biases the study towards finding a positive effect of the carbohydrate supplement.

The above discussion is included because it is a contemporary viewpoint of an existing body of research. It is also an example that even the most accepted viewpoints should be continually challenged by critically evaluating

> **Key point 2.10**
>
> *Specific criticism about research into carbohydrate supplementation during sport and exercise highlights the importance of critically and objectively reviewing research to fully evaluate its veracity.*

the research. In doing so, we will gain a better insight and understanding of exactly what we do know, what grey areas exist, how well we can trust the existing viewpoint, and what more we need to learn.

Hopefully, the discussions above are making you aware that it is far too simple to sum up the influence of carbohydrate on sport and exercise fatigue in a single statement or mechanism. Disagreement between studies could be due to things like the mode and intensity of exercise, training status and muscle fibre type distribution of the participants, and pre-exercise muscle glycogen stores. For example, we know that during cycling blood glucose levels and total carbohydrate oxidation rates progressively decline prior to fatigue much more than they do during running. This means that the mechanisms by which carbohydrate may exert beneficial effects on fatigue may differ between cycling and running-based research.

2.2.3.2.4 GLYCOGEN AND SPORT AND EXERCISE FATIGUE: A BRIEF SUMMARY

The above discussions give a lot of information without many clear answers, which, while frustrating, is an accurate picture of the current state of knowledge in this field. While it would be tempting to bury our heads in the sand and stick with the comfortable and familiar theory that glycogen depletion leads to an energy crisis in the muscle that causes fatigue, we cannot do this as we would be ignoring a lot of other research findings. Here is what we do know:

1 Depletion of muscle glycogen is, in some way or ways, associated with the development of fatigue during sport and exercise.
2 Depletion of muscle glycogen does not lead to whole-muscle ATP depletion. However, localised glycogen depletion within the muscle may lead to localised ATP depletion, which could disrupt specific steps of the excitation-contraction coupling process and contribute to fatigue.
3 Currently, it appears that localised muscle glycogen depletion may interfere with the ATP-dependent process of calcium movement into and out of the muscle cell, which would interfere with muscles' ability to produce force.
4 During prolonged sport and exercise, depletion of muscle and liver glycogen may lead to hypoglycaemia. The role of hypoglycaemia on fatigue may be peripheral (less uptake of glucose into the muscle) or central (reduced uptake of glucose by the brain).

> **Key point 2.11**
>
> *The importance of glycogen during sport and exercise is well known, and the literature into carbohydrate supplementation is wide-ranging. Despite this, our knowledge is far from complete, and the links between glycogen, carbohydrate supplementation, and fatigue still require more study.*

2.2.4 Free fatty acids

Approximately 90% of fat stores are in the form of triglycerides in adipose cells located at various sites around the body. However, there is a small but important store of intramuscular triglycerides. Adipose and muscle triglycerides can be oxidised for fuel during sport and exercise. Adipose triglyceride stores are broken down via lipolysis, a process regulated by specific hormone-sensitive lipases that yields one glycerol and three fatty acid molecules from each triglyceride molecule. Glycerol and fatty acids move into the blood, where glycerol can be taken up by the liver and used to form triglyceride or converted to glucose. Free fatty acids can enter the muscle via a family of fatty acid transporter proteins and the protein fatty acid translocase (FAT/CD36). Once inside the muscle cell, fatty acids are converted to acyl-CoA and enter the mitochondria via the carnitine shuttle. Once inside the mitochondria the fatty acids can undergo β-oxidation, whereby carbon units in the form of acetyl-CoA are removed from the fatty acyl-CoA molecule. Two carbon units are removed for each cycle of β-oxidation. These acetyl-CoAs can then enter the Krebs cycle and contribute to aerobic ATP resynthesis. Fat cannot generate ATP anaerobically.

> **Key point 2.12**
>
> *Fat is stored as triglyceride and can be broken down into fatty acids, taken up by the muscles, and undergo β-oxidation before being used to generate energy aerobically in the Krebs cycle.*

Fat stores are abundant, even in lean individuals (approximately 60,000–100,000 Kcal in an average young adult male, or enough energy to run at 9 minutes per mile for over 800 miles – theoretically of course!), therefore fatty acid depletion is not a cause of fatigue even during very long duration sport and exercise. However, fat metabolism can still influence fatigue during sport and exercise. The contribution of lipids to energy expenditure increases with the duration of activity. One of the goals of aerobic training is to improve the body's ability to metabolise fat as a fuel source, due to limited available glycogen stores. Endurance training can increase the rate of appearance of free fatty acids in the blood, suggesting greater lipolysis, and their rate of disappearance from the blood, suggesting greater uptake by the liver/skeletal muscles.[59] Other studies confirm increased oxidation of free fatty acids during sport and exercise following endurance training,[60–62] increased intensity at which maximal fat oxidation occurs,[63] and that sparing of muscle glycogen can occur when the ability to oxidise fatty acids is enhanced.[64] These metabolic improvements likely relate to training-induced increases in fatty acid transport protein content and localisation at the sarcolemma and mitochondria.[65] Development of a metabolic profile where fatty acid oxidation could delay muscle glycogen depletion may delay fatigue, particularly during prolonged sport and exercise. However, muscle glycogen sparing is not consistently observed with increased fatty acid oxidation.

In recent years, some interesting research has suggested that training in a fasted state (i.e. with purposely low muscle and/or liver glycogen stores) may be more beneficial for improving fat oxidation compared with training with an abundance of available glycogen. Training in the fasted state may cause a greater disturbance in energy homeostasis within the muscle, triggering adaptations such as increased activity of key enzymes involved in β-oxidation that enable

> **Key point 2.13**
>
> *Training in a fasted state may enable metabolic adaptations that allow the muscle to better oxidise fat for energy, potentially sparing muscle glycogen and delaying fatigue. However, the benefit of training in a fasted state on sport and exercise performance is equivocal.*

the muscle to use more free fatty acids.[63] Interestingly, training in a fasted state may also stimulate better oxidative metabolism of carbohydrate, suggesting an overall stimulus to oxidative metabolism. Training while fasted also results in lower blood insulin and greater blood epinephrine concentrations, which facilitates greater lipolysis and opportunity for fatty acid oxidation. Therefore, training in a fasted state may enable athletes to alter their metabolic responses to sport and exercise and, perhaps, delay fatigue.[66] However, while training in a fasted state may enable muscle glycogen sparing (both acutely and as a result of chronic adaptations),[67] training in a fasted state and then undertaking an exercise session with sufficient carbohydrate stores causes the body to shift back to preferentially utilising carbohydrate, even with an improved potential for fat oxidation.[59] As a clear link between training in a fasted state and improved sport and exercise performance has not been made,[67,68] more research is required before its efficacy as a tool for counteracting fatigue during sport and exercise can be properly examined.

2.3   Summary

- ATP is the most important source of chemical energy in the body and must constantly be replenished from food energy sources, predominantly carbohydrates and fats.
- Significant whole-muscle ATP depletion is not observed during sport and exercise, regardless of the intensity or duration.
- Significant ATP depletion can occur at specific locations within muscle fibres, which may contribute to fatigue.
- Depletion of PCr stores is associated with fatigue during single short duration maximal exercise efforts, and repeated efforts with short recovery durations. However, PCr depletion does not fully explain the fatigue observed during these forms of exercise.
- While muscle glycogen depletion is associated with fatigue during sport and exercise, the exact mechanisms behind this association are still under debate.

- It is unlikely that muscle glycogen depletion causes whole-muscle ATP depletion. However, depletion of specific intramuscular glycogen storage depots may cause localised ATP depletion that could affect specific excitation-contraction coupling processes such as calcium release from the sarcoplasmic reticulum.
- Blood glucose is a primary CNS fuel. During prolonged sport and exercise, development of hypoglycaemia due to liver glycogen depletion may contribute to the development via reduced brain glucose uptake.
- Hypoglycaemia may also impair muscle glucose uptake and reduce carbohydrate oxidation, thereby impairing muscle function. However, the evidence for hypoglycaemia as a common or consistent cause of fatigue is weak.
- Carbohydrate supplementation studies have reinforced the importance of carbohydrate availability to sport and exercise performance but have not yet clarified the mechanisms behind carbohydrate efficacy. Many of the commonly cited mechanisms for performance improvement with carbohydrate supplementation, such as muscle glycogen sparing, are open to significant debate.
- Carbohydrate supplementation research has come under critical scrutiny, and this should be considered prior to evaluating the role of supplementation research in developing our knowledge of carbohydrate and its links to sport and exercise performance and fatigue.
- Fatty acid availability is not a direct factor in the development of fatigue. However, practices such as endurance training and training in a fasted state may promote metabolic adaptations that allow the muscle to oxidise more fat during sport and exercise, thereby sparing muscle glycogen and delaying fatigue, particularly during prolonged activity. However, the research findings have not been consistent, and more work is required in this area.

To think about...

You are the coach of a national level Olympic-distance triathlete (1,500 metre swim; 40 km cycle; 10 km run, approximate duration 2 hours). You would like to develop your athlete's metabolic response to exercise so that you can be sure they are as 'fuel efficient' as possible.

Based on the content of this chapter, what strategies would you put in place during training and competition to ensure that your athlete's fuel use was optimal for performance in this event? As you think about this, also think about the justification for your decisions. What prompted you to make each decision? Are your decisions supported by the research? Remember, the onus is on avoidance of fatigue......

Test yourself

Answer the following questions to the best of your ability. Try to understand the information gained from answering these questions before you progress with the book.

1 Describe the importance of ATP to energy provision during sport and exercise.
2 Summarise the potential differences between whole-muscle ATP depletion and individual fibre ATP depletion during sport and exercise.
3 What is the potential role of PCr in fatigue during the following types of exercise: a single maximal-intensity effort; repeated maximal efforts with short recoveries; prolonged exercise that includes bursts of maximal effort with short recoveries?
4 What does our current knowledge indicate about the link between muscle glycogen depletion and ATP resynthesis during sport and exercise?
5 How might hypoglycaemia, in some sport and exercise situations, potentially contribute to fatigue?
6 Briefly outline the important considerations we must make when interpreting results of carbohydrate supplementation research and how these results influence our understanding of carbohydrate and fatigue.
7 Explain how altering the metabolism of free fatty acids during sport and exercise may contribute to improved sport and exercise performance and, potentially, delay fatigue.

References

1 Noakes TD, St Clair Gibson A. Logical limitations to the "catastrophe" models of fatigue during exercise in humans. *Br J Sports Med.* 2004;38(5):648–649.
2 Gaitanos GC, Williams C, Boobis LH, Brooks S. Human muscle metabolism during intermittent maximal exercise. *J Appl Physiol (1985).* 1993;75(2):712–719.
3 Baldwin J, Snow RJ, Gibala MJ, Garnham A, Howarth K, Febbraio MA. Glycogen availability does not affect the TCA cycle or TAN pools during prolonged, fatiguing exercise. *J Appl Physiol (1985).* 2003;94(6):2181–2187.
4 Gibala MJ, Gonzalez-Alonso J, Saltin B. Dissociation between muscle tricarboxylic acid cycle pool size and aerobic energy provision during prolonged exercise in humans. *J Physiol.* 2002;545(2):705–713.
5 Westerblad H, Bruton JD, Katz A. Skeletal muscle: energy metabolism, fiber types, fatigue and adaptability. *Exp Cell Res.* 2010;316(18):3093–3099.
6 Hargreaves M, Spriet LL. Skeletal muscle energy metabolism during exercise. *Nat Metab.* 2020;2(9):817–828.
7 Cheng AJ, Place N, Westerblad H. Molecular basis for exercise-induced fatigue: the importance of strictly controlled cellular Ca(2+) handling. *Cold Spring Harb Perspect Med.* 2018;8(2):1–19.

8 Karatzaferi C, de Haan A, Ferguson RA, van Mechelen W, Sargeant AJ. Phospho-creatine and ATP content in human single muscle fibres before and after maximum dynamic exercise. *Pflugers Arch.* 2001;442(3):467–474.

9 Jeneson JA, Schmitz JP, van Dijk JH, Stegeman DF, Nicolay K. Exercise ability is determined by muscle ATP buffer content, not Pi or pH. *The FASEB Journal.* 2010;24:801.833.

10 Bogdanis GC, Nevill ME, Lakomy HKA, Boobis LH. Muscle metabolism during repeated sprint exercise in man. *J Physiol.* 1994;475:25P–26P.

11 Casey A, Constantin-Teodosiu D, Howell S, Hultman E, Greenhaff PL. Metabolic response of type I and II muscle fibers during repeated bouts of maximal exercise in humans. *Am J Physiol.* 1996;271(1 Pt 1):E38–E43.

12 Bogdanis GC, Nevill ME, Boobis LH, Lakomy HK, Nevill AM. Recovery of power output and muscle metabolites following 30 s of maximal sprint cycling in man. *J Physiol.* 1995;482(Pt 2):467–480.

13 Billaut F, Bishop D. Muscle fatigue in males and females during multiple-sprint exercise. *Sports Med.* 2009;39(4):257–278.

14 Bogdanis GC, Nevill ME, Boobis LH, Lakomy HK. Contribution of phosphocreatine and aerobic metabolism to energy supply during repeated sprint exercise. *J Appl Physiol (1985).* 1996;80(3):876–884.

15 Mendez-Villanueva A, Edge J, Suriano R, Hamer P, Bishop D. The recovery of repeated-sprint exercise is associated with PCr resynthesis, while muscle pH and EMG amplitude remain depressed. *PLoS ONE.* 2012;7(12):e51977.

16 Harris RC, Hultman E, Kaijser L, Nordesjo LO. The effect of circulatory occlusion on isometric exercise capacity and energy metabolism of the quadriceps muscle in man. *Scand J Clin Lab Invest.* 1975;35(1):87–95.

17 Trump ME, Heigenhauser GJ, Putman CT, Spriet LL. Importance of muscle phosphocreatine during intermittent maximal cycling. *J Appl Physiol (1985).* 1996;80(5):1574–1580.

18 Kreider RB, Kalman DS, Antonio J, et al. International Society of Sports Nutrition position stand: safety and efficacy of creatine supplementation in exercise, sport, and medicine. *J Int Soc Sports Nutr.* 2017;14:18.

19 Clarke H, Kim DH, Meza CA, Ormsbee MJ, Hickner RC. The evolving applications of creatine supplementation: Could creatine improve vascular health? *Nutrients.* 2020;12(9):1–23.

20 Balsom PD, Ekblom B, Soerlund K, Sjodln B, Hultman E. Creatine supplementation and dynamic high-intensity intermittent exercise. *Scand J Med Sci Sports.* 1993;3(3):143–149.

21 Birch R, Noble D, Greenhaff PL. The influence of dietary creatine supplementation on performance during repeated bouts of maximal isokinetic cycling in man. *Eur J Appl Physiol Occup Physiol.* 1994;69(3):268–276.

22 Barnett C, Hinds M, Jenkins DG. Effects of oral creatine supplementation on multiple sprint cycle performance. *Aust J Sci Med Sport.* 1996;28(1):35–39.

23 Cox G, Mujika I, Tumilty D, Burke L. Acute creatine supplementation and performance during a field test simulating match play in elite female soccer players. *Int J Sport Nutr Exerc Metab.* 2002;12(1):33–46.

24 Dawson B, Cutler M, Moody A, Lawrence S, Goodman C, Randall N. Effects of oral creatine loading on single and repeated maximal short sprints. *Aust J Sci Med Sport.* 1995;27(3):56–61.

25 McKenna MJ, Morton J, Selig SE, Snow RJ. Creatine supplementation increases muscle total creatine but not maximal intermittent exercise performance. *J Appl Physiol (1985).* 1999;87(6):2244–2252.

26 Mohr M, Krustrup P, Bangsbo J. Match performance of high-standard soccer players with special reference to development of fatigue. *J Sports Sci.* 2003;21(7):519–528.

27 Spencer M, Lawrence S, Rechichi C, Bishop D, Dawson B, Goodman C. Time-motion analysis of elite field hockey, with special reference to repeated-sprint activity. *J Sports Sci.* 2004;22(9):843–850.

28 Duthie G, Pyne D, Hooper S. Applied physiology and game analysis of rugby union. *Sports Med.* 2003;33(13):973–991.

29 Sirotic AC, Coutts AJ, Knowles H, Catterick C. A comparison of match demands between elite and semi-elite rugby league competition. *J Sports Sci.* 2009;27(3):203–211.

30 Krogh A, Lindhard J. The relative value of fat and carbohydrate as sources of muscular energy: with appendices on the correlation between standard metabolism and the respiratory quotient during rest and work. *Biochem J.* 1920;14(3–4):290–363.

31 Levine S, Gordon B, Derick C. Some changes in the chemical constituents of blood following a marathon race: with special reference to the development of hypoglycaemia. *J Am Med Assoc.* 1924;82:1778–1779.

32 Bergstrom J, Hultman E. A study of the glycogen metabolism during exercise in man. *Scand J Clin Lab Invest.* 1967;19(3):218–228.

33 Bergstrom J, Hermansen L, Hultman E, Saltin B. Diet, muscle glycogen and physical performance. *Acta Physiol Scand.* 1967;71(2):140–150.

34 Febbraio MA, Dancey J. Skeletal muscle energy metabolism during prolonged, fatiguing exercise. *J Appl Physiol (1985).* 1999;87(6):2341–2347.

35 Parkin JM, Carey MF, Zhao S, Febbraio MA. Effect of ambient temperature on human skeletal muscle metabolism during fatiguing submaximal exercise. *J Appl Physiol (1985).* 1999;86(3):902–908.

36 Vissing J, Haller RG. The effect of oral sucrose on exercise tolerance in patients with McArdle's disease. *N Engl J Med.* 2003;349(26):2503–2509.

37 Williams JH, Batts TW, Lees S. Reduced muscle glycogen differentially affects exercise performance and muscle fatigue. *ISRN Physiol.* 2012 (2013):1–9.

38 Ortenblad N, Nielsen J, Saltin B, Holmberg HC. Role of glycogen availability in sarcoplasmic reticulum Ca2+ kinetics in human skeletal muscle. *J Physiol.* 2011;589(Pt 3):711–725.

39 Vigh-Larsen JF, Ortenblad N, Spriet LL, Overgaard K, Mohr M. Muscle glycogen metabolism and high-intensity exercise performance: a narrative review. *Sports Med.* 2021;51(9):1855–1874.

40 Nielsen J, Ortenblad N. Physiological aspects of the subcellular localization of glycogen in skeletal muscle. *Appl Physiol Nutr Metab.* 2013;38(2):91–99.

41 Jensen R, Ortenblad N, Stausholm MH, et al. Heterogeneity in subcellular muscle glycogen utilisation during exercise impacts endurance capacity in men. *J Physiol.* 2020;598(19):4271–4292.

42 Ortenblad N, Westerblad H, Nielsen J. Muscle glycogen stores and fatigue. *J Physiol.* 2013;591(18):4405–4413.

43 Chin ER, Allen DG. Effects of reduced muscle glycogen concentration on force, Ca2+ release and contractile protein function in intact mouse skeletal muscle. *J Physiol.* 1997;498(Pt 1):17–29.

44 Duhamel TA, Green HJ, Perco JG, Ouyang J. Comparative effects of a low-carbohydrate diet and exercise plus a low-carbohydrate diet on muscle sarcoplasmic reticulum responses in males. *Am J Physiol Cell Physiol.* 2006;291(4): C607–C617.

45 Nielsen J, Schroder HD, Rix CG, Ortenblad N. Distinct effects of subcellular glycogen localization on tetanic relaxation time and endurance in mechanically skinned rat skeletal muscle fibres. *J Physiol.* 2009;587(Pt 14):3679–3690.

46 Nybo L, Moller K, Pedersen BK, Nielsen B, Secher NH. Association between fatigue and failure to preserve cerebral energy turnover during prolonged exercise. *Acta Physiol Scand.* 2003;179(1):67–74.

47. Matsui T. Exhaustive endurance exercise activates brain glycogen breakdown and lactate production more than insulin-induced hypoglycemia. *Am J Physiol Regul Integr Comp Physiol.* 2021;320(4):R500–R507.

48 Nybo L. CNS fatigue and prolonged exercise: effect of glucose supplementation. *Med Sci Sports Exerc.* 2003;35(4):589–594.

49 Coyle EF, Coggan AR, Hemmert MK, Ivy JL. Muscle glycogen utilization during prolonged strenuous exercise when fed carbohydrate. *J Appl Physiol (1985).* 1986;61(1):165–172.

50 Coggan AR, Coyle EF. Reversal of fatigue during prolonged exercise by carbohydrate infusion or ingestion. *J Appl Physiol (1985).* 1987;63(6):2388–2395.

51 Felig P, Cherif A, Minagawa A, Wahren J. Hypoglycaemia during prolonged exercise in normal men. *New Engl J Med.* 1982;306:895–900.

52 Claassen A, Lambert EV, Bosch AN, Rodger l M, St Clair Gibson A, Noakes TD. Variability in exercise capacity and metabolic response during endurance exercise after a low carbohydrate diet. *Int J Sport Nutr Exerc Metab.* 2005;15(2): 97–116.

53 Karelis AD, Smith JW, Passe DH, Peronnet F. Carbohydrate administration and exercise performance: what are the potential mechanisms involved? *Sports Med.* 2010;40(9):747–763.

54 De Bock K, Derave W, Ramaekers M, Richter EA, Hespel P. Fiber type-specific muscle glycogen sparing due to carbohydrate intake before and during exercise. *J Appl Physiol (1985).* 2007;102(1):183–188.

55 Hargreaves M, Costill DL, Coggan A, Fink WJ, Nishibata I. Effect of carbohydrate feedings on muscle glycogen utilization and exercise performance. *Med Sci Sports Exerc.* 1984;16(3):219–222.

56 Tsintzas OK, Williams C, Boobis L, Greenhaff P. Carbohydrate ingestion and glycogen utilization in different muscle fibre types in man. *J Physiol.* 1995;489(Pt 1):243–250.

57 Tsintzas K, Williams C, Constantin-Teodosiu D, et al. Phosphocreatine degradation in type I and type II muscle fibres during submaximal exercise in man: effect of carbohydrate ingestion. *J Physiol.* 2001;537(Pt 1):305–311.

58 Cohen D. The truth about sports drinks. *Br Med J.* 2012;345:1–8.

59 Friedlander AL, Casazza GA, Horning MA, Usaj A, Brooks GA. Endurance training increases fatty acid turnover, but not fat oxidation, in young men. *J Appl Physiol (1985).* 1999;86(6):2097–2105.

60 Friedlander AL, Casazza GA, Horning MA, Buddinger TF, Brooks GA. Effects of exercise intensity and training on lipid metabolism in young women. *Am J Physiol.* 1998;275(5):E853–E863.

61 Martin WH, 3rd, Dalsky GP, Hurley BF, et al. Effect of endurance training on plasma free fatty acid turnover and oxidation during exercise. *Am J Physiol.* 1993;265(5 Pt 1):E708–E714.

62 Phillips SM, Green HJ, Tarnopolsky MA, Heigenhauser GF, Hill RE, Grant SM. Effects of training duration on substrate turnover and oxidation during exercise. *J Appl Physiol (1985).* 1996;81(5):2182–2191.

63 Van Proeyen K, Szlufcik K, Nielens H, Ramaekers M, Hespel P. Beneficial metabolic adaptations due to endurance exercise training in the fasted state. *J Appl Physiol (1985).* 2011;110(1):236–245.

64 De Bock K, Derave W, Eijnde BO, et al. Effect of training in the fasted state on metabolic responses during exercise with carbohydrate intake. *J Appl Physiol (1985).* 2008;104(4):1045–1055.

65 Talanian JL, Holloway GP, Snook LA, Heigenhauser GJ, Bonen A, Spriet LL. Exercise training increases sarcolemmal and mitochondrial fatty acid transport proteins in human skeletal muscle. *Am J Physiol Endocrinol Metab.* 2010;299(2): E180–188.

66 Aird TP, Davies RW, Carson BP. Effects of fasted vs fed-state exercise on performance and post-exercise metabolism: A systematic review and meta-analysis. *Scand J Med Sci Sports.* 2018;28(5):1476–1493.

67 Howard EE, Margolis LM. Intramuscular Mechanisms Mediating Adaptation to Low-Carbohydrate, High-Fat Diets during Exercise Training. *Nutrients.* 2020;12(9):1–16.

68 Impey SG, Hearris MA, Hammond KM, et al. Fuel for the Work required: a theoretical framework for carbohydrate periodization and the glycogen threshold hypothesis. *Sports Med.* 2018;48(5):1031–1048.

3 Metabolic acidosis

3.1 Introduction

Metabolic acidosis (a reduction in the normal pH of a fluid or tissue by endogenous production of acidic substances) represents an area of confusion with regard to sport and exercise fatigue. Many coaches, athletes, and students (and academics) hold the view that the development of acidosis, primarily via lactic acid accumulation, is a key cause of fatigue. As usual, however, it is a little more complicated. This chapter will discuss acidosis from the perspective of lactic acid, lactate, and hydrogen production. The links between these factors and fatigue will be evaluated, and recent research that challenges these links will be discussed. While reading this chapter, it is important to remember that most of the knowledge is still being added to, and the topic remains fiercely debated among academics and researchers. Therefore, the information is not the final word on the topic of metabolic acidosis but is a summary of where our knowledge currently sits.

> **Key point 3.1**
>
> *Although our knowledge of the processes involved in metabolic acidosis has developed significantly, the exact causes of metabolic acidosis, and its role in fatigue during sport and exercise, are still keenly debated.*

3.2 The role of metabolic acidosis in sport and exercise fatigue: a brief history

As the title of this section indicates, this is a brief history of lactate, lactic acid, and metabolic acidosis. For a more detailed history, see the excellent article by Ferguson *et al.*[1]. Lactate was discovered in 1780, and some rudimentary initial findings about the potential link between lactate and physical exertion in animals were published during the 18th century.[1] However, the belief that

DOI: 10.4324/9781003326137-5

lactic acid is produced in human skeletal muscles during exercise and that accumulation of lactic acid causes fatigue can be traced back to research carried out in the early 1900s. By electrically stimulating muscle preparations, researchers reported that the muscles produced lactic acid.[1] When these muscle preparations were incubated in nitrogen or oxygen (O_2) rich environments at different temperatures following stimulation, lactic acid concentrations increased more in the nitrogen incubation compared with the O_2 incubation. In other words, lactic acid concentrations were lowest in muscles that were exposed to O_2. Based on these findings, it was concluded that increases in lactic acid concentration were greatest under anaerobic conditions, slower in normal air, and completely absent in a pure O_2 environment.[2] It was also concluded that "*lactic acid is spontaneously developed under anaerobic conditions in muscle*" and "*fatigue due to contractions is accompanied by an increase in lactic acid*".[2] Therefore, it appears these early authors were stating that increases in lactic acid caused fatigue in skeletal muscles. However, this is incorrect, as the authors did not state that lactic acid *causes* fatigue; they merely documented the production of lactic acid and the occurrence of muscle fatigue. No cause-and-effect relationship was implied.[2] This distinction is crucial, as these initial findings may have been misinterpreted to mean that lactic acid has a causative role in muscle fatigue;[2] an interpretation that still influences our views of sport and exercise fatigue today.

Following the early documentation of lactic acid production in skeletal muscle, other researchers reported increased blood lactate concentrations when people exercised to fatigue and described the biochemistry of glycolysis and its supposed production of lactic acid.[3,4] Perhaps inevitably, given earlier findings and understanding of biochemistry at the time, the conclusion was made that during intense work, muscles contract in the absence of an adequate O_2 supply (in "anaerobiosis"), thereby producing lactic acid which causes muscle acidosis that leads to fatigue. All these connections were assumed to be cause-and-effect,[4] and the belief that lactic acid production causes acidosis and muscle fatigue was born.

Since this early work, many studies have been published that appear to support the link between lactic acid production, acidosis, and fatigue. In the 1970s, a linear relationship was found between lactate accumulation and loss of muscle force in frogs[5] and later, in human thigh muscle.[6] These studies also indicated that the decline in muscle force and the increase in muscle acidity followed a similar time course, suggesting that they may influence one another.[7] Both acidosis and the decline in muscle force production occur more slowly following a period of physical training, and in slow twitch (predisposed to aerobic metabolism) compared with fast twitch (predisposed to anaerobic metabolism) muscles. These studies appear to provide evidence for a role of lactic acid in muscle fatigue. However, these studies used correlation analysis to associate acidosis with fatigue. While correlations do show the association between two variables, they cannot evidence a cause-and-effect relationship between them. Simply put, while acidosis and fatigue may correlate, it cannot be said that acidosis *causes* fatigue. Indeed, much of the research that showed a correlation between lactic acid and fatigue also showed relationships between other metabolic measures and fatigue.[7]

3.2.1 How might lactic acid cause fatigue?

Two main hypotheses were posed for how lactic acid production may cause fatigue. Firstly, reduced muscle pH may impair muscle contraction via a decline in muscle force production and muscle shortening velocity (Section 3.3.3.1). Intramuscular acidosis was thought to do this by reducing sarcoplasmic reticulum calcium (Ca^{2+}) release[8] and Ca^{2+} sensitivity.[9] Secondly, intramuscular acidosis could cause

Key point 3.2

Potential causes of lactic acid-induced fatigue included impaired isometric muscle force and contraction velocity, and inhibition of glycolysis due to a reduction in intramuscular pH.

fatigue by inhibiting glycolysis (Section 3.3.3.3).[10-13] This hypothesis was developed through observation of reduced activity of key enzymes that regulate glycolysis during exercise that causes notable reductions in muscle pH. Both of these theories gain some support from research that shows making the blood more alkaline can enable better maintenance of work and power during intermittent high-intensity exercise.[14-16] However, there is a counter-argument to the suggestion that acidosis inhibits glycolysis (Section 3.3.3.3).

3.3 Metabolic acidosis and fatigue: the counter-view

The large amount of interest and research effort spent examining metabolic acidosis during sport and exercise and its role in fatigue has not brought all the answers, and metabolic acidosis remains a hotly debated topic. However, these efforts have generated knowledge that now provides us with a more detailed and nuanced view of the role of metabolic acidosis in fatigue.

An important question to answer when discussing the biochemistry of lactic acid is "*What does the body produce during sport and exercise – lactic acid or lactate*"? Reading lay articles, or even scientific papers on the subject, you will often see that the terms lactic acid and lactate are used interchangeably as though they mean the same thing. Importantly, they do not. Lactic acid is, as the name suggests, an acidic compound that has the potential to release a proton (hydrogen ion, H^+) into a solution, thereby making that solution more acidic (Figure 3.1). Conversely, lactate does not have this ability. As lactate does not donate H^+, it does not directly make its environment more acidic.

During sport and exercise, ATP is resynthesised via glycolysis (Figure 3.2) and oxidative phosphorylation. Glycolysis is always active regardless of the intensity of sport/exercise or the extent of the oxidative contribution to ATP

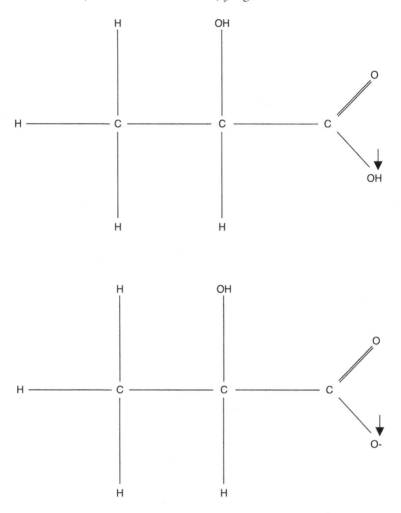

Figure 3.1 The chemical structure of lactic acid (top) and lactate (bottom). Lactic acid has a proton (hydrogen ion) that dissociates and moves into the surrounding solution, increasing its acidity. However, it is lactate and not lactic acid that is produced in muscle during sport and exercise. Lactate does not contain a hydrogen ion; therefore, it does not release hydrogen and cannot directly increase the acidity of its environment.

resynthesis. This is because carbohydrate needs to be converted to pyruvate, which is then converted to acetyl CoA for entry into the Krebs cycle. The conversion of carbohydrate to pyruvate occurs via glycolysis (Figure 3.2). Specific stages of glycolysis, particularly those involving ATP hydrolysis, produce H⁺ (Equation 3.1 and Figure 3.2). A greater flux (activity) of glycolysis will lead to greater H⁺ production. During intense sport and exercise, the mitochondria are not able to metabolise all of the pyruvate that is produced in glycolysis (in other words, the activity of the mitochondria lags behind the activity of glycolysis).[17] To prevent pyruvate accumulation, which would inhibit glycolysis and thereby impair both anaerobic and oxidative ATP resynthesis, pyruvate can be converted, via the lactate dehydrogenase reaction, to lactate (Figure 3.2).[17] This is crucial: lactate, not lactic acid, is produced via glycolysis.[18] The lactate dehydrogenase reaction also consumes H^+ and regenerates the H^+ carrier molecule nicotinamide adenine dinucleotide (NAD^+), which is able to take up H^+ from the cytosol and transport it into the electron transport chain where it plays a critical role in oxidative ATP resynthesis. The conversion of pyruvate to lactate, involving use of NADH and H^+ and the production of NAD^+, is summarised in the following equation:

$$\text{Pyruvate} + \text{NADH} + H^+ \xrightleftharpoons{\text{Lactate dehydrogenase}} \text{Lactate} + NAD^+ \qquad (3.1)$$

Where NADH is the reduced form of NAD^+ (meaning it has H^+ attached to it), and NAD^+ the oxidised form (it does not have H^+ attached to it and is therefore ready to accept H^+).

High energy demands can cause H^+ to be produced at greater rates than it can be removed by NAD^+.[19,20] In this situation, NAD^+ may become saturated with H^+ ions.[19] This saturation could lead to H^+ accumulation in the cytosol that, if unchecked, could reduce intramuscular acidity to the extent that the function of the tissue may be compromised (Section 3.3.3). The lactate dehydrogenase reaction acts as a buffer against this cellular H^+ accumulation by consuming H^+ and recycling NAD^+ in the process of converting pyruvate to lactate.[4] Simply put, the production of lactate is alkalinising to the cell, not acidifying. Lactate may also facilitate H^+ removal from the cell via monocarboxylate (MCT) transporters present in cell membranes (Section 3.3.1). These transporters also serve to remove H^+ from the cell, meaning that the removal of lactate from the muscle also removes H^+.[21]

As already discussed, lactate does not directly make the internal environment more acidic; therefore, its production cannot directly contribute to intramuscular acidosis. This would appear to clarify the issue and suggest that the lack of lactic acid production during sport and exercise means that lactic acidosis cannot be considered a cause of fatigue. However, it is possible that the production of lactate, as a strong acid anion (negatively charged ion), may cause a reduction in cell strong ion difference (the difference in concentration of positively and negatively charged ions).

Key point 3.3

Lactate, not lactic acid, is produced in glycolysis. Lactic acid has the potential to directly make its environment more acidic by releasing a hydrogen ion, whereas lactate does not. This has important implications for the role of lactate/lactic acid in fatigue.

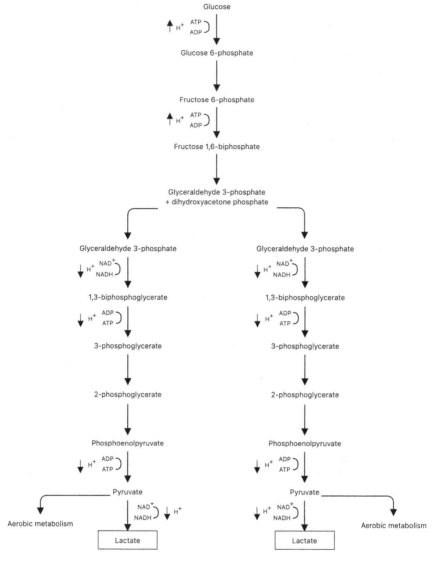

Figure 3.2 A simplified view of glycolysis, showing the metabolism of a glucose molecule to pyruvate for entry into the Krebs cycle (aerobic metabolism). Also
highlighted are the reactions of glycolysis that produce hydrogen (H^+) and
those that consume or remove.

Reducing the strong ion difference (i.e. increasing the concentration of anions)
creates the need to balance this with an increased concentration of positively
charged ions (cations) in order to maintain electroneutrality.[18] This is accom-
plished in large part via the production of H^+ from the hydrolysis of water
into its constituents (HO^- and H^+).[7,18] Therefore, lactate production may still

indirectly cause some intramuscular acidosis. However, the impact of this on sport and exercise fatigue has not been quantified.

As stated above and shown in Figure 3.2, lactate, not lactic acid, is produced in glycolysis. Lactic acid is not present in the body[7] as the acid dissociation constant of lactic acid is lower than the normal pH of body tissues and fluids. This means that lactic acid would dissociate into lactate and H^+. The relationship between these two ions, in terms of how they are produced and what effect they have on their environment and on one-another, is crucial to understanding the counter-argument to the lactic acidosis hypothesis. We have discussed (and will continue to do so) lactate, and we have mentioned H^+; specifically, that it can make the environment in which it is placed more acidic. Let us discuss this further.

A H^+ ion is essentially a hydrogen atom that has donated its single electron in an oxidation reaction. The structure of a hydrogen atom is a nucleus containing a single proton, and a single electron "spinning" around that nucleus. If the hydrogen atom loses its electron, all that remains is a single proton. That is why H^+ ions are also referred to as protons. The plus sign in H^+ refers to the fact that the ion is now positively charged (a cation) as it only contains a proton. Hydrogen ions (protons) are acidic (an acid is any substance that donates protons) and therefore make the solution they are placed in (water, blood, or intracellular fluid) more acidic.

A traditional viewpoint is that production of lactate is also associated with production of H^+ ions, which causes a reduction in the pH of the intramuscular environment. Simply put, this view states that production of lactate is a cause of acidosis. However, this view has been challenged by numerous researchers who state that lactate has no involvement in H^+ production (and vice versa), and that in fact H^+ is produced during glycolysis from the hydrolysis of ATP (Figure 3.2).[4,22,23] This would appear to absolve lactate from any role in the development of acidosis during sport and exercise. However, as with most topics in this book, the picture is not black and white, as other researchers contend that lactate production does cause acidosis by altering the strong ion difference (as discussed above), and that the coincidental production of lactate and H^+ during sport and exercise is, essentially, the production of lactic acid.[18,24,25] Some of the confusion may relate to the experimental designs used by research studies in this topic. Some studies use small amounts of human tissue in a laboratory environment in an attempt to artificially re-create the internal environment of the body (termed *in vitro* research), whereas other studies actually use an entire, living human or animal (*in vivo* research). It is extremely difficult to replicate the complex functioning of animal tissue *in vitro*; therefore, this type of research may not produce a full picture of biochemical processes. A good example is that some *in vitro* research examining the role of pH reduction on muscle

> **Key point 3.4**
>
> *A H^+ ion is a hydrogen atom that has donated its single electron, leaving behind a single proton. Hydrogen ions are acidic and will make the solution they are placed in more acidic.*

function carried out ex-
periments at tissue tem-
peratures notably lower
than that of an intact,
in vivo muscle. Acid-
base regulation is influ-
enced by temperature,
and studies conducted
at temperatures much
nearer to normal physi-
ological temperatures

Key point 3.5

*The production of lactate does not directly pro-
duce H^+ and therefore does not directly make
its environment more acidic. However, lactate
production may alter the strong ion difference,
thereby indirectly causing H^+ production.*

have reported less effect of reduced pH on muscle function (see Section 3.3.3).
Also, looking at the complex biochemical reactions underpinning metabolic
processes in isolation may limit our understanding of exactly what is going on,
as these reactions are interdependent and influence one another.[4] It is therefore
more appropriate to study them as a group event – something that is very difficult to do. The key message is that the methods used by researchers should be
considered when reading research into the biochemistry of metabolic acidosis.
Regardless of the exact cause of its production, what is important is that accumulation of H^+ can reduce the pH of the muscle and blood. This pH reduction
(acidosis) has long been considered a cause of muscle fatigue during intense
sport and exercise (see Section 3.3.3).

3.3.1 Lactate: misconceptions and benefits

Lactate remains a misunderstood substance for many. The most important
misconception is that lactate is directly responsible for fatigue during sport
and exercise. However, there are other common misconceptions, as well as
some important benefits, of lactate production that should be addressed. As
already mentioned, study of the myriad roles of lactate continues unabated,
meaning that our knowledge in this area continues to develop. As a result,
what we thought we knew can change. The following is accurate at the time of
writing, but readers should try to stay abreast of new developments.

1 Lactate is a waste product that serves no useful purpose.

This is an often repeated, and probably not much thought about, statement. As a general rule, the body does not "waste" much of its energy or
resources. Even things that appear at first to be wasteful (for example: the
large amount of metabolic energy that is released as heat) actually serve
an important role (this heat keeps us warm and regulates our body temperature, enabling our body systems to function optimally). Therefore,
it does not make sense to view lactate as an unwanted fatigue-inducing
agent; a by-product that through some flawed metabolic evolution has to
be tolerated and its damaging effects minimised. Indeed, this view is no
longer relevant, for at least two reasons. The first is that lactate production

can actually reduce acidosis within skeletal muscle, potentially enhancing or at least maintaining function and improving sport and exercise performance. The traditional interpretation that lactate accumulation is the cause of fatigue is erroneous, and a classic example of the misapplication of the cause-and-effect phenomenon. Larger amounts of lactate are detected during periods of high-intensity work when some performance decrement may also be seen; however, lactate production is high due to its role in buffering excess pyruvate and H^+ and is not itself directly impairing performance.

The benefit of lactate production is further evidenced by observations made in patients with McArdle's disease, which is a genetic condition characterised by an inability to break down glycogen via glycolysis, and therefore an inability to produce lactate. People with this condition actually fatigue more quickly during sport and exercise than people who do produce lactate, providing some evidence that lactate production is beneficial to performance.

The second reason why lactate is not simply a waste product is that it is a fuel source during and after sport and exercise. Approximately 75% of all lactate produced during sport and exercise is used as muscle fuel.[26] The use of lactate as a fuel is facilitated by the presence of specialised MCT proteins present in the sarcolemma and the mitochondria of muscle fibres which facilitate the transport of lactate from fibre to fibre, and into the mitochondria for conversion back to pyruvate and subsequent oxidation. Lactate is also converted to glucose post-sport and exercise in the liver in a process called gluconeogenesis, which helps to replenish our finite carbohydrate stores.[27] We also now know that the brain, previously thought to exclusively use glucose as a fuel source, uses lactate to generate energy at rest but particularly during sport and exercise that causes pronounced increases in arterial blood lactate concentration.[28-30]

The functional importance of lactate is being further understood by studies investigating its ergogenic effects as a supplement during sport and exercise. In particular, supplementation with lactate during high-intensity, short-duration exercise has been shown to significantly improve performance.[31] The primary mechanism behind this performance improvement appears to be an alkalinising effect of lactate on the blood, as lactate is buffered to bicarbonate, and bicarbonate is a primary blood-based acid buffering system. Therefore, lactate consumption may increase the pH gradient between the muscle and blood, which would facilitate the movement of H^+ out of the muscle and into the blood, where it could then be buffered by bicarbonate. However, as with most sports supplements that show potentially beneficial effects, there is also research that reports no benefit of lactate supplementation on performance.[32,33]

2 Lactate causes muscle soreness, pain, and other uncomfortable symptoms during and after sport and exercise.

There is no convincing evidence that lactate directly contributes to the uncomfortable muscular sensations typically felt during and in the hours and days after hard and/or unaccustomed sport and exercise. The unpleasant muscle symptoms sometimes felt during sport and exercise, such as soreness and burning, are likely due to stimulation of pain-generating (nociceptive) free nerve endings in the muscle (termed group III and IV muscle afferents; also see Section 3.3.3.4) by biochemical substances such as H^+, and by mechanical stress associated with contraction.[30] Small studies in humans have suggested that the combined presence of high concentrations of lactate, ATP, and protons similar to that seen during intense sport and exercise can cause sensations of muscle pain; however, high concentrations of any of these metabolites individually do not appear to cause pain.[34] If lactate does indirectly increase H^+ concentration as a result of shifts in the strong ion difference (Section 3.3), this is one mechanism whereby lactate could potentially be indirectly implicated in the development of muscle soreness/pain during sport and exercise. However, the evidence does not currently support this as a strong contributor to sport and exercise-induced muscle soreness/pain.

As the lactate produced during sport and exercise is removed from muscle within approximately 1 hour after cessation of activity,[35] it cannot be the cause of delayed onset muscle soreness. The exact cause(s) of delayed onset muscle soreness are unknown, but it is likely due to a pathway effect involving micro-trauma of the muscle architecture that leads to inflammation, intramuscular oedema (swelling), and the hormone-mediated sensitisation of free nerve endings in the muscle.[36-38]

3.3.2   Is there any way that lactate can be a cause of sport and exercise fatigue?

The above sections have hopefully helped you to see how as our understanding of lactate has developed; this knowledge has moved us away from considering lactate as a performance limiting metabolite. However, there are contentions in the literature that lactate may still make some contribution to fatigue during sport and exercise. These contentions mostly revolve around debate on the extent to which lactate contributes to acidosis. You could be forgiven for thinking that a sound application of biochemical principles to this question would provide a conclusive answer but take a look at the citations at the end of this sentence to see that is not the case![4,23-25,39-41] As a result of this ongoing debate, it is currently difficult to answer the question "is there any way that lactate can be a cause of sport and exercise fatigue?" so I will answer it with a caveat.

Lactate could potentially contribute to fatigue *if* the production of lactate in some way contributes to increased acidosis. As Ferguson et al.[1] say in their excellent review, "*it remains feasible that [lactate] has a small (perhaps ~5%) but potentially*

Key point 3.6

Many of the enduring myths about the negative aspects of lactate can be dispelled; however, it is plausible that lactate still makes a small but meaningful contribution to sport and exercise fatigue.

significant deleterious effect in intact systems such as perfused skeletal muscle and heart and intact humans." While I appreciate you may be frustrated not to get a clear answer, this uncertainty is reflective of our current state of knowledge in this area. As Ferguson *et al.*[1] state, the quote from Fletcher and Hopkins[2] still appears to have relevance today: "*there is hardly any important fact concerning the [lactate] formation in muscle which, advanced by one observer, has not been contradicted by some other.*"

An additional challenge when trying to interpret the impact of acidosis on fatigue is that there is still no agreement on exactly what are the major source(s) of H⁺ production during sport and exercise! The contention that glycolysis is a source of H⁺ is dispelled by Pesi *et al.*,[42] who balanced the equations for the chemical reactions of glycolysis to demonstrate no net H⁺ production (and, in fact, some H⁺ consumption). Robergs *et al.*[4] state that it is ATP hydrolysis at intensities above that which can be met by oxidative metabolism that is a key source of H⁺. However, Ferguson *et al.*[1] argue that this could only be true if we observe a decreasing concentration of ATP in this scenario, which we invariably do not (Ferguson *et al.*[1] then go on to implicate lactate production as a significant contributor to the strong ion difference and, therefore, to H⁺ production). More questions, fewer answers!

3.3.3 The impact of hydrogen production on muscle function

This section focuses on the primary potential mechanisms of acidosis on muscle function. For quantitative descriptions of the magnitude of decrement in isometric and dynamic muscle force and muscle velocity associated with acidosis, the reader is referred to Debold[43] and Debold *et al.*[44]

3.3.3.1 Sarcoplasmic reticulum calcium release, calcium binding to troponin C, and myofilament calcium sensitivity

Originally, it was thought that metabolic acidosis caused a reduction in muscle force by reducing the rate of Ca^{2+} release from the sarcoplasmic reticulum. The release of Ca^{2+} is crucial for muscle contraction, and if insufficient Ca^{2+} is released, then the muscle may contract with less force. However, it appears that the normal processes of Ca^{2+} release from the sarcoplasmic reticulum are not impaired, even when muscle pH levels are as low as 6.2 (from a normal resting pH of ~7.1).[33] It therefore appears that the influence of acidosis on Ca^{2+} movement from its intramuscular storage site is minimal.[45]

Once Ca^{2+} has been released from the sarcoplasmic reticulum, it must bind with troponin C, part of a complex of three proteins

Key point 3.7

Intramuscular acidosis can impair the Ca^{2+} sensitivity of the myofilaments and the rate at which ATP detaches from the myosin head.

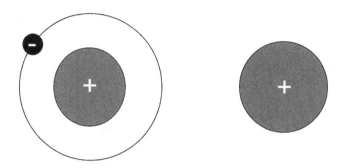

Figure 3.3 A hydrogen atom (left), composed of a single proton (positive charge, +) and a single electron (negative charge, -). The loss of the single electron in an oxidation reaction leaves the single positively charged proton remaining (right). This single proton is referred to by the abbreviation H^+.

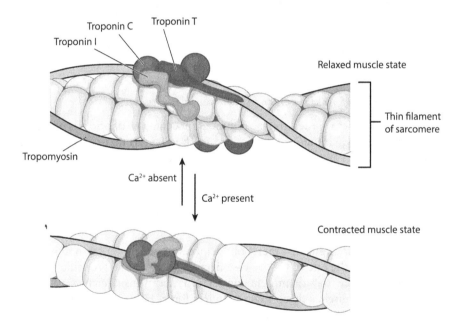

Figure 3.4 In a relaxed muscle (top of picture), the protein tropomyosin blocks the myosin binding sites on actin, preventing actin and myosin from interacting. When calcium binds to troponin C (bottom of picture), it causes a shape change in the troponin complex that pushes tropomyosin away from the myosin binding sites, allowing actin and myosin to interact and muscle contraction to take place. Note that myosin is not shown in this figure.

that play a crucial role in initiating cross-bridging of the two primary contractile filaments, actin and myosin (figure 3.4). This cross-bridging is necessary for muscle contraction. If Ca^{2+} cannot bind to troponin C, then actin and myosin cannot interact and muscle contraction will not occur. At low intramuscular pH, H^+ competes with Ca^{2+} to bind to troponin C,[19] and for this reason, it was thought that intramuscular H^+ accumulation would reduce muscle force. However, the depressive effect of H^+ on cross-bridge force production persists even when sufficient Ca^{2+} is present to saturate troponin C binding sites, suggesting that the influence of H^+ on cross-bridge force is at least partly independent of any potential role of H^+ in impaired Ca^{2+}-binding to troponin C.[46,47] Another potential way that acidosis could impair contractile force is by slowing the rate at which ADP dissociates from the myosin head, which would essentially reduce the ability of myosin to move actin.[44,48] Further advances in this area now indicate that other metabolites, such as inorganic phosphate (Pi), may have more of an impact than H^+ on contractile function,[45] and it is likely that Pi and H^+ synergistically impair muscle force by reducing the Ca^{2+} sensitivity of the myofilaments (meaning that more Ca^{2+} is required to activate the myofilaments)[43,44,49] (see Chapter 5 for more information on Ca^{2+} and Pi). Therefore, acidosis currently remains implicated in impaired muscle contraction, but be prepared for more research to come!

3.3.3.2 Muscle membrane excitability

Research into the effect of H^+ on the excitability of skeletal muscle (the ability of the electrical signal to move across the muscle membrane and into the muscle to stimulate Ca^{2+} release) is a good example of how H^+ can exert positive effects on muscle function. During repeated muscle contractions, potassium (K^+) is lost from the intramuscular environment and accumulates in the extracellular environment (this will be discussed in more detail in Chapter 5). Accumulation of K^+ in the extracellular space can impair the excitability of the muscle fibre, reducing contraction force. Intramuscular acidity can help to maintain muscle fibre excitability and force production during repeated contractions. The most likely mechanism at play here is that acidosis inhibits sarcolemmal chloride (Cl^-) channels. Chloride channels account for the majority of passive sarcolemmal conductance, meaning that they help to keep the muscle membrane at its resting electrical potential (essentially, they inhibit depolarisation).[45] The acidosis-induced inhibition of Cl^- channels therefore facilitates depolarisation, which helps to counteract the reduced excitability caused by extracellular K^+ accumulation.[45,50]

> **Key point 3.8**
>
> Acidosis may help to maintain muscle membrane excitability and force production, perhaps by counteracting the force-depressing effects of extracellular potassium accumulation via inhibition of muscle membrane chloride channels.

3.3.3.3   *The rate of glycolysis*

Significant relationships have been reported between reduced muscle pH and reduced power output or work performed during maximal intermittent sport and exercise.[51-53] It has been suggested that intramuscular acidosis may negatively affect the function of key enzymes involved in glycolysis (primarily phosphofructokinase and glycogen phosphorylase).[54] Enzymes function optimally at the normal pH of the tissue in which they are located; reducing this pH may impair enzyme function and, in the case of glycolysis, reduce the ability of the muscle to replenish ATP.[55] There is evidence to show that during intense maximal intermittent sport and exercise, particularly consisting of short repeated bouts of work, the contribution of glycolysis to energy requirement progressively declines.[13,55,56] Some studies have implicated acidosis as a primary inhibitor of glycolysis in these situations,[54,55,57] which is reinforced by research showing that making the blood more alkaline appears to enable greater removal of H^+ from the working muscle, leading to improved sport and exercise performance. However, some studies have found no effect of increased blood alkalinity on performance.[13,53,58] Discrepancies in results may be due to the exercise intensity and duration, use of short recovery durations between exercise bouts; and the *in vivo* buffer capacity of research participants. As a result, this research alone should not be used to form a conclusion about the effect of acidosis on the rate of glycolysis.

Some authors have found no influence of acidosis on muscle glycolytic rate[41,59] and have suggested that muscle pH reductions typically found during sport and exercise have no effect on glycolysis. This view is further supported by the following observations:

1   The time course of muscle force recovery after intense sport and exercise is much faster than the time course of pH recovery.
2   People are able to produce high muscle force/power under conditions of acidosis.
3   No significant correlations have been found between recovery of muscle pH and recovery of sprint performance.[60]
4   Some studies in skinned muscle fibres (meaning fibres that have had their surface membrane removed mechanically or chemically) suggest that acidosis has a lesser influence on muscle fatigue than previously thought.[61]

Clearly, there is conflict in the literature regarding the effects of acidosis on the function of glycolysis. Methodological differences probably have a part to play in this conflict (e.g. differences in the mode, duration, and intensity of exercise, the

> **Key point 3.9**
>
> *The suggestion that acidosis inhibits glycolytic enzymes and therefore slows the rate of glycolysis is controversial, with some research demonstrating no associations between muscle pH and muscle force production or high-intensity sport and exercise performance.*

intracellular environment created within muscle tissue, use of *in vivo* and *in vitro* experimental models). However, our knowledge of sport and exercise physiology continues to develop and become more nuanced. This greater depth of knowledge is making us more aware of the extent of the interactive effects of different "fatigue agents", and how the effects of changes in the rate of production/accumulation of one of these agents may be exacerbated (e.g. H^+ and Pi) or attenuated (e.g. K^+ and H^+) by changes in the rate of production/accumulation of another agent. We probably should not be surprised by this, as the physiology of the body is highly interactive. This interactivity may mean that the absolute impact of any single potential fatigue agent, such as H^+ accumulation/acidosis, may be less than we previously thought.[62]

3.3.3.4 *Central nervous system drive*

High-intensity sport and exercise can lead to large amounts of H^+ moving from the muscle into the blood. If H^+ enters the blood at too high a rate, it can exceed the buffering capacity of the blood and an extracellular (i.e. blood) acidosis can develop. Extracellular acidosis can desaturate arterial haemoglobin, termed the Bohr effect.[63] Desaturation of arterial haemoglobin can impair O_2 delivery to the brain.[64–66] This may in turn induce a level of cerebral hypoxia that could contribute to central fatigue.[7,64,67–69] Indeed, fatigue of a central origin has been shown to occur within a few seconds of maximal force production.[70] Therefore, the blood alkalinising effect of substances such as sodium bicarbonate may attenuate arterial haemoglobin desaturation and attenuate reductions in central nervous system drive.[7] This suggestion has support from studies showing that blood acidosis increases ratings of perceived exertion (RPE) and reduces exercise tolerance, and that ingestion of bicarbonate attenuates increases in RPE.[64,71]

> **Key point 3.10**
>
> *Extracellular acidosis can lead to arterial haemoglobin desaturation, which in turn can impair oxygen delivery to the brain, inducing a cerebral hypoxia that could contribute to the development of central fatigue.*

> **Key point 3.11**
>
> *Accumulation of H^+ in the muscle interstitial space can stimulate group III/IV afferents, leading to reduced voluntary central nervous system drive and/or compromised responsiveness of motor cortical cells.*

Increasing H^+ concentration may also contribute to reduced central drive via a mechanism independent of cerebral deoxygenation. Accumulation of H^+

in the interstitial space of skeletal muscles can stimulate metabolically sensitive group III/IV afferents.[72] These afferents are specialised sensory neurons that project back to the central nervous system, relaying information about the metabolic status of the muscle. In this situation, the brain interprets the muscles as being in a metabolically challenged situation, and the response is a reduction in motor neuron output mediated by inhibition of voluntary central nervous system drive and/or compromised responsiveness of motor cortical cells (those involved in generating the electrical signal for coordinated skeletal muscle movement).[72-74] This response is an attempt to ease the metabolic challenge by reducing the force-producing capacity of the muscles.

3.3.4 *Lactate, hydrogen, acidosis, and fatigue: a brief summary*

Explaining the potential influence of metabolic acidosis on sport and exercise fatigue is tricky, not least because there is still much ongoing debate on the topic. Regarding lactate, here are some key things to remember:

1 Lactate, not lactic acid, is produced in the muscles during intense sport and exercise.
2 Lactate and lactic acid should not be thought of as the same thing: they are different substances.
3 Lactate is produced *in response to* the muscle becoming more acidic due to production of H^+. Lactate production is *not* a primary cause of muscle acidity.
4 Lactate production likely *reduces* muscle acidity by consuming H^+.
5 Lactate is an important source of fuel for exercising muscles and the brain.

Lactate may indirectly contribute to fatigue, perhaps by contributing to H^+ production via water hydrolysis. However, the possible contribution of lactate to fatigue in sport and exercise is small. During intense sport and exercise, fatigue would occur sooner if lactate were not produced.

Based on current research evidence, it appears that metabolic acidosis stemming from H^+ production does play a role in fatigue during sport and exercise, although this role may be smaller, or at least more synergistic, than previously thought. There is evidence that a reduced pH can actually increase muscle force production and help to maintain muscle excitability in some situations. However, H^+ production may impact performance in ways other than direct muscle impairment, such as by reducing central nervous system drive and increasing effort perception. Therefore, H^+ should still be considered in discussions on sport and exercise fatigue, just not as the "go to" culprit for all things fatigue-related.

3.4 Summary

• Research conducted in the early 1900s on muscle preparations claimed to identify the production of lactic acid under anaerobic conditions and elevated lactic acid concentration at the point of muscle fatigue.

- This research may have been misinterpreted to mean that lactic acid production causes muscle fatigue.
- Lactic acid was suggested to contribute to fatigue by impairing isometric muscle force production and muscle shortening velocity, and by inhibiting glycolysis via reduced activity of important glycolytic enzymes.
- An important distinction is that lactate, not lactic acid, is produced via glycolysis at rest and during sport and exercise.
- Hydrogen ions are hydrogen atoms that have lost their single electron, leaving behind a single proton. Hydrogen ions are acidic and make the solution they are placed in more acidic.
- Lactate does not release H^+ ions, meaning that lactate does not directly make the environment more acidic.
- Lactate may indirectly increase H^+ production by contributing to a reduction in the strong ion difference, thereby leading to the hydrolysis of water. However, the functional relevance of this to sport and exercise fatigue is unknown.
- Lactate is an important source of fuel for skeletal muscles and the brain and acts as a H^+ buffer. Therefore, lactate production serves to reduce tissue acidity, in opposition to the traditional perspective.
- It is feasible that lactate may play a small role in sport and exercise fatigue.
- Hydrogen production may contribute to fatigue by negatively impacting the interaction between Ca^{2+} and the myofilaments, slowing the rate at which ADP dissociates from the myosin head, reducing central nervous system drive via arterial haemoglobin desaturation and associated declines in cerebral O_2 delivery, and stimulating group III/IV afferents in the muscle interstitium, leading to reduce voluntary central nervous system drive and/or compromised responsiveness of motor cortical cells.

To think about...

The production of lactate rather than lactic acid and the beneficial roles of lactate production during sport and exercise (as a fuel source and metabolic buffer) have been known for quite some time. Despite this wealth of scientific research, it is still common to hear many athletes, coaches, sports commentators (many of whom are former elite athletes) and sport and exercise science students place the blame for sore, tired muscles and impaired performance on "lactic acid build up".

Why is there still such a reliance on outdated explanations for a particular phenomenon? Is it because people feel more comfortable with established explanations that the majority believe to be correct, despite evidence to the contrary? Or is it because the findings and messages produced by scientific research are not getting through to the people who can learn from them and make use of them? If the messages aren't getting through, why not? How do you think that scientists and researchers should make themselves heard?

Test yourself

Answer the following questions to the best of your ability. Try to understand the information gained from answering these questions before you progress with the book.

1 How did the perception develop that an increased production of lactic acid contributed to fatigue during sport and exercise?
2 What are the two primary ways in which lactic acid production was thought to contribute to sport and exercise fatigue?
3 What is the difference between a lactic acid molecule and a lactate molecule? What is the importance of this difference for the development of acidosis?
4 What is the difference between a hydrogen atom and a proton? What is the importance of this difference for the development of acidosis?
5 List the main misconceptions about, and benefits of, lactate that were discussed in the chapter.
6 What are the main ways in which acidosis is thought to impair sport and exercise performance?

References

1   Ferguson BS, Rogatzki MJ, Goodwin ML, Kane DA, Rightmire Z, Gladden LB. Lactate metabolism: historical context, prior misinterpretations, and current understanding. *Eur J Appl Physiol.* 2018;118(4):691–728.
2   Fletcher WM, Hopkins FG. Lactic acid in amphibian muscle. *J Physiol.* 1907;35(4):247–309.
3   Hill AV, Lupton H. Muscular exercise, lactic acid, and the supply and utilization of oxygen. *Q J Med.* 1923;16:135–171.
4   Roberts RA, Ghiasvand F, Parker D. Biochemistry of exercise-induced metabolic acidosis. *Am J Physiol Regul Integr Comp Physiol.* 2004;287(3):R502–R516.
5   Fitts RH, Holloszy JO. Lactate and contractile force in frog muscle during development of fatigue and recovery. *Am J Physiol.* 1976;231:R502–R516.
6   Spriet LL, Soderlund K, Bergstrom M, Hultman E. Skeletal muscle glycogenolysis, glycolysis, and pH during electrical stimulation in men. *J Appl Physiol (1985).* 1987;62(2):616–621.
7   Cairns SP. Lactic acid and exercise performance: culprit or friend? *Sports Med.* 2006;36(4):279–291.
8   Lamb GD, Recupero E, Stephenson DG. Effect of myoplasmic pH on excitation-contraction coupling in skeletal muscle fibres of the toad. *J Physiol.* 1992;448:211–224.
9   Fitts RH. The cross-bridge cycle and skeletal muscle fatigue. *J Appl Physiol (1985).* 2008;104(2):551–558.
10 Balsom PD, Seger JY, Sjodin B, Ekblom B. Physiological responses to maximal intensity intermittent exercise. *Eur J Appl Physiol Occup Physiol.* 1992;65(2):144–149.
11 Brooks S, Nevill ME, Meleagros L, et al. The hormonal responses to repetitive brief maximal exercise in humans. *Eur J Appl Physiol Occup Physiol.* 1990;60(2):144–148.

12 Christmass MA, Dawson B, Arthur PG. Effect of work and recovery duration on skeletal muscle oxygenation and fuel use during sustained intermittent exercise. *Eur J Appl Physiol Occup Physiol.* 1999;80(5):436–447.

13 Gaitanos GC, Williams C, Boobis LH, Brooks S. Human muscle metabolism during intermittent maximal exercise. *J Appl Physiol (1985).* 1993;75(2):712–719.

14 Bishop D, Edge J, Davis C, Goodman C. Induced metabolic alkalosis affects muscle metabolism and repeated-sprint ability. *Med Sci Sports Exerc.* 2004;36(5): 807–813.

15 Bishop D, Claudius B. Effects of induced metabolic alkalosis on prolonged intermittent-sprint performance. *Med Sci Sports Exerc.* 2005;37(5):759–767.

16 Lavender G, Bird SR. Effect of sodium bicarbonate ingestion upon repeated sprints. *Br J Sports Med.* 1989;23(1):41–45.

17 Jeukendrup AE. Performance and endurance in sport: can it all be explained by metabolism and its manipulation? *Dialogues Cardiovasc Med.* 2012;17(1): 40–45.

18 Lindinger MI, Kowalchuk JM, Heigenhauser GJ. Applying physicochemical principles to skeletal muscle acid-base status. *Am J Physiol Regul Integr Comp Physiol.* 2005;289(3):R891–R894; author reply R904–R910.

19 Keyser RE. Peripheral fatigue: high-energy phosphates and hydrogen ions. *PMR.* 2010;2(5):347–358.

20 Proia P, Di Liegro CM, Schiera G, Fricano A, Di Liegro I. Lactate as a metabolite and a regulator in the central nervous system. *Int J Mol Sci.* 2016;17(9):1–20.

21 Glancy B, Kane DA, Kavazis AN, Goodwin ML, Willis WT, Gladden LB. Mitochondrial lactate metabolism: history and implications for exercise and disease. *J Physiol.* 2021;599(3):863–888.

22 Brooks GA. What does glycolysis make and why is it important? *J Appl Physiol* 2010;108:1450–1451.

23 Robergs RA. Lingering construct of lactic acidosis. *Am J Physiol.* 2005;289: R904–R910.

24 Boning D, Strobel G, Beneke R, Maassen N. Lactic acid still remains the real cause of exercise-induced metabolic acidosis. *Am J Physiol Regul Integr Comp Physiol.* 2005;289(3):R902–R903; author reply R904–R910.

25 Boning D, Maassen N. Last word on point:counterpoint: lactic acid is/is not the only physicochemical contributor to the acidosis of exercise. *J Appl Physiol (1985).* 2008;105(1):368.

26 Brooks GA. Lactate: link between glycolytic and oxidative metabolism. *Sports Med.* 2007;37(4–5):341–343.

27 Brooks GA. Cell-cell and intracellular lactate shuttles. *J Physiol.* 2009;587(Pt 23):5591–5600.

28 Ide K, Schmalbruch IK, Quistorff B, Horn A, Secher NH. Lactate, glucose and O2 uptake in human brain during recovery from maximal exercise. *J Physiol.* 2000;522(Pt 1):159–164.

29 Quistorff B, Secher NH, Van Lieshout JJ. Lactate fuels the human brain during exercise. *FASEB J.* 2008;22(10):3443–3449.

30 Caldwell HG, Gliemann L, Ainslie PN. *Exercise Metabolism.* Switzerland: Springer; 2022.

31 Morris DM, Shafer RS, Fairbrother KR, Woodall MW. Effects of lactate consumption on blood bicarbonate levels and performance during high-intensity exercise. *Int J Sport Nutr Exerc Metab.* 2011;21(4):311–317.

32 Russ AE, Schifino AG, Leong C. Effect of lactate supplementation on VO2peak and onset of blood lactate accumulation: A double-blind, placebo-controlled trial. *Acta Gymnica*. 2019;49(2):51–57.

33 Painelli Vde S, da Silva RP, de Oliveira OM, Jr., et al. The effects of two different doses of calcium lactate on blood pH, bicarbonate, and repeated high-intensity exercise performance. *Int J Sport Nutr Exerc Metab*. 2014;24(3):286–295.

34 Pollak KA, Swenson JD, Vanhaitsma TA, et al. Exogenously applied muscle metabolites synergistically evoke sensations of muscle fatigue and pain in human subjects. *Exp Physiol*. 2014;99(2):368–380.

35 Monedero J, Donne B. Effect of recovery interventions on lactate removal and subsequent performance. *Int J Sports Med*. 2000;21(8):593–597.

36 Aminian-Far A, Hadian MR, Olyaei G, Talebian S, Bakhtiary AH. Whole-body vibration and the prevention and treatment of delayed-onset muscle soreness. *J Athl Train*. 2011;46(1):43–49.

37 Lewis PB, Ruby D, Bush-Joseph CA. Muscle soreness and delayed-onset muscle soreness. *Clin Sports Med*. 2012;31(2):255–262.

38 Hotfiel T, Freiwald J, Hoppe MW, et al. Advances in delayed-onset muscle soreness (DOMS): part I: pathogenesis and diagnostics. *Sportverletz Sportschaden*. 2018;32(4):243–250.

39 Boning D, Maassen N. Point: Lactic acid is the only physicochemical contributor to the acidosis of exercise. *J Appl Physiol (1985)*. 2008;105(1):358–359.

40 Lindinger MI, Heigenhauser GJ. Counterpoint: lactic acid is not the only physicochemical contributor to the acidosis of exercise. *J Appl Physiol (1985)*. 2008;105(1):359–361; discussion 361–352.

41 Lamb GD, Stephenson DG. Point: counterpoint: lactic acid accumulation is an advantage/disadvantage during muscle activity. *J Appl Physiol*. 2006;100(4):1410–1412.

42 Pesi R, Balestri F, Ipata PL. Anaerobic glycolysis and glycogenolysis do not release protons and do not cause acidosis. *Curr Metabolomics Syst Biol*. 2020;7(1):6–10.

43 Debold EP. Decreased myofilament calcium sensitivity plays a significant role in muscle fatigue. *Exerc Sport Sci Rev*. 2016;44(4):144–149.

44 Debold EP, Fitts RH, Sundberg CW, Nosek TM. Muscle fatigue from the perspective of a single crossbridge. *Med Sci Sports Exerc*. 2016;48(11):2270–2280.

45 Cheng AJ, Place N, Westerblad H. Molecular basis for exercise-induced fatigue: the importance of strictly controlled cellular $Ca(2^+)$ handling. *Cold Spring Harb Perspect Med*. 2018;8(2):1–19.

46 Debold EP, Dave H, Fitts RH. Fiber type and temperature dependence of inorganic phosphate: implications for fatigue. *Am J Physiol Cell Physiol*. 2004;287(3): C673–C681.

47 Metzger JM, Moss RL. Calcium-sensitive cross-bridge transitions in mammalian fast and slow skeletal muscle fibers. *Science*. 1990;247(4946):1088–1090.

48 Debold EP, Beck SE, Warshaw DM. Effect of low pH on single skeletal muscle myosin mechanics and kinetics. *Am J Physiol Cell Physiol*. 2008;295(1):C173–C179.

49 Jarvis K, Woodward M, Debold EP, Walcott S. Acidosis affects muscle contraction by slowing the rates myosin attaches to and detaches from actin. *J Muscle Res Cell Motil*. 2018;39(3–4):135–147.

50 Lindinger MI, Cairns SP. Regulation of muscle potassium: exercise performance, fatigue and health implications. *Eur J Appl Physiol*. 2021;121:721–748.

51 Bishop D, Edge J, Goodman C. Muscle buffer capacity and aerobic fitness are associated with repeated-sprint ability in women. *Eur J Appl Physiol.* 2004;92(4–5): 540–547.

52 Krustrup P, Mohr M, Steensberg A, Bencke J, Kjaer M, Bangsbo J. Muscle metabolites during a football match in relation to a decreased sprinting ability. Fifth World Congress of Soccer and Science; 2004; Lisbon, Portugal.

53 Messonnier L, Denis C, Feasson L, Lacour JR. An elevated sarcolemmal lactate (and proton) transport capacity is an advantage during muscle activity in healthy humans. *J Appl Physiol (1985).* 2006.10.1152/japplphysiol.00807.2006

54 Parolin ML, Chesley A, Matsos MP, Spriet LL, Jones NL, Heigenhauser GJ. Regulation of skeletal muscle glycogen phosphorylase and PDH during maximal intermittent exercise. *Am J Physiol.* 1999;277(5):E890–E900.

55 Spriet LL, Lindinger MI, McKelvie RS, Heigenhauser GJ, Jones NL. Muscle glycogenolysis and H+ concentration during maximal intermittent cycling. *J Appl Physiol (1985).* 1989;66(1):8–13.

56 McCartney N, Spriet LL, Heigenhauser GJ, Kowalchuk JM, Sutton JR, Jones NL. Muscle power and metabolism in maximal intermittent exercise. *J Appl Physiol (1985).* 1986;60(4):1164–1169.

57 Korzeniewski B, Rossiter HB. Each-step activation of oxidative phosphorylation is necessary to explain muscle metabolic kinetic responses to exercise and recovery in humans. *J Physiol.* 2015;593(24):5255–5268.

58 Katz A, Costill DL, King DS, Hargreaves M, Fink WJ. Maximal exercise tolerance after induced alkalosis. *Int J Sports Med.* 1984;5(2):107–110.

59 Bangsbo J, Madsen K, Kiens B, Richter EA. Effect of muscle acidity on muscle metabolism and fatigue during intense exercise in man. *J Physiol.* 1996;495(Pt 2):587–596.

60 Girard O, Mendez-Villanueva A, Bishop D. Repeated-sprint ability – part I: factors contributing to fatigue. *Sports Med.* 2011;41(8):673–694.

61 Karatzaferi C, Franks-Skiba K, Cooke R. Inhibition of shortening velocity of skinned skeletal muscle fibers in conditions that mimic fatigue. *Am J Physiol Regul Integr Comp Physiol.* 2008;294(3):R948–R955.

62 Fitts RH. The role of acidosis in fatigue: pro perspective. *Med Sci Sports Exerc.* 2016;48(11):2335–2338.

63 Volianitis S, Bredmose PP, Nielsen HB, Stromstad M, Quistorff B, Secher NH. Bicarbonate infusion attenuates arterial desaturation during maximal exercise. *FASEB J.* 2016;30(1):lb685–lb685.

64 Nielsen HB, Bredmose PP, Stromstad M, Volianitis S, Quistorff B, Secher NH. Bicarbonate attenuates arterial desaturation during maximal exercise in humans. *J Appl Physiol (1985).* 2002;93(2):724–731.

65 Secher NH, Seifert T, Van Lieshout JJ. Cerebral blood flow and metabolism during exercise: implications for fatigue. *J Appl Physiol (1985).* 2008;104(1):306–314.

66 Raberin A, Meric H, Mucci P, Lopez Ayerbe J, Durand F. Muscle and cerebral oxygenation during exercise in athletes with exercise-induced hypoxemia: a comparison between sea level and acute moderate hypoxia. *Eur J Sport Sci.* 2020;20(6):803–812.

67 Knicker AJ, Renshaw I, Oldham AR, Cairns SP. Interactive processes link the multiple symptoms of fatigue in sport competition. *Sports Med.* 2011;41(4):307–328.

68　Nybo L, Secher NH. Cerebral perturbations provoked by prolonged exercise. *Prog Neurobiol.* 2004;72(4):223–261.

69　Amann M, Calbet JA. Convective oxygen transport and fatigue. *J Appl Physiol (1985).* 2008;104(3):861–870.

70　Gandevia SC, Allen GM, Butler JE, Taylor JL. Supraspinal factors in human muscle fatigue: evidence for suboptimal output from the motor cortex. *J Physiol.* 1996;490(Pt 2):529–536.

71　Swank A, Robertson RJ. Effect of induced alkalosis on perception of exertion during intermittent exercise. *J Appl Physiol (1985).* 1989;67(5):1862–1867.

72　Hureau TJ, Broxterman RM, Weavil JC, Lewis MT, Layec G, Amann M. On the role of skeletal muscle acidosis and inorganic phosphates as determinants of central and peripheral fatigue: A (31) P-MRS study. *J Physiol.* 2022;600(13): 3069–3081.

73　Amann M, Wan HY, Thurston TS, Georgescu VP, Weavil JC. On the influence of group III/IV muscle afferent feedback on endurance exercise performance. *Exerc Sport Sci Rev.* 2020;48(4):209–216.

74　Sidhu SK, Weavil JC, Thurston TS, et al. Fatigue-related group III/IV muscle afferent feedback facilitates intracortical inhibition during locomotor exercise. *J Physiol.* 2018;596(19):4789–4801.

4 Environmental stress

4.1 Introduction

Sport and exercise takes place in ever-more varied locations around the world, both at the professional/elite and recreational levels thus exposing participants to potentially hostile environmental conditions. In fact, many event locations are specifically chosen for their hostile environments. For example, the Marathon Des Sables (6 day, 250 km run through the Sahara Desert, average temperature 30°C, peak temperature >50°C), the StrathPuffer (24-hour mountain bike race in the Scottish Highlands in January, significant snow and ice under-wheel, prolonged exposure to sub-zero temperatures, snow and/or rainfall), and mountain climbing (exposure to very cold temperatures, significant snowfall, and the effects of altitude). Events in environments such as this place strain on many body systems and physiological processes above and beyond that experienced in more neutral environments.

This chapter will follow a similar approach to Chapter 3, as certain aspects of environmental stress are as much a cause of fatigue during sport and exercise as acidosis in the minds of many. The chapter will address dehydration and hyperthermia (as caused primarily by environmental conditions) and sport and exercise undertaken at altitude (real or simulated). The concepts of dehydration and hyperthermia are often linked as though one cannot exist without the other. This is not the case. Therefore, the chapter will address them as separate issues but will combine them as necessary. The classical mechanisms of dehydration-induced fatigue will be highlighted, along with other less well-known potential mechanisms. The evolution of knowledge regarding dehydration and fatigue will then be discussed, culminating in an overview of current thinking on this topic.

The section on hyperthermia will follow a similar approach. Classical theories will be discussed, including the concept of a 'critical' core temperature that once attained impairs sport and exercise performance. The link between dehydration and hyperthermia will also be highlighted, as will the potential roles of dehydration and hyperthermia, alone and in combination, on sport and exercise fatigue. By the end of the chapter, the reader should have a greater

DOI: 10.4324/9781003326137-6

critical understanding of the potential influence that these two commonly cited factors have on sport and exercise fatigue.

The potential impact of altitude on fatigue processes will be drawn from the literature investigating acute hypoxia, both real and simulated. This is in keeping with the rest of this book, which discusses fatigue in more acute contexts. Professional or mass participation sport and exercise events at the upper range of high altitude are almost non-existent, for obvious logistical and safety reasons.

The wealth of data on human performance in the environments introduced above could alone fill several books. Therefore, this chapter will at times provide overviews of topics, with signposting to further resources where appropriate. The focus will be retained as much as possible on how these environmental conditions may influence predominantly physiological fatigue processes during sport and exercise.

4.2   Dehydration and fatigue

4.2.1   Defining terms

Before progressing, it is useful to define some of the key terms that will be used throughout this chapter. *Hydration* or *euhydration* refers to an appropriate body water content for an individual. It is the absence of

> **Key point 4.1**
>
> *The terms dehydration and hypohydration do not mean the same thing. Dehydration is the process of losing water from the body; hypohydration is the end result of this water loss.*

hyper or hypohydration. *Hyperhydration* refers to a state of excess body water content. Hyperhydration can be a potentially serious condition and will be discussed in this chapter. The dynamic process of losing body water is termed *dehydration*. Finally, a state of insufficient body water content is termed *hypohydration*. Dehydration and hypohydration are closely related but do not mean the same thing. For example, during sport and exercise, a person loses fluid, primarily through sweat. At the end of sport and exercise, they may have lost a volume of fluid that is equivalent to 1.5% of their body mass (BM). Therefore, through the process of dehydration, the person has become hypohydrated by 1.5%. Dehydration is the process of body water loss; hypohydration is the result of this loss.

4.2.2   The importance of water in the body

Despite having no caloric value, water is one of the most important nutrients for life, second only to oxygen (O_2). A person can survive for several weeks without consuming food and can survive losses of up to 40% of their BM in fat, carbohydrate, and protein. However, a matter of days without water, or a water loss of only 9%–12% of BM, can be fatal. Our reliance on water is due to its prevalence in the body and the number of important roles that it carries out to enable optimal function. When euhydrated, water comprises approximately 60% of the BM of an adult male and 50% of an adult female (this figure is partly dependent on body composition; lean tissue contains much more water than fat (approx. 73% versus 10%). Approximately two thirds of body water content is contained inside our cells (intracellular fluid), with the other third outside (extracellular fluid).

Water is the medium in which most of the life preserving processes in cells, tissues, and organ systems occur (Table 4.1). The importance of water means it is critical to ensure an appropriate water balance, defined as the balance between water intake and water loss (Figure 4.1). Most of the factors highlighted in Table 4.1 are important during sport and exercise as well as at rest. Therefore, it is easy to see why body water content and its loss during sport and exercise has been considered for so long a critical determinant of performance.

Table 4.1 Important functions of water within the human body

1 Forms the fluid portion of blood, allowing the transport of nutrients, waste products, oxygen, and immune cells to all parts of the body.
2 Maintains appropriate blood volume; crucial for function of the cardiovascular system.
3 Plays a role in metabolic reactions.
4 Acts as a solvent for proteins, glucose, vitamins and minerals.
5 Plays an important role in maintenance of electrolyte balance.
6 Forms the fluid portion of sweat, allowing thermoregulation to occur.
7 Transports heat from deeper regions of the body to the skin surface, further assisting thermoregulation.
8 Helps to lubricate joints.
9 Major constituent of spinal and eye fluid.

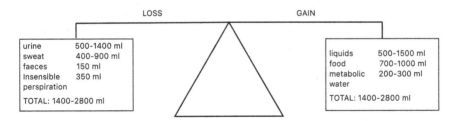

Figure 4.1 Typical daily water loss and gain for an average adult. The figures for water loss and gain will be influenced by diet, fluid ingestion, body mass, body composition, environmental conditions, and level of physical activity/sport/exercise. The scale can tip to the left (negative water balance; greater water loss than gain: dehydration/hypohydration) or to the right (positive water balance, greater water gain than loss: hyperhydration).

A complication when trying to understand concepts associated with water balance is that most of the factors that influence water balance (levels of exercise/sport/physical activity, sweat rate, body composition, diet, fluid intake) are individual. As a result, water losses and requirements differ significantly between people. One of the most important factors influencing water balance is sweat loss during physical activity/sport and exercise. The influence of physical activity on body water loss has led to the recommendation that water requirements should be calculated with reference to the amount of daily physical activity someone is engaged in. It is recommended that normal adults should consume 1–1.5 ml of water for every kcal expended, and athletes should consume 1.5 ml of water for every kcal expended. Therefore, an athlete who expends 4,000 kcal per day would require 6,000 ml, or 6 L, of water (from food and fluid sources combined) per day. However, as you will see as you read this chapter, current fluid intake recommendations for athletes and the general population are being challenged.

> **Key point 4.2**
>
> *Body water balance is influenced by factors that vary greatly between people. As a result, water requirements can vary significantly from person to person.*

4.2.3   *Classical mechanism of dehydration-induced performance decrement*

During sport and exercise, sweat rate greatly increases. Sweating is the main way that the body dissipates heat produced from the increase in energy metabolism during sport and exercise. The fluid portion of sweat comes predominantly from blood plasma, which is the liquid portion of the blood in which the red and white cells and platelets are suspended. The loss of fluid from blood plasma causes a decrease in plasma volume. Reduced plasma volume means that less blood enters the heart in each cardiac cycle (termed reduced cardiac filling pressure). Reduced cardiac filling pressure contributes to a reduction in stroke volume (the volume of blood pumped from the heart in each beat) and cardiac output ($\dot{Q}$; the volume of blood pumped from the heart per minute), meaning that heart rate has to increase to maintain appropriate blood and O_2 delivery to working tissue. This reduction in cardiac efficiency may in itself lead to impaired sport and exercise performance,

> **Key point 4.3**
>
> *Dehydration may contribute to performance decrement directly by reducing cardiac efficiency and indirectly by contributing to the development of hyperthermia.*

with an approximate increase in heart rate of 3–5 beats per minute for every 1% loss of BM due to dehydration.[1] However, if water loss and sport/exercise continue, reduced plasma volume may lead to competition for blood flow between core organs/tissues and the skin (termed circulatory stress). This competition could lead to reduced skin blood flow, impairing evaporative heat loss and leading to an increase in core body temperature (hyperthermia). Therefore, according to the classical theory, dehydration may impair performance directly through alterations in cardiac efficiency, and indirectly by contributing to the development of hyperthermia. An overview of the classical theory of dehydration-induced performance decrement is in Figure 4.2.

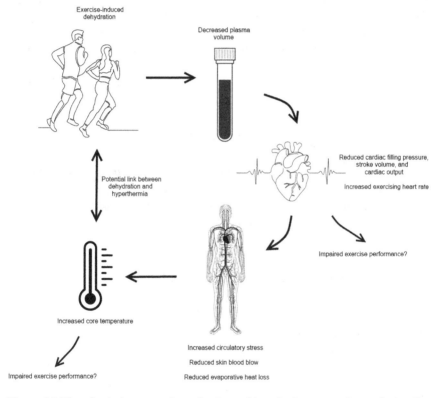

Figure 4.2 The classical proposed mechanism of impaired sport and exercise performance with dehydration. Body water loss decreases plasma volume, leading to reduced cardiac filling pressure, stroke volume and cardiac output. This impaired cardiac efficiency means that heart rate has to increase to maintain appropriate blood and oxygen delivery to working tissue. Elevated heart rate could in itself lead to impaired performance. However, if water loss continues, reduced plasma volume may lead to competition for blood flow between the core organs and tissues and the skin (circulatory stress). This competition could lead to reduced skin blood flow, impairing evaporative heat loss and leading to an increase in core body temperature.

4.2.4   Other potential mechanisms of dehydration-induced performance decrement

Dehydration can alter metabolic function by increasing liver glucose output and the reliance on carbohydrate metabolism via increased oxidation of muscle glycogen, which leads to greater blood lactate concentration at a given intensity.[2,3] The greater reliance on carbohydrate oxidation when hypohydrated may be due to an increased sympathoadrenal response, decreased cellular energy status, and increased muscle temperature.[3-5] Greater reliance on carbohydrate oxidation could contribute to fatigue via glycogen depletion (see Chapter 2).

Perceived exertion during sport and exercise may increase when hypohydrated compared to the same intensity in a euhydrated state.[1] Similarly, cognitive function (vision, attention, memory, etc.) may be impaired when hypohydrated.[6] The impact on these parameters will depend in part on the extent of hypohydration. If hypohydration does alter the perception of effort and mental processes during sport and exercise, this could contribute to decreased performance by altering factors such as motivation, decision-making, and pacing strategies. The impact of various factors, including hypohydration on perceptual responses to sport and exercise, will be discussed in this chapter and Chapter 6. Causes of fatigue attributable to dehydration can be central or peripheral in origin and are further discussed in Section 4.7 and summarised in Figure 4.3.

> **Key point 4.4**
>
> *Dehydration may contribute to performance decrement, directly or indirectly, by altering the perception of effort, cognitive function, and energy metabolism.*

4.3   Dehydration and sport and exercise fatigue: research issues

There is an abundance of research showing that dehydration during sport and exercise can lead to performance decrements.[7,8] The potential negative consequences of dehydration discussed in Sections 4.2.3 and 4.2.4 have informed published guidelines for fluid intake during sport and exercise. The guidelines recommend that people should develop customised fluid replacement programmes that enable them to begin sport

> **Key point 4.5**
>
> *Early research established an apparent 'threshold' hypohydration level of 2% body mass, above which aerobic sport and exercise performance is impaired. This threshold has become established as a cornerstone of fluid intake recommendations and guidelines.*

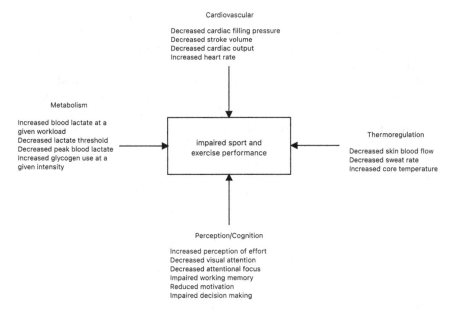

Cardiovascular

Decreased cardiac filling pressure
Decreased stroke volume
Decreased cardiac output
Increased heart rate

Metabolism

Increased blood lactate at a
given workload
Decreased lactate threshold
Decreased peak blood lactate
Increased glycogen use at a
given intensity

impaired sport and
exercise performance

Thermoregulation

Decreased skin blood flow
Decreased sweat rate
Increased core temperature

Perception/Cognition

Increased perception of effort
Decreased visual attention
Decreased attentional focus
Impaired working memory
Reduced motivation
Impaired decision making

Figure 4.3 A summary of the factors associated with dehydration that could contribute to impaired sport and exercise performance.

and exercise euhydrated and that prevent excessive fluid losses during sport and exercise.[9] An obvious question is: what is classed as 'excessive' fluid losses? Early literature that provided the foundation for study into hydration and sport and exercise identified an apparent 'threshold' fluid decrement of 2% of a person's BM, above which aerobic performance appeared to be impaired.[8–10] Over the years, this 2% dehydration threshold has become firmly established as a principle on which fluid intake recommendations are based.

However, it is important to consider how research was carried out so that we can better interpret its results. Some of the earlier studies investigating fluid balance and sport and exercise performance are regularly cited as classic papers in the field and support the notion that dehydration impairs performance. A limitation of some of these studies is the manner in which dehydration was 'achieved'. Some studies required people to sit for extended periods of time in a hot environment without drinking anything.[9] Some studies required participants to complete prolonged exercise in a hot environment with limited fluid intake, followed by a further period of rest (sometimes with restricted fluid intake) *then* undertake another exercise session.[11,12] Some studies also used diuretics to stimulate fluid loss by increasing urine output.[13] These approaches essentially ensure that a person *begins* exercise in a hypohydrated state, rather than losing fluid and potentially becoming hypohydrated *during* exercise. None of these approaches would routinely be carried out by a person preparing to undertake sport and exercise in the real world. Using these study designs, it also may not be possible to separate the effects of hypohydration on performance from possible effects of the procedures used to achieve hypohy-dration.[9] Due to this concern, it has been suggested that only studies in which hypohydration develops during sport and exercise provide a valid measure of the effects of hypohydration.[9,14]

If research is carried out with the aim of studying the effect of fluid restriction on sport and exercise performance, then it is probable that the people taking part in that research will know that they are going to have to exercise with no fluid intake, or a greatly reduced fluid intake compared to that they would normally choose to consume. This foreknowledge may give the participants a different mind-set about the activity they are about to do, perhaps making them anticipate a poorer performance.[9] In fact, it has been shown that when people are aware at the beginning of exercise that their fluid intake is going to be restricted, they begin exercise at a lower intensity than when they are able to drink *ad libitum*.[15] This shows that the negative influence of performance attributed to hypohydration can, depending on the research approach taken, be due to other factors.

Many research participants come from what is termed a 'convenience' sample, meaning a group of people to which the researchers have easy access. As a result, participants are often not of a high athletic ability. Athletes may differ in many ways, physiologically and psychologically, from convenience participants. Therefore, results produced from research using convenience samples may not be relevant to different groups of people such as competitive athletes. Using heterogeneous samples could cloud understanding of hydration and sport and exercise performance, as it is known that there is a very large inter-individual variability in tolerance to different extents of hypohydration.[14]

Perhaps, the most important consideration to make when interpreting de-hydration research is the type of exercise undertaken. Much of the research used fixed intensity exercise, and/or protocols requiring participants to exercise to exhaustion. These are understandable choices, as this form of exercise allows researchers to control for many factors that can influence study results. However, protocols requiring exercise to exhaustion can be unreliable.[16,17] If performance in these tests varied to a great extent, it may over-state the influence of factors such as dehydration on performance, or it could have the opposite effect and mask the effects of such interventions. Also, fixed-intensity exercise (whether to exhaustion or not) is not representative of the majority of real-world sport and exercise scenarios. In most competitive sports, the aim is to complete a set distance in the fastest possible time, rather than perform for as long as possible. Real-world sport and exercise is also usually self-paced, meaning the athlete has the choice of whether

Key point 4.6

The way in which research into dehydration and sport/exercise performance is carried out should be considered when interpreting the results of such research.

to increase or decrease intensity at any time. Therefore, while fixed-intensity exercise allows only one of two choices (keep going vs. stop), self-paced exercise allows continual changes in effort that could affect performance.[17]

Key point 4.7

Studies using self-paced sport and exercise demonstrate that fluid loss does not impair performance. A review of the literature further states that dehydration only impairs performance during fixed-workload exercise.

The issues with some previous research into the effects of dehydration on sport and exercise performance are further highlighted when we consider more recent investigations. A number of recent studies have shown that dehydration does not impair performance lasting from 60 minutes to more than 4 hours, in both normal and warm environments, despite participants losing 1.7%–3.1% of their pre-activity BM.[18-21] These losses exceed that stated by earlier research to impair performance (i.e. the 2% 'threshold'), so why was performance not impaired? To explain the likely reasons, it would be useful to summarise each of the studies in turn and then bring this information together into a final summary.

4.3.1 Marino et al.[19]

These authors found that ingesting no fluid during 60 minutes of self-paced high-intensity cycling in moderate (hypohydration 1.7% BM) or warm (hypohydration 2.1% BM) conditions did not impair performance compared with consuming enough fluid to maintain BM. Interestingly, the authors provided evidence to suggest that the neuromuscular system altered muscle recruitment in response to different hydration levels, thereby enabling a similar performance level despite differences in hydration status.

4.3.2 Nolte et al.[20]

This study was a little different to some of the other hydration research, as it investigated the relationship between fluid intake and time to complete a 14.5-km march in soldiers. Interestingly, no relationship between fluid intake and march time, or BM loss and march time, was found. Furthermore, the soldiers' hydration status was maintained despite BM losses of around 2%.

4.3.3 Zouhal et al.[21]

This study investigated the relationship between BM change (as an indicator of hydration) and marathon finishing time. The authors found that the greater the BM loss, the faster the marathon finishing time. Put another way, the people who lost more weight, and therefore were perhaps more hypohydrated, tended to perform better than those who maintained a stable hydration status or who drank more fluid than they lost during the run.

4.3.4   *Dion et al.*[18]

These authors reported that the time to complete a half-marathon was not different when people either drank enough water to maintain BM or drank according to the dictate of their thirst (in other words, they drank as much water as they wanted to when they felt thirsty). People drank about four times as much water and lost an average of 3.1% BM, when drinking to thirst. However, there was no difference in performance, sweat loss, sweat rate, body temperature, or heart rate between the trials.

4.3.5   *Overall Summary*

The research studies discussed above, and others that have found either no effect or a minimal effect of dehydration on sport and exercise performance,[22–24] have one thing in common: they all used self-paced, real-world sport and exercise (meaning the studies were either conducted in natural situations, or natural sport and exercise was well replicated in a laboratory setting). As discussed above, self-paced sport and exercise gives the participant more options about how they regulate their performance, making it more appropriate to test the influence of factors such as dehydration on performance. In fact, an analysis of a subset of dehydration research showed that dehydration only impairs sport and exercise performance when fixed-workload exercise (which does not mimic real-world sport and exercise) is used.[25]

> **Key point 4.8**
>
> *Reduced body mass during sport and exercise does not necessarily mean that a person's hydration status has been negatively affected. Body mass loss does not necessarily equate with fluid loss.*

Another interesting point from the above studies is that a BM loss of, say, 2% during sport and exercise does not necessarily mean that a person has become notably hypohydrated. For example, participants in the study by Nolte *et al.*[20] lost on

> **Key point 4.9**
>
> *Only people with specific characteristics may show improved performance with high levels of body mass loss. Therefore, intentional body mass loss should not be recommended as a general strategy for improving performance.*

average 1.98% of their BM. Yet according to urinary measures, the hydration status of those participants was not affected. This suggests that BM changes may not accurately reflect body water loss. During sport and exercise, additions can be made to total body water content by production of water from aerobic energy metabolism, and the release of water from the breakdown of stored muscle and liver glycogen.[26] Similarly, BM losses can occur through substrate oxidation, independent of fluid loss. Therefore, processes are at work during sport and exercise that can reduce BM but at the same time increase total body water content. As a result, BM loss can decrease by as much as 1%–3% without notable dehydration occurring.[26]

The fact that BM loss can occur during sport and exercise without the onset of hypohydration suggests that it may not be necessary to drink sufficient fluid to prevent BM loss. In fact, some researchers suggest that the athletes who finish races fastest tend to be the athletes who drink more to the dictates of their own thirst rather than in an attempt to prevent BM loss,[21] and that drinking to thirst is potentially the most effective hydration strategy during most sport and exercise scenarios.[14,18] Body mass loss without hypohydration would actually be beneficial from a performance perspective as the athlete would have less mass to transport during their event, enabling them to compete at a given intensity while expending less effort and energy. In support of this suggestion, it is frequently observed that the fastest finishers in endurance activities are often those who lose the most BM during the event.[8,21,27] Therefore, should we recommend that people taking part in endurance sport and exercise actually aim to lose BM, thereby making the activity 'easier'? Certainly not. As one study puts it:

> …the possibility remains that high levels of body weight loss in **certain unique individuals** might enhance exercise performance simply as the result of a lesser body weight that needs to be transported.
> (bold highlighting by the author of this book)[21]

This statement draws attention to the fact that a lot of the research that has found a relationship between BM loss and improved performance during endurance sport and exercise has used participants who are either well-trained, experienced endurance athletes, well acclimated to the environmental conditions in which the study took place, or all of these things. These factors may allow them to respond to BM loss differently than individuals who do not have these characteristics. It is also important to note that some of the relationships between BM loss and endurance performance, while statistically significant, are actually quite small. For

Key point 4.10

There is some evidence that performance is not different with body mass losses less than or greater than 2% BM.

example, in their study of 643 marathon runners Zouhal *et al.*[21] reported a correlation coefficient of *r* = 0.21 between BM change and marathon finishing time. Statistically, this correlation was significant and suggested that greater BM loss led to a faster finishing time. However, this correlation indicates that only 4% of the change in marathon finishing time was shared with changes in BM during the event. Indeed, restricting fluid during sport and exercise probably does not provide a performance benefit, but neither does consuming more fluid than would be ingested under normal conditions.[18] Therefore, drinking according to thirst may be the most effective strategy.

There is evidence that dehydration-induced BM loss during sport and exercise does not impair performance. There is also evidence against the long-held belief that dehydration increases cardiovascular and thermoregulatory strain during sport and exercise, and that this leads to impaired performance (Figure 4.2). During self-paced sport and exercise, increases in core temperature and heart rate associated with dehydration do not appear to influence performance,[18,28,29] ratings of perceived exertion, or heat stress.[18]

It is often difficult to see the 'big picture' regarding research findings in a given area, particularly one as large as hydration and sport and exercise performance. Luckily, a recent meta-analysis has made the job easier.[30] This analysis reviewed 13 studies that used 60-minute cycle time trials under real-world conditions. None of the studies reported a statistically significant negative effect of dehydration on performance. Other important findings from this meta-analysis were:

- Hypohydration during exercise by an average of about 2.2% BM does not impair performance, and in fact may cause a performance improvement (albeit trivial).
- Drinking to thirst increases power output during cycle time trials by an average of about 5% compared to drinking below thirst, and by an average of about 2.5% compared to drinking more than dictated by thirst alone.
- The probability that drinking to thirst alone confers a general advantage during cycle time trials is 98% compared to drinking below thirst, and 62% compared to drinking above thirst.
- There is no relationship between percentage change in BM and percentage change in power output during cycling exercise.
- Both exercise duration and intensity are more important determinants of performance than dehydration.
- There is no significant difference in performance between exercise that results in a BM loss of less than 2% or a BM loss of more than 2%.
- It is not dehydration itself that is responsible for performance decrements during sport and exercise, but rather drinking insufficiently to satisfy thirst. Therefore, drinking 'ahead' of thirst in order to prevent BM loss and performance decrement, as has become a much-believed dogma, is not necessary.
- Following thirst sensation during real-word sport and exercise is the most effective way to maximise performance.

The study of Goulet[30] is an excellent summary of research findings about the *real-world* effect of dehydration on endurance sport and exercise performance. However, it is important to note that Goulet[30] only reviewed studies that involved 1 hour of cycle

Key point 4.11

Research suggests that neither under- nor over-drinking during sport and exercise will significantly improve performance. Therefore, drinking to thirst may be the most effective strategy.

exercise in trained cyclists or endurance-trained people. As was mentioned earlier, a particular set of characteristics may be required for notable BM loss not to impair performance. This should be considered when applying the findings of this study to other populations.

4.4   Dehydration and fluid intake during sport and exercise in the heat

A potentially crucial distinction to make when evaluating the possible impact of dehydration on sport and exercise performance is the environmental conditions. The research discussed in Section 4.3 almost exclusively investigated fluid losses in thermoneutral conditions. Perhaps unsurprisingly, the risk of encountering a state of hypohydration is greater when sport and exercise, particularly aerobic sport and exercise, is undertaken in hot conditions,[31] and when skin temperature is raised (Section 4.7.3) and when fluid losses are > 3% BM.[31]

You may have noted that the fluid loss 'threshold' in the previous sentence was 3%, not 2% as discussed in Section 4.3. This greater 'threshold' may be in part due to the concern that lower levels of hypohydration may actually be within normal euhydrated fluctuations in body water content, meaning the results of research investigating smaller fluid losses could not confidently be attributed to the process of dehydration or the state of hypohydration.[14] In line with this concern, a recent review interpreted the existing hypohydration evidence to mean that "when hypohydration is present (*possibly* > 2% BM), endurance cycling performance in the heat is compromised, *at least when all typical physiological and perceptual symptoms [of hypohydration] are present*"[14] (emphases added by the author of this book). This is an interesting interpretation, as it shows that a review of evidence conducted within the last 5 years still needs to emphasise uncertainty in the required extent

Key point 4.12

Even recent reviews of the evidence suggest caution and highlight the inter-individual differences associated with the physiological and perceptual impacts of hypohydration.

of hypohydration for performance decrement and highlights the likely inter-individual differences that should be considered when evaluating the physiological and perceptual impact of a given degree of hypohydration. This caveated interpretation does not align with the broader perspective of dehydration and hypohydration as a definitive and universally accepted/understood contributor to sport and exercise fatigue, even in elevated ambient temperatures.

While no one is arguing that hydration is unimportant for health, daily physical function, and sport and exercise performance, the body of evidence available to us shows that as with most other topics in sport and exercise science, hydration is not as simple or clear-cut as we used to think. We are now aware that there is a significant individual aspect to hydration in sport and

Key point 4.13

Athletes and practitioners should understand the risks of dehydration/hypohydration in their specific situations.

exercise, influenced by factors including but not limited to age, sex, body composition, and ethnicity, that will govern how rapidly someone loses fluid during sport and exercise and what extent of fluid loss can be tolerated before performance decrement may occur. Not only this, but characteristics of the sport/exercise such as duration and intensity, environmental conditions (heat, humidity, wind, etc.), mode of activity (running, cycling, rowing, swimming, etc.), and any clothing/protective equipment requirements, will also influence the dynamics of hydration. These points emphasise why Burke[31] recommends that athletes and practitioners should focus on understanding the risks associated with dehydration and hypohydration in their own scenarios rather than seeking a 'universal truth' about hydration and sport and exercise performance.

Several research syntheses into dehydration and hypohydration during sport and exercise in the heat have been published in recent years. These publications have acknowledged the inherent challenges in researching this area and the limitations of some published work and have encouraged a more bespoke approach to hydration practices during sport and exercise in the heat. The greatest consensus from these publications revolves around the following points:

- In thermoneutral conditions, drinking according to the dictates of thirst may be adequate; particularly if the activity is at most moderate-intensity and no longer than ~60–90 minutes.[14,31-33]
- If sport and exercise takes place in the heat, particularly if the activity is intense and/or prolonged (~ >90 minutes), a more guided fluid intake practice may be more appropriate.[14,31-33]
- Guided fluid intake practices should still consider the individual athlete, activity intensity and duration, ambient conditions, and the nature of the sport (rules, clothing requirements, fluid intake opportunities, etc.).[14,31-33]

Less consensus is available on the 'threshold' of fluid loss associated with performance depletion, perhaps due again to greater awareness of the interindividual variability in tolerance to fluid loss. Furthermore, Periard

> **Key point 4.14**
>
> *Guided fluid intake may be more appropriate if sport and exercise is taking place in the heat, particularly if the activity is prolonged and/or intense.*

et al.[33] make a good point that potential dehydration-induced performance decrement does not function like a switch where an athlete immediately transitions from no performance decrement to significant performance decrement. Rather, it is a progressive process that may not occur until relatively late into an activity. Not only can this make it challenging to accurately assess the impact of dehydration on performance,[33] but it also argues against the logic of assigning critical hypohydration 'thresholds'.

Hopefully, the above discussion brings a little clarity to the topic of dehydration and sport and exercise performance in the heat, even if the clarity brought is a greater awareness of the lack of clarity in the area! Speaking about lack of clarity, this section will finish with a good example of the debate that remains ongoing regarding drink to thirst and guided drinking strategies during sport and exercise in both thermoneutral and hot conditions. Kenefick[32] published a review that made, among others, the following points:

- Guided fluid intake is a better option than drinking to thirst during sport and exercise lasting > 2 hours.
- Guided drinking is a better option during high-intensity activity that stimulates high sweat rates.
- Guided drinking should be employed when endurance performance is a primary concern (e.g. during competitive events).
- Guided drinking should be used when carbohydrate intake of ≥ 1 g.min^{-1} in the form of a carbohydrate solution is required.

Subsequently, Goulet[34] published a commentary paper providing evidence he believed contradicted each of the claims made in the Kenefick[32] paper. Briefly, Goulet[34] claimed:

- There are no published randomised controlled trials that have compared guided drinking and drinking to thirst during sport and exercise > 2 hours, and there is observational data that contradicts the recommendation of Kenefick[32].
- There are no published data that support guided drinking over drinking to thirst during high-intensity activity with high sweat rates, and again there is data showing no performance advantage of guided drinking over drinking to thirst during this type of activity.

- There are no published data to support the contention that guided drinking should be used when endurance performance is a concern.

Key point 4.15

There is ongoing debate about the relevance of guided drinking vs. drinking to thirst in different sport and exercise situations.

- There is no supporting evidence, and there is potentially contradictory evidence, regarding the use of guided drinking when > 1 g.min^{-1} of carbohydrate intake is required.

As exasperating as these conflicting perspectives can sometimes be, it is important that you are aware of them as a natural part of sport and exercise science. Such conflict and debate also serve to remind us that not only do we need to continue producing high-quality science to further our knowledge, but we also need to embrace the uncertainty that comes from studying human beings in diverse and often chaotic sport and exercise scenarios. Should dehydration be considered a potential fatigue agent during sport and exercise in thermoneutral and hot conditions? Yes. Is it as ubiquitous as used to be thought? No (certainly not for thermoneutral conditions). Is dehydration and sport and exercise performance complex, multi-faceted, individualised, and resistant to catch-all thresholds and recommendations? Yes!

4.5   Hyperhydration during sport and exercise

Sections 4.3 and 4.4 introduced the debate about guided drinking vs. drinking to thirst. There is another issue that suggests drinking to thirst may sometimes be a more appropriate and, perhaps, safer option: hyperhydration (defined in Section 4.2.1).

There are several potential issues with hyperhydration. Firstly, hyperhydration will increase BM which may be detrimental to performance, particularly during weight-bearing sport and exercise. Secondly, there have been many instances of people reporting a variety of gastrointestinal symptoms of differing severities when trying to drink more than they would through choice during sport and exercise, usually to prevent BM loss. Clearly, gastrointestinal problems will hamper sport and exercise performance. However, a potentially more serious consequence of hyperhydration is the development of *hypervolemia* (abnormal increases in blood plasma volume) or *hyponatraemia* (an abnormally low blood sodium level).

Firstly, it is important to note that modest hypervolaemia is a normal, desirable chronic

Key point 4.16

The prevalence of hyponatraemia during endurance sport and exercise is higher than originally thought.

adaptation to endurance training. Increases in plasma volume, and hence blood volume, contribute to the improved cardiac (greater stroke volume, maximal $\dot{Q}$, and lower heart rate) and thermoregulatory (increased sweating sensitivity and sweat rate) function characteristic of improved fitness.[35] However, excessive hypervolaemia can be detrimental to performance and, more importantly, health. Increased body water content can occur for many reasons:

- Protein breakdown, which increases both plasma proteins and plasma volume.[36]
- Increased plasma volume due to increased plasma sodium concentration.[37]
- Retention of sodium due to increased activity of aldosterone.[38]
- Increased plasma volume due to increased activity of vasopressin.[39]
- Impairment of renal function due to dehydration.[40]

However, a common cause of increased body water content is, of course, fluid overload via excessive fluid intake. The potential causes of hypervolaemia help to explain why most cases of hypervolaemia during sport and exercise occur during ultra-endurance activities (for example, running races lasting anything greater than a marathon distance)[41–43] as shorter duration activities give less time to generate these potential causes (unless, perhaps, in highly abnormal environmental conditions). As previously mentioned, hypervolaemia increases a person's BM, which can be detrimental to performance as the person has to transport this increased mass for the duration of the activity. However, a more serious potential consequence of hypervolaemia is the development of hyponatraemia, defined as an abnormally low serum sodium concentration (< 135 mmol.L) either during or up to 24 hours after sport and exercise.[44]

The prevalence of hyponatraemia during endurance sport and exercise ranges from approximately 13%–51% of participating athletes, much higher than previously thought.[45,46] While hyponatraemia is more likely to occur during very long duration activities, it has been reported in rowers, open-water swimmers, and rugby players.[46] Features of hyponatraemia can range from no or minimal symptoms such as weakness, dizziness, headache, nausea, and vomiting, to serious symptoms including fluid accumulation in the brain (cerebral oedema), altered mental function, seizures, fluid accumulation in the lungs (pulmonary oedema), coma, and death.[45] The severity of symptoms is dependent in part on the rate and extent of the drop in extracellular sodium content.[45]

> **Key point 4.17**
>
> *The primary cause of sport and exercise-associated hyponatraemia is over-drinking. High sweat sodium concentrations can also increase the risk of hyponatraemia, as less fluid intake is required to dilute blood sodium to dangerous levels.*

There are multiple potential risk factors for development of hyponatraemia during endurance sport and exercise[47,48]:

- The composition of ingested fluids.
- Low BM index.
- Longer exercise time.
- Type of activity (higher risk in swimming vs. running vs. cycling).
- Lack of endurance experience.
- Environmental conditions, particularly ambient temperature.
- Geographical location of the activity (highest prevalence in the USA, lowest prevalence in Africa, Asia, and Oceania).
- Use of nonsteroidal anti-inflammatory drugs.
- Female sex.[47]

However, studies have established that the strongest risk factor for development of hyponatraemia is excessive fluid intake during sport and exercise.[45,47,49] This highlights a clear link between hypervolaemia and hyponatraemia. It is also important

> **Key point 4.18**
>
> *Fluid intake guidelines that encourage high rates of fluid ingestion can place athletes at increased risk of developing hyponatraemia. In situations where guidelines to restrict excessive fluid intake have been implemented, cases of hyponatraemia have fallen.*

to consider sweat composition as a potential risk factor for hyponatraemia. Production of salty sweat (sweat with a high sodium content) reduces the amount of over-drinking necessary to cause hyponatraemia.[49]

We now know that the primary risk factor for hyponatraemia is over-drinking during sport and exercise, and that sweat sodium content can also influence the risk of developing hyponatraemia. Sweat composition is different between individuals, and appropriate fluid intake during sport and exercise is dependent on many factors such as body size, activity intensity, sweat rate, and environmental conditions, all of which are individual and/or highly variable. Therefore, it is easy to see how fluid intake guidelines that encourage athletes to drink as much as is tolerable during sport and exercise or to drink specific absolute volumes without accounting for individual modulating factors could place an athlete at significant risk of developing hyponatraemia. These same reasons make it unfeasible to produce universal guidelines for the prevention of hyponatraemia. However, general recommendations have been made, the key one being that athletes should drink according to thirst and no more than 400–800 ml.hour.[45] This rate of fluid intake is much lower than that shown to produce hyponatraemia (up to 1,500 ml.hour).[45] Implementation of guidelines to restrict excessive fluid intake is associated with reductions in the number of cases of sport and exercise hyponatraemia.[50,51]

4.6 Hyperthermia

4.6.1 How hot is too hot?

Hyperthermia is an abnormally high core body temperature. Normal core body temperature is between 36°C and 37.5°C; however, the specific value will differ slightly depending on the location of measurement (rectal, oesophageal, tympanic, etc.). Technically, hyperthermia is therefore a body temperature greater than 37.5°C. However, there are different severities of hyperthermia, depending on the core temperature reached.

Hyperthermia and fever (as part of an illness) both involve an elevated core temperature, but they are not the same thing as they have different causes and are regulated in different ways. A fever occurs when specific immune cells produced in response to infection release substances that stimulate the hypothalamus to raise core temperature. Essentially, normal core temperature is now considered too cold, and the hypothalamus raises core temperature to a new, higher set point. This process is analogous to raising the temperature setting on a thermostat. Conversely, hyperthermia occurs when core body temperature rises without direct prior stimulation of the temperature control regions in the brain, usually because of an imbalance between heat production and heat dissipation.

> **Key point 4.19**
>
> *Normal core temperature is between 36°C and 37.5°C. Technically, hyperthermia is any core temperature above this range. Hyperthermia can differ in severity depending on factors, including the core temperature reached.*

4.6.2 Development of hyperthermia during sport and exercise

Hyperthermia can develop whenever body heat production exceeds body heat loss. A classic cause of hyperthermia during sport and exercise was described in Section 4.2.3 and Figure 4.2. Fundamentally, core temperature will increase when body heat gain from muscle metabolism, radiation (usually from the sun), and convection (if air temperature is higher than skin temperature) is greater than heat loss via conduction, convection, radiation, and evaporation (by far the most important method of heat loss during sport and exercise). Therefore, it is no surprise that the development of hyperthermia is most common in situations where dissipation of body heat is impaired. This includes sport and exercise in the heat and/or humidity, with insufficient air flow, while wearing excessive clothing, without sufficient shading, or a combination of these factors. The most challenging environment in which to maintain normal body temperature is when it is both hot and humid. Sport and exercise in the heat leads to warmer skin temperatures (Section 4.7.3). While this is beneficial for evaporative heat loss, it reduces the temperature difference between the body core and skin, and between the skin and ambient air, thereby making it more difficult to transfer heat from the core to the skin, and then to the surrounding air. When humidity is added into the equation, evaporative heat loss is greatly impaired as sweat on the surface of the skin cannot easily vaporise into the air due to the high ambient moisture already present (particularly when humidity levels exceed about 60%). Therefore, sport and exercise in hot and humid conditions significantly impairs all body heat loss avenues, increasing the likelihood of body heat gain. Continued activity in a situation of net body heat gain will lead to a progressive increase in core temperature, potentially exacerbating the previously mentioned cardiac and circulatory stresses.

4.7   Hyperthermia, combined hyperthermia and hypohydration, and fatigue: research findings

This section will highlight the potential mechanisms explaining the role of hyperthermia, and hyperthermia combined with hypohydration, in impaired sport and exercise performance (Figure 4.4). The reader is referred to the excellent review of Periard et al.,[52] the content of which related to the impact

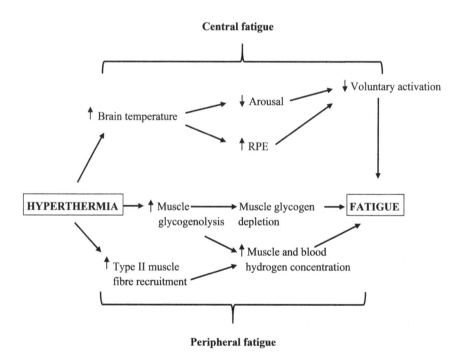

Figure 4.4 Potential causes of hyperthermia-induced fatigue during sport and exercise. The causes of fatigue are characterised as central or peripheral in origin. Redrawn from Cheung SS, Sleivert GG. *Exerc Sport Sci Rev.* 2004;32:100–106.

of hyperthermia, alone and in conjunction with hypohydration, on the performance of different types of sport and exercise will be an excellent accompaniment to this section.

4.7.1 *Peripheral fatigue associated with hyperthermia, and combined hyperthermia and hypohydration*

Exercising in the heat increases blood flow to the skin to enable heat transfer from the body tissues to the surrounding environment. In a situation of high blood demand from both the working muscle and the skin, the required $\dot{Q}$ may not be met,[53] particularly if $\dot{Q}$ is already reduced due to an attenuated stroke volume caused by decreased plasma volume (i.e. dehydration; Figure 4.2).[54] Therefore, impaired cardiovascular function is a potential cause of fatigue during sport and exercise in the heat. Indeed, during activity that requires the athlete to exercise at their maximum rate of O_2 consumption ($\dot{V}O_2max$) blood flow to the working muscle is reduced, indicating a failure of the cardiovascular system to deliver O_2 at the required rate.[52,55] When combined hyperthermia and hypohydration are present, $\dot{Q}$ is reduced at intensities above approximately 60% $\dot{V}O_2max$.[56] This reduction in $\dot{Q}$ has the potential to reduce blood flow and therefore O_2 delivery to working muscles and the brain. However, during prolonged submaximal sport and exercise in the heat, muscle blood flow and therefore O_2 delivery and uptake remain similar to activity carried out at the same intensity in a normal temperature, yet performance in the heat is still impaired.[57,58] Cardiovascular impairments which reduce O_2 delivery to working muscles occur at lower absolute intensities in the presence of heat stress due to more rapid reductions in $\dot{Q}$ and mean arterial pressure.[52]

It is well known that hypohydration delays the onset of sweating during sport and exercise.[59,60] During sport and exercise in the heat, sweat rate has been shown to decrease in proportion to the extent of hypohydration[61] and combined hyperthermia and hypohydration reduces the amount of skin blood flow at a given core temperature. Potential mechanisms for these impairments include reduced responsiveness of neural structures that regulate evaporative heat loss, inhibition of regions of the hypothalamus, and impaired function of sweat glands.[52] These data demonstrate that a combination of hyperthermia and hypohydration may be a potent driver of fatigue during sport and exercise, due primarily to impaired thermoregulation.

During prolonged submaximal sport and exercise in the heat muscle glycogen use and anaerobic metabolism are elevated compared with thermoneutral conditions.[62-64] Specific mechanisms behind this altered metabolic response involve increased muscle temperature, reduced muscle energy status, and an increased sympathoadrenal response, all of which can stimulate key enzymes involved in glycogenolysis and glycolysis.[52,65,66] While hyperthermia is a potent contributor to increased carbohydrate metabolism during sport and exercise,[52] this is not considered a primary cause of fatigue during sport and exercise in the heat, certainly during intense activity lasting ~60–90 minutes as the rate of muscle glycogen depletion over this duration is not sufficient to limit performance.[52,67] Conversely, more prolonged sport and exercise in the heat could be susceptible to performance limitations related to increased glycogenolytic and glycolytic rates.[52]

When hyperthermia is combined with hypohydration during sport and exercise, muscle blood flow and hence O_2 delivery can decline due to impaired $\dot{Q}$ as discussed earlier. Reduced O_2 delivery may alter the metabolic response of the muscle and manifest as a more 'anaerobic' metabolic environment, evidenced by the association between reduced muscle blood flow, impaired substrate delivery, and 'anaerobic' metabolite accumulation.[52] However, it appears unlikely that hypohydration further increases the rate of muscle glycogenolysis; increased glycogenolysis seems to be driven by hyperthermia (systemic and local).[52]

> **Key point 4.20**
>
> *Potential causes of peripheral fatigue with hyperthermia, and hyperthermia with hypohydration, include impaired cardiovascular function leading to reduced blood flow to working muscle, delayed sweating, reduced sweat rate, increased muscle glycogen breakdown, and impaired muscle contraction.*

Exercise-induced hyperthermia, up to a core temperature of approximately 41°C and muscle temperature of approximately 42°C, does not impair the ability of muscles to contract.[54,68] Direct electrical stimulation of the motor neurons (Section 1.3.1) of skeletal muscles shows that the muscles are able to produce the same amount of force when hyperthermic compared to normal temperature.[57]

4.7.2   Central fatigue associated with hyperthermia, and combined hyperthermia and hypohydration

As mentioned in Section 4.7.1, hyperthermia does not directly impair the ability of muscles to contract. Similarly, hyperthermia does not appear to impair the ability of a person to voluntarily contract their muscle for a short period of time (a few seconds). However, sustained voluntary muscle force production deteriorates significantly when hyperthermia is present (Figure 4.5). Reduced ability to generate muscle force despite no

> **Key point 4.21**
>
> *There is good evidence to show that hyperthermia reduces the ability to produce muscle force despite no change in the ability of the muscle itself to produce force. This suggests that central factors may be more important than peripheral factors in hyperthermia-induced fatigue.*

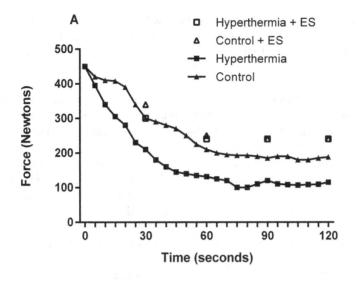

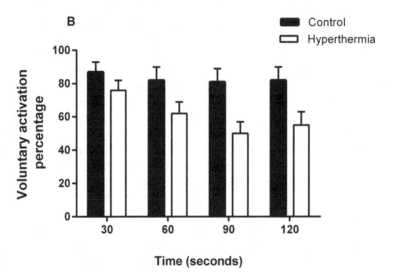

Figure 4.5 Force production from the thigh muscle during a 2 minute maximal knee extension during hyperthermia (core temperature of 40°C) and control (core temperature of 38°C; A). Participants were asked to make a maximal effort for the entire 2 minutes. Electrical stimulation (ES) of the muscle was applied every 30 seconds during the contraction. Electrical stimulation showed that the ability of the muscle to contract was not influenced by hyperthermia (A). However, participants were not able to voluntarily maintain the level of force production that the muscle was capable of, or that they could maintain in the control trial (B). This suggests that the causes of reduced force production in the hyperthermia trial were central in origin. Re-drawn from: Nybo L, Nielsen B. *J Appl Physiol*. 2001;91:1055–1060.

change in the ability of the muscle itself to produce force suggests that central factors may be important in the development of fatigue with hyperthermia. However, the role of peripheral factors should not be overlooked. Sensory feedback from working muscles and skin may modify central alterations in neuromuscular recruitment.[54]

During prolonged sport and exercise in hyperthermia, a progressive reduction in cerebral blood flow relative to thermoneutral conditions is observed.[52,69] Reduced cerebral blood flow may be due to increased cutaneous blood flow, decreased $\dot{Q}$ and arterial pressure, and decreased arterial CO_2 pressure due to hyperventilation (hypocapnia).[70,71] When hyperthermia is combined with hypohydration, reductions in cerebral blood flow are exacerbated.[52] However, reduced cerebral blood flow does not appear to impair central neural drive as the brain is able to increase O_2 extraction, resulting in a maintenance or even increase in cerebral metabolism in hyperthermic and hyperthermic/hypohydrated vs. thermoneutral states.[69,72] Nevertheless, there do appear to be changes in cerebral activity during prolonged sport and exercise in the heat. Specifically, activity in brain regions associated with attention, mental readiness, focus, wakefulness, and arousal declines.[73,74] These alterations are also associated with increased core temperature and rating of perceived exertion.[75] Together, these changes indicate that prolonged sport and exercise in a hyperthermic state may induce central alterations that make it more challenging for people to maintain attention and arousal. However, whether or not these alterations are linked to reduced cerebral blood flow is currently unknown.[52]

During sport and exercise in the heat, the temperature of blood in the jugular vein (the main vein that brings blood from the head to the heart) drops slightly, meaning the temperature difference between jugular venous blood and blood in the aorta (the main blood vessel leading away from the heart) is reduced.[54,55] This implies that the brain is storing heat during sport and exercise in hot temperatures. Indeed, average brain temperature increases in line with aortic blood temperature, remaining at least 0.2°C warmer than core temperature.[55]

The role of brain temperature on sport and exercise fatigue is interesting. In animals, increasing brain temperatures without increasing core temperature reduces the ability and willingness to continue exercising.[76] These behavioural responses are similar to those seen in people during sport and exercise in hyperthermic states. However, it is difficult to confirm that increased brain temperature has the same effect in humans because it is very difficult to selectively cool or warm a human brain without altering core temperature.[55] This difficulty is one of the reasons why there is still debate around the role of brain temperature and the benefits of a 'cooler brain' on human fatigue.[77,78] It is possible that increased brain temperature may stimulate areas of the hypothalamus to reduce motor activity,[52,55] but this suggestion needs further investigation.

Research has demonstrated that reductions in voluntary skeletal muscle activation occur alongside increases in core temperature.[79,80] However, it is important to note that such impairments in voluntary activation appear to occur only during sustained isometric muscle contractions, not dynamic contractions,[52] reducing the validity of the findings with regard to most sporting situations. Furthermore, the research is not conclu-

Key point 4.22

During exercise in hyperthermia, brain blood flow decreases, brain temperature increases, and brain regions linked to arousal, focus, and attention are impaired.

sive. In some studies, there has been no additive impact of hyperthermia on voluntary skeletal muscle activation above and beyond the impact of exercise itself,[81] whereas others have shown that hyperthermia and exercise combine to increase the rate of decline in voluntary activation.[52,82] It appears that the nature of the hyperthermic stimulus (e.g. passive or active (exercise-induced) hyperthermia) and the demands of the sport/exercise, particularly with regard to muscle contraction characteristics, should be considered when evaluating the potential direct impact of hyperthermia on central neural drive.

Section 4.7.1 discussed how prolonged sport and exercise in the heat is associated with increased muscle glycogenolysis and anaerobic metabolism. Anaerobic metabolism is associated with production of metabolites (see Chapters 2, 3, and 5 for more detail) that stimulate group IV muscle afferents (referred to in Chapters 2, 3, and 5, and discussed in more detail in Chapter 6). Such afferent stimulation can result in reduced corticospinal excitability and hence reduced voluntary muscle activation (i.e. central fatigue) in an effort to limit the extent of peripheral fatigue. However, the relevance of this potential fatigue mechanism to sport and exercise in the heat is questionable. In fact, the relative impact of group IV afferent stimulation on reduced muscle activation may even decline during sport and exercise in the heat, where there is a greater relative impact of more direct temperature and O_2 delivery-related impairments to central nervous system (CNS) function.[52,83]

4.7.3   *High core temperature or high skin temperature?*

Early research observed that during sport and exercise in the heat people voluntarily stopped exercise at a very similar core temperature (approximately 40°C), despite the many factors (motivation, training status, heat acclimatisation, hydration, etc.) that can influence performance in the heat.[84–86] Fatigue at, or very close to, this core temperature occurred despite differences in initial core temperature and the rate of heat storage during activity. Attainment of high core temperature was associated with reduced CNS drive, leading to the suggestion that attainment of a critical core temperature is a safety brake to prevent development of catastrophic hyperthermia, or is perhaps the threshold for a progressive reduction in performance.[54,87,88] This belief, termed the critical core temperature hypothesis, became the mainstay by which impaired performance in the heat was explained, and was rarely questioned.[89]

Much of the research that supports the critical core temperature hypothesis used methods that raised not only core temperature but also that of the muscle and skin. This is an important point, as raising the temperature of the skin narrows the temperature gradient between the core and skin. Narrowing this gradient means that a greater skin blood flow is required to dissipate core body heat. As discussed earlier in this chapter, elevated skin blood flow may impair cardiovascular function via reduced cardiac filling pressure, likely modulated by increases in heart rate and associated reductions in stroke volume.[90] Increased skin blood flow due to elevated skin temperatures may also reduce brain blood flow and O_2 delivery,[69] although this may not in itself induce a central fatigue response.[91] Therefore, research that increases core and skin temperature together will find it very difficult to confidently separate and identify the effects of increases in core or skin temperature independently. It is also worth considering that a core temperature of 40°C is much lower than what would be required for cellular damage to occur, and that the CNS appears able to tolerate temperatures of more than 41°C for several hours without damage.[92] This questions the relevance of a critical core temperature of 40°C.

High skin temperatures alone can impair sport and exercise performance independent of changes in core temperature. Some studies have shown high skin temperature to cause fatigue at modest core temperatures (approximately 38°C) and with no difference in heart

Key point 4.23

Most research that identified a 'critical' core temperature limiting performance in the heat used protocols that also caused elevated core and skin temperature. Therefore, the role of increased core temperature in isolation cannot be determined.

Key point 4.24

The 'critical' core temperature of approximately 40°C is much lower than the temperature required to cause cellular damage. Therefore, the relevance of this temperature as a limiting factor in sport and exercise performance should be questioned.

Key point 4.25

Research shows that performance can be maintained with a core temperature greater than the proposed 'critical' temperature of 40°C. This argues for the presence of other factors that limit sport and exercise performance in the heat.

Table 4.2 Estimated skin blood flow requirements during prolonged high-intensity running at different body core and skin temperatures. From: Sawka et al[61]

Core temp. (°C)	Skin temp. (°C)	Temp. gradient (°C)	Skin blood flow (litres per minutes)
38	30	8	1.1
38	32	6	1.5
38	34	4	2.2
38	36	2	4.4
39	30	9	1.0
39	32	7	1.3
39	34	5	1.8
39	36	3	2.9

At any given skin temperature, increased core temperature increases the temperature gradient between the core and the skin, and there is a reduction in skin blood flow. At any given core temperature, increasing the skin temperature reduces the temperature gradient between the core and the skin, and there is an increase in skin blood flow.

rate response compared to a control trial. Other studies have shown the onset of fatigue with high skin temperatures at core temperatures lower than 38.5°C but with a higher heart rate relative to exercise intensity, indicating cardiovascular strain (Table 4.2).[90,93,94] These studies appear to show that high skin temperatures can contribute to negative physiological responses at core temperatures much lower than those associated with the critical core temperature hypothesis.[89] Furthermore, high skin temperature can exacerbate the negative consequences of hypohydration on performance.[90,95] Therefore, sport and exercise in the heat, where both hyperthermia and hypohydration are a possibility, could be particularly susceptible to performance decrements from high skin temperature. Indeed, this is a main way in which high skin temperature is thought to impair sport and exercise in the heat: increasing the demand for skin blood flow, reducing central blood volume, $\dot{Q}$ and, hence, $\dot{V}O_2$max (although it may not surprise you to know that there is still debate about the specific mechanism(s) at play, with some suggestion that cardiac impairment with increased skin temperature is related more to direct temperature-related increases in heart rate and reduced stroke volume rather than blood volume-redistribution mechanisms, and that skin temperature may only reduce $\dot{V}O_2$max if elevated core temperature is also present).[90] Because of reduced $\dot{V}O_2$max, relative intensity will increase, making the activity feel harder, altering metabolic response to the activity, and eventually causing activity cessation. The change in cardiovascular demand due to increased skin temperature would be exacerbated in the presence of hypohydration, where cardiovascular integrity may already be compromised.

Further argument against the critical core temperature hypothesis comes from research showing that endurance performance can be maintained despite core temperatures much higher than the 40°C 'cut-off' temperature. Researchers have reported no difference in running speed during an 8 km time trial when core temperature was below or above 40°C.[87] Similar findings have been reported over longer distance running, with no association between high core temperature and performance.[96,97] Interestingly, in the studies that found no effect of high core temperature on performance, skin temperatures were only cool to warm.

The above discussions clearly demonstrate that potential causes of fatigue during sport and exercise in the heat go a lot further than the attainment of a critically high core temperature. In fact, the critical core temperature hypothesis has received strong challenge in recent years. Current knowledge now identifies a range of potential causes of hyperthermia-related fatigue, including high core temperature, high skin temperature, reduced brain blood flow and electrical activity, and increased brain temperature. While the field has moved on notably in the last decade, the exact cause(s) of fatigue during sport and exercise in the heat are unknown. This is mainly due to the difficulty in measuring some known factors of hyperthermia-associated fatigue, most notably brain temperature, in exercising human. However, what is now clear is that hyperthermia-induced fatigue is not an all-or-nothing event that occurs upon reaching a critical core temperature, but is instead a progressive, integrated occurrence involving both peripheral feedback and central processes.[55]

4.8   Hypoxia

This section is titled 'hypoxia' rather than 'altitude', as much of the data investigating performance limitations related to O_2 availability has artificially induced varying degrees of hypoxia in a controlled environment, rather than conducting the work at elevated altitudes. The research has been carried out in this way due to logistical issues of travelling to altitude, and the obvious ethical and safety issues associated with acutely exposing people to real-world altitude without prior acclimation/acclimatisation.

As with hyperthermia and hydration, the body of work investigating aspects of human performance in hypoxic situations could receive multiple books worth of attention. In keeping with the overall aim of this book, discussion of hypoxia will focus on the *acute* limitations to sport and exercise performance in people who did not grow up and do not live at altitude.

As altitude will be discussed in this section it is important to ask the question: how high above sea level do you have to go (or do you have to simulate) before you are at 'altitude'? There are subtly different definitions based on where you look, but common thresholds found in the literature[98–100] are:

- Moderate altitude: > 1,500 m
- High altitude: > 2,500 m
- Very high altitude: > 3,500 m

Key point 4.26

Altitude can be classified as moderate, high, or very high; however, the physiological responses to altitude occur on a sliding, non-linear scale with individual differences.

At the extremes of land altitude, the highest of which is the peak of Mount Everest at 8,849 m, there is a region known as the death zone. Commonly defined as an elevation of > 8,000 m, it is called the death zone as it is extremely dangerous. At this altitude, muscle power output can be depressed to the point where activity becomes impossible, body heat generation can fall precipitously which significantly increases the risk of hypothermia, and the low barometric pressure induces hypoxia and high-altitude illness.[101,102] For most, survival at this altitude would be measured in hours. Emphasising this, more than 80% of all deaths that have occurred on Mount Everest have occurred in the death zone.[103]

Despite the categorisation of different altitudes as described above, it is inappropriate to consider the human response to altitude (or hypoxia) as categorised and predictable. The altitude at which symptoms of exposure begin to develop is different amongst individuals; while symptoms are rare at moderate altitudes, they will occur for some.[100] The severity of symptoms/performance limitations does not change in a stepwise/categorical fashion, but more on a sliding and non-linear scale. The only constant is that progressive increases in altitude will elicit progressively more severe symptoms/limitations in everyone.

4.8.1   Acute hypoxia: performance impact

There are three main methods of acute hypoxic exposure; (1) Hypobaric hypoxia, whereby increasing terrestrial elevation reduces the ambient barometric pressure, meaning less O_2 is inhaled per breath (i.e. the air is 'thinner'); (2) Simulated hypobaric hypoxia, whereby barometric pressure is artificially reduced in a specialised chamber, and (3) Normobaric hypoxia, whereby the concentration of O_2 in the air is reduced to simulate altitude with no changes in barometric pressure. Different forms of hypoxia may elicit different physiological and performance limitations, but before discussing this it is important to contextualise the sport and exercise performance decrements associated with acute hypoxic exposure.

Deb *et al.*[104] conducted the most recent review of the effects of acute hypoxic exposure on sport and exercise performance. The authors split sport and exercise into different categories (time trials, time-to-exhaustion tests, intermittent sprinting, short-duration sprinting) and different durations (< 2 minutes, 2–10 minutes, and > 10 minutes). The relationship between acute hypoxia and sport and exercise performance lasting > 2 minutes was curvilinear. Across all categories of sport and exercise, there was a ~17% negative effect of acute hypoxia on performance, with a 6.5% reduction for every 1,000 m of elevation. Time-trial performance declined by 16.2%, time

Key point 4.27

Acute hypoxia causes significant decrements in time-trial performance, time to exhaustion, intermittent sport and exercise, and sport and exercise lasting > 2 minutes.

to exhaustion by 44.5%, intermittent exercise by 5.6%, and sprint performance by 2.9%. There was no statistically significant effect of acute hypoxia on performance < 2 minutes, an 18% reduction in performance lasting 2–10 minutes (14% reduction per 1,000 m of altitude), and a ~27% reduction in performance lasting >10 minutes (18% reduction per 1,000 m of altitude).

The data of Deb *et al.*[104] is the most comprehensive and current synthesis of the effects of acute hypoxia on different sport and exercise demands. However, the analysis did not discriminate between the effects of different types of acute hypoxic exposure. The best available overall evidence we have for the differential effects of hypobaric and normobaric hypoxia on aspects of sport and exercise performance comes from Treml *et al.*[105] These authors found that some underlying physiological mechanisms that may explain fatigue in acute hypoxia potentially differ depending on the type

> **Key point 4.28**
>
> *The type of acute hypoxia (hypobaric and normobaric) can influence sport and exercise performance and the underlying mechanisms behind performance decrement.*

of acute hypoxic exposure (particularly simulated normobaric vs. hypobaric hypoxia); this data will be discussed in Section 4.8.2. There may also be differences in fluid retention parameters between hypoxia types, but these data are primarily from resting studies.[105,106] Regarding sport and exercise performance, larger time-trial performance decrements have been found in acute hypobaric vs. normobaric hypoxia.[107,108]

Brain function and cognitive performance can also be impaired in acute hypoxia. In particular, executive function, attention, episodic memory, and information processing may be impaired.[109,110] Interestingly, performing sport and exercise in acute hypoxia can significantly improve cognitive function (depending on the characteristics of the individual and the hypoxia itself), particularly attention, information processing, and memory, but not executive function.[111,112] Moderate-intensity sport and exercise is more effective than high-intensity sport and exercise at improving cognitive function in acute hypoxia, meaning that the benefit may not be felt by people undertaking high-intensity training or competing.[111] Cognitive impacts of acute altitude are not a focus of this chapter unless they contribute to fatigue *per se*, so the interested reader is referred to Jung *et al.*[111] for an excellent overview of the area.

4.8.2   *Acute hypoxia: potential mechanisms underlying performance impairment*

It probably comes as no surprise that the determinants of fatigue in acute hypoxia are complex.[113] One of the most potent physiological drivers behind reduced performance in acute hypoxia seems to be the reduction in arterial

O_2 saturation (SaO_2). Reduced SaO_2 has been identified as a key predictor of the cognitive impairment sometimes observed in hypoxia,[114] although the mechanisms behind this are

> **Key point 4.29**
>
> *The reduction in arterial O_2 saturation with acute hypoxia is a key physiological driver behind reduced performance.*

not yet understood.[112] Reduced SaO_2 can also challenge the ability to maintain convective-diffusive O_2 delivery from the lungs to the working muscle tissue, meaning that the delivery and ultimately the utilisation of O_2 may be impaired. This mechanism is one of the ways in which $\dot{V}O_2$max may decrease in acute hypoxia (more on this in Section 4.8.2.2).[115] Comprehensive statistical modelling has confirmed that SaO_2 is a significant performance moderator in acute hypoxia, with a 4.5% reduction in time to exhaustion, 1.3% reduction in time-trial performance, 2.4% reduction for sport and exercise lasting 2–10 minutes, and 2.8% reduction for sport and exercise lasting > 10 minutes, for every 1% reduction in SaO_2.[104] Interestingly, SaO_2 is a more important performance moderator in trained vs. untrained individuals.[104] Due to the broad underlying effects of reduced SaO_2, mitigating its reduction in hypoxia is critical for attenuating performance impairments, particularly in trained people.[104]

4.8.2.1 *Resting and exercising cardiovascular responses*

Maximum heart rate (HRmax), representing the upper ceiling of cardiac performance during sport and exercise, declines with acute normobaric and hypobaric hypoxic exposure.[105,115,116] It appears that HRmax begins to decline as soon as altitude starts to increase, and that the reduction in HRmax with increasing altitude is roughly linear.[116] However, there are large inter-individual and inter-study differences.[116] Similar to SaO_2, it appears that more highly trained people display a relatively greater reduction in HRmax with acute hypoxic exposure.[116] However, there appears to be no effect of age or sex on the reduction in HRmax.[117,118] Reductions in SaO_2 have been linked to reductions in HRmax,[116,119] however this association is quite weak and suggests that other causative mechanisms exist for a declining HRmax. What these mechanisms may be is currently unknown. It is unlikely that alterations in autonomic nervous system activity have an acute effect on HRmax (conversely, it is likely that this is the major contributor to reduced HRmax with chronic hypoxic exposure).[116,120] There could be direct hypoxia-related changes to the electrical activity of the heart that are associated with reductions in HRmax.[116,121] Regardless of the specific causative mechanisms, reductions in HRmax of 5 and 7.5 beats per minute may be expected at 2,500 m and 3,500 m elevation, respectively.[116] This would have the effect of lowering the upper ceiling of functional cardiac performance, and hence high-intensity sport and exercise performance. As a result, reduced HRmax is identified as a performance-limiting factor at altitude.[116] Interestingly, this effect may differ depending on the type of hypoxia, with HRmax reduced to a larger extent in normobaric vs. hypobaric hypoxia, although a similar rate of decline with increasing elevation is seen in both hypoxia types.[105]

It is important to highlight an ongoing (at the time of writing) debate around the effect of acute hypoxia on HRmax. Prevailing opinion is that HRmax declines with chronic exposure to hypoxia, but also with acute exposure.[116] If this is indeed the case, it would stand to reason that maximum cardiac output ($\dot{Q}$max) would also decline with acute hypoxic exposure, as maximal stroke volume is at least maintained with hypoxic exposure.[115,116,122] However, recent mathematical modelling for predicting cardiovascular responses during exercise at acute altitude reported that acute hypoxia does not limit HRmax, or therefore $\dot{Q}$max.[123] These findings were challenged on the basis of flawed assumptions about known physiological responses to altitude.[122] The original authors of the mathematical modelling rebutted this by stating that Richalet and Hermand[122] based their argument on findings from chronic altitude exposure, whereas the modelling of Lloyd *et al.*[123] focused on acute exposure to hypoxia.[124] While the mathematical model presented by Lloyd *et al.*[123] will continue to be refined,[124] this contemporary exchange in the literature is an interesting view into the ongoing debates about the effects of acute and chronic hypoxia on physiological function and performance. It is also important to weigh up predictions from modelling against what we currently understand based on direct observation of humans performing in hypoxic environments.

Cardiovascular responses to submaximal sport and exercise are certainly influenced by acute hypoxia. As has already been discussed, in acute hypoxia SaO_2 declines. This decline requires a higher $\dot{Q}$ in order to preserve O_2 transport to working tissues (essentially, the body needs to pump more blood to the working tissue because that blood is now carrying less O_2). The higher $\dot{Q}$ is achieved by increasing HR.[121,125] The extent of the increase in $\dot{Q}$ is related to the severity of hypoxia.[121] The main mechanism behind the increase in HR in acute hypoxia is likely related to increased sympathetic and reduced parasympathetic autonomic activity, mediated by activation of peripheral chemoreceptors in response to reduced SaO_2.[121,125,126] Exercising stroke volume is unchanged in acute hypoxia due to an increased end-systolic volume modulated by changes in myocardial mechanics during the systolic and diastolic phases of heart contraction.[125,127,128] The combination of increased HR and maintained stroke volume serves to increase $\dot{Q}$.

While HRmax likely declines with acute hypoxic exposure, resting HR likely increases.[115] Of course, resting HR represents the lower limit of cardiac function. So, with resting HR

Key point 4.30

Maximum heart rate may decrease and resting heart rate may increase with acute hypoxia. This reduces the functional heart rate reserve available to the athlete.

increasing and HRmax decreasing, the functional HR reserve of an individual decreases. Simply put, there is less cardiac 'capacity' to respond to sport and exercise challenges. Increased resting

> **Key point 4.31**
>
> *For a given submaximal intensity, a higher $\dot{Q}$ is required to compensate for the lower SaO_2. Higher $\dot{Q}$ is achieved by increasing heart rate.*

HR could be due to increased sympathetic and decreased parasympathetic activity[121] and again may be influenced by hypoxia type, with resting HR higher in hypobaric vs. normobaric hypoxia.[116]

4.8.2.2 Submaximal $\dot{V}O_2$ and $\dot{V}O_2$max

Earlier, it was mentioned that acute hypoxia reduces $\dot{V}O_2$max, by 6%–7% per 1,000 m increase in altitude.[115] Much of the decrement in $\dot{V}O_2$max can be explained by the mechanisms discussed above,

> **Key point 4.32**
>
> *$\dot{V}O_2$max is reduced in acute hypoxia, likely due to elevated $\dot{Q}$ and heart rate and potentially reduced maximum heart rate.*

namely the reduction in SaO_2 and potentially HRmax and the required increase in HR and $\dot{Q}$ to preserve O_2 delivery to working tissue. In this situation, $\dot{Q}$ and HR will reach their maximum values at a lower $\dot{V}O_2$ than in normoxia, thereby reducing $\dot{V}O_2$max. Despite the well-documented ability of the cardiovascular system to significantly increase muscle blood flow in response to reduced SaO_2,[129,130] the lower $\dot{Q}$ at $\dot{V}O_2$max in hypoxia has been linked to a significant reduction in muscle blood flow that also makes a large contribution to the reduction in $\dot{V}O_2$max in hypoxia (although the extent of the contribution may depend on the severity of hypoxia).[131] Interestingly, the mode of sport/exercise and the type of hypoxia may play a role in $\dot{V}O_2$max reductions. The absolute decline (not the rate of decline) in $\dot{V}O_2$max has been shown to be larger for treadmill running and cycling in normobaric hypoxia vs. hypobaric hypoxia, and $\dot{V}O_2$max (as well as SaO_2) declines more during hypoxic running vs. cycling.[105] These activity mode-related differences may be related to some of the known normoxic physiological differences between sports like running and cycling.[105] It is worth reiterating that there is complexity in the influences of the multiple potential physiological mechanisms, characteristics of the hypoxic environment, and nature of the sport/exercise on ultimate performance impairments.

In contrast to $\dot{V}O_2$max, submaximal $\dot{V}O_2$ at a given absolute power/speed is similar in acute hypoxia vs. normoxia.[116,132,133] Combined with reduced $\dot{V}O_2$max, this means that a given absolute power/speed performed at altitude will require a greater fraction of $\dot{V}O_2$max compared with normoxia. Given what we know about the potential influence of different intensity domains on fatigue processes (Section 8.2.1), this is likely a prominent contributor to fatigue during sport and exercise in acute hypoxia.

A key physiological marker, or threshold, in sport and exercise physiology, is the critical power (or critical speed for running events). The critical power is the highest metabolic rate that can be achieved using solely oxidative metabolism and represents the boundary between heavy and severe-intensity sport and exercise (Section 8.2.1.3). The critical power has important implications for sport and exercise tolerance and ultimately performance, with tolerable sport and exercise duration decreasing as the intensity increases above critical power. The power-duration relationship that underpins the critical power concept[134] is retained in acute hypoxia,[113] but reduced SaO_2 and potentially reduced muscle O_2 delivery, coupled with the reduction in $\dot{V}O_2$max, will cause critical power to be reached at a lower absolute intensity[135-137] and mean that the potentially fatigue-inducing processes that occur when exercising above the critical power (Section 8.2.1.3) will also begin at a lower intensity. Critical power declines with increasing hypoxia in a curvilinear manner from low altitude (simulated or real) onwards.[138]

A second parameter intimately linked to the critical power is the W' (W prime). Historically, this has been interpreted as the 'anaerobic' analogy of the critical power, originally thought to represent the finite anaerobic energy store that a participant was able to utilise when exercising above critical power.[134] While this is largely accurate, as always the underlying physiology is more complex.[139] We now know that manipulating things such as inspired O_2 can alter W'. The W' declines with hypoxia, but only

> **Key point 4.33**
>
> *In acute hypoxia, intensity at critical power is reduced. The W' can decline with hypoxia, but only at elevations above 4,250 metres.*

when hypoxia exceeds that associated with an altitude of 4,250 m (very high altitude).[138] Possible mechanisms for the reduced W' in severe hypoxia include reduced muscle and venous O_2 concentration which would reduce the availability of readily accessible O_2 for use above critical power,[135,140] redistribution of blood flow to respiratory muscles,[113,140] and reduced central motor drive.[138]

Regardless of the specific mechanisms behind hypoxia-related impairments to critical power and W', these impairments help to explain the known performance impairments during time to exhaustion and time-trial activity that were summarised in Section 4.8.1. This section also stated that sport and exercise lasting < 2 minutes was not impaired in hypoxia, which conflicts with the potentially negative impact of hypoxia on W'. However, only two studies analysed by Deb *et al.*[104] investigated activities lasting < 2 minutes at simulated altitudes greater than the 4,250 m suggested to impair W'.

Another crucial physiological marker is the lactate threshold, which demarks the transition from the moderate to the heavy-intensity domain (Section 8.2.1.2). As with the transition from heavy- to severe-intensity activity, mov-

Key point 4.34

Lactate threshold will occur at a lower absolute intensity in acute hypoxia, which could negatively impact on fatigue at a given absolute intensity.

ing from the moderate to the heavy-intensity domain exerts notable influence on the potential physiological underpinnings of performance and fatigue (Section 8.2.1.2). Similar to critical power, the relationship between power/speed and the lactate threshold is retained in acute hypoxia so that lactate threshold occurs at an almost identical percentage of peak power/speed/$\dot{V}O_2$max in acute hypoxia and normoxia.[141] The key difference, as with critical power, is that as peak power/speed/$\dot{V}O_2$max is reduced in acute hypoxia, the lactate threshold will occur at a lower absolute intensity. This also means that a given absolute intensity performed in hypoxia will elicit a greater blood lactate response than in normoxia.[142] The influence of acute hypoxia on lactate threshold and critical power demonstrates that the transition from moderate- to heavy- to severe-intensity activity will happen at lower absolute intensities, which for a given absolute intensity will lead to a shorter time to fatigue, or will necessitate the lowering of intensity (and therefore a lower performance level) to accomplish the task (for more detail on the role of intensity domains on fatigue, see Chapter 8).

4.8.2.3 *Substrate use*

The multitude of cardiovascular and metabolic alterations associated with sport and exercise in acute hypoxia leads to the question: is substrate use altered during sport and exercise in acute hypoxia? Once again, there are conflicting data here. Some research shows an increased reliance on carbohydrate metabolism in acute hypoxia, mediated perhaps by increased sympathetic hormone-stimulated increases in glycogenolysis and gluconeogenesis.[143] Conversely, other research has suggested increased fat oxidation in acute hypoxia, perhaps via increased activity of transcription factors that inhibit the conversion of pyruvate to acetyl-coA.[144] The most recent synthesis of evidence in the field found no consistent change in carbohydrate or fat metabolism during sport and exercise in hypoxia compared

Key point 4.35

There appears to be no consistent change in fuel metabolism during sport and exercise in acute hypoxia.

with intensity-matched normoxic activity.[145] Factors that may influence fuel use in hypoxia include the severity, duration, and type of hypoxic exposure (hypobaric hypoxia may affect substrate use more than normobaric hypoxia), intake (or not) of a pre-activity meal, and activity intensity.[145]

4.8.2.4   Central fatigue

Section 4.8.1 discussed how cognitive function can be impaired in acute hypoxia, but that sport and exercise may potentially override this impairment. But what of central fatigue in hypoxia? It appears that acute hypoxia may differentially influence the

> **Key point 4.36**
>
> *Central fatigue may be exacerbated during sport and exercise in acute hypoxia due mainly to impaired O_2 delivery to the brain. This may be a more important fatigue mechanism in severe hypoxia.*

ability to voluntarily activate skeletal muscles depending on the duration of the contraction with performance of short (3 seconds) contractions associated with impaired voluntary activation, but not long (20 seconds) contractions.[146] A possible explanation here is that longer duration contractions may give sufficient time for redirection of blood flow and O_2 delivery to the motor cortex, spinal cord, and neurons innervating the contracting muscle, allowing greater voluntary activation.[146,147] The study of McKeown *et al.*[146] used isolated contractions of a single muscle group, which may have influenced the findings. However, findings from whole-body sport and exercise are similar and show that central fatigue is exacerbated during sport and exercise in acute hypoxia, due predominantly to impaired O_2 delivery to the brain.[148,149] Although, the extent of the impact of hypoxia on central fatigue may depend on the severity of hypoxia, the intensity of the activity, and the mode of activity as a greater contribution of central fatigue has not been found in repeated-sprint activity compared with constant load activity.[150] The influence of hypoxia severity is supported by evidence showing that peripheral mechanisms are dominant performance limiters at low and moderate hypoxia, but as hypoxia becomes more severe central mechanisms become dominant, likely related to brain hypoxic effects on voluntary activation and effort perception.[151,152]

4.8.2.5   Respiratory considerations

Unsurprisingly, a key response to acute hypoxia is an increase in ventilation facilitated by the effects of reduced SaO_2 on peripheral chemoreceptors.[115,153] which is exacerbated by sport and exercise.[153] While ventilation does not appear to limit $\dot{V}O_2$max in acute hypoxia,[113] acute hypoxia can exacerbate diaphragmatic and abdominal muscle fatigue during prolonged sport and exercise.[154]

The increased work done by the respiratory muscles due to the increased ventilatory demand may also elicit a metaboreflex, mediated perhaps by inorganic phosphate and/or hydrogen ion production,[154] that increases blood flow to the respiratory muscles at the expense of blood flow to the working skeletal muscles,

> **Key point 4.37**
>
> *Acute hypoxia may exacerbate diaphragmatic and abdominal muscle fatigue and increase work done by the respiratory muscles, which may reduce blood flow to the working muscles and exacerbate peripheral fatigue.*

thereby exacerbating peripheral fatigue.[155] This finding, along with evidence that unloading the respiratory muscles during acute hypoxic exercise (via use of an assisted breathing machine) significantly increases time to exhaustion, suggests that respiratory muscle work and/or fatigue may be a significant contributor to sport and exercise fatigue in acute hypoxia. However, the influence of respiratory muscle work/fatigue on fatigue in acute hypoxia may depend on factors such as activity intensity and the extent of the reduction in SaO_2.

4.9   Summary

- Research investigating hydration and sport and exercise performance is primarily concerned with the concepts of euhydration, hyperhydration, dehydration, and hypohydration.
- Dehydration and hypohydration are not the same. Dehydration is the dynamic process of body water loss, and hypohydration is the end result of this water loss (the extent of body water loss).
- Water is critical for life and for sport and exercise performance, due to its abundance in the body and its involvement in many cellular, tissue, and organ system processes.
- Hydration status is commonly assessed by quantifying body water balance, defined as the balance between water intake and water loss.
- Dehydration can reduce blood plasma volume, meaning less blood enters the heart during each cardiac cycle. This can decrease stroke volume and $\dot{Q}$, and increase heart rate. Furthermore, competition for blood flow between the skin and the core organs may develop, impairing evaporative heat loss and increasing the risk of hyperthermia.
- Dehydration may increase muscle glycogen use at a given intensity, which could contribute to fatigue via glycogen depletion. However, increased muscle glycogen use with dehydration may also depend on the presence of hyperthermia.
- Dehydration may increase effort perception and impair aspects of cognitive function during exercise.

- Early hydration research identified an apparent threshold fluid decrement of 2% of BM, above which aerobic performance appeared to be impaired. However, this research was subject to limitations.
- A number of recent studies that attempted to address the limitations of the earlier research have shown little or no performance decrement, and perhaps a small performance enhancement, during endurance sport and exercise with hypohydration greater than 2% BM.
- The rate of dehydration may be higher during sport and exercise in the heat, but there remains uncertainty around the required extent of hypohydration for performance decrement. Also, inter-individual differences should be considered.
- Guided fluid intake is recommended during sport and exercise taking place in the heat, particularly if the activity is intense and/or prolonged. However, debate in this area is ongoing.
- Excessive fluid intake during sport and exercise appears to be the most important risk factor for the development of hypervolaemia and hyponatraemia. Strategies to reduce excessive fluid intake are associated with fewer incidences of hyponatraemia.
- Hyperthermia is an abnormally high core temperature (normal core temperature ranges from 36–37.5°C).
- Hyperthermia can develop any time body heat production is greater than body heat dissipation. The most challenging environment for maintenance of body temperature is when it is hot and humid.
- Potential peripheral factors associated with hyperthermia-induced fatigue include reduced blood and O_2 delivery to working muscles due to reduced central blood volume (which is exacerbated with combined hyperthermia and hypohydration), and increased muscle glycogen use.
- Hypohydration can delay the onset of sweating and reduce sweat rate during sport and exercise.
- It appears that central alterations due to hyperthermia (increased core temperature, increased brain temperature, reduced brain blood and O_2 delivery, reduced activity of brain regions associated with attention, focus, and arousal, suppression of motor output) may exert more of an influence on hyperthermia-induced fatigue during sport and exercise.
- The concept of a 'critical' core temperature of approximately 40°C that, once reached, causes fatigue during sport and exercise appears to be false.
- A high skin temperature may be more important than high core temperature in contributing to hyperthermia-induced fatigue during sport and exercise. High skin temperatures require a higher skin blood flow, which may impair cardiac function, reduce $\dot{V}O_2$max, and increase relative intensity, causing the athlete to fatigue earlier.
- Fatigue during sport and exercise in the heat is a progressive occurrence that likely involves both peripheral feedback and central processes.
- The physiological and cognitive responses to acute hypoxia can be thought of as occurring on a sliding and non-linear scale. However, progressive increases in altitude will cause progressive impairments for everyone.

- Acute hypoxia causes significant impairments in time-trial and time-to-exhaustion activity, and sport and exercise lasting > 2 minutes.
- Normobaric and hypobaric hypoxia may exert different effects on physiology and ultimately on sport and exercise performance.
- Acute hypoxia can impair executive function, attention, episodic memory, and information processing. Moderate-intensity activity can ameliorate these effects.
- The reduction in SaO_2 is a key contributor to impaired performance in acute hypoxia.
- Acute hypoxia may reduce HRmax and raise resting heart rate, reducing the functional heart rate reserve.
- Submaximal $\dot{Q}$ is increased with acute hypoxia in an attempt to counter the reduced SaO_2. Increased $\dot{Q}$ is achieved via increasing heart rate.
- Acute hypoxia reduces $\dot{V}O_2$max, meaning that a given activity intensity will require a higher fraction of $\dot{V}O_2$max compared with normoxia.
- Both critical power and lactate threshold occur at lower absolute intensities in acute hypoxia, with potentially crucial consequences for sport and exercise tolerance.
- There appears to be no consistent change in substrate use with acute hypoxia. A number of confounding factors may play a role in this lack of consistency.
- Central fatigue may be exacerbated during sport and exercise in acute hypoxia, due mainly to impaired brain O_2 delivery.
- Greater diaphragmatic, abdominal, and other respiratory muscle fatigue may contribute to fatigue during sport and exercise in acute hypoxia.

To think about...

The incidence of major sporting events being hosted in countries with extreme environmental conditions is increasing. Research an example of a sporting event that has taken place in one of the environments discussed in this chapter (heat, altitude, or a combination of the two). Then think about the following:

A. Do you think holding an event in such an environment is fair to all nations/teams taking part, or does it favour those from countries that regularly experience these conditions?
B. Are there any ethical issues (from a sporting, medical, or health perspective) associated with hosting competitions in these conditions?
C. What about the sponsors, employees, and fans of these teams – what thoughts might they have about the situation? And would these thoughts differ based on the specific region/country in which the event is hosted?

Test yourself

Answer the following questions to the best of your ability. Try to understand the information gained from answering these questions before you progress with the book.

1 Define and differentiate between the terms dehydration, hypohydration, and hyperhydration.
2 Briefly explain the 'classical' mechanism of dehydration-induced performance decrement.
3 What are the other ways in which dehydration may impair sport and exercise performance?
4 What are the key limitations with some of the hydration research that has been used to justify the 2% of BM dehydration threshold?
5 Summarise the key issues involved in the current debate around drinking to thirst vs. guided drinking.
6 Define and briefly explain the terms hypervolaemia and hyponatraemia.
7 What are the primary possible causes of peripheral and central fatigue associated with hyperthermia?
8 What are the key arguments against the critical core temperature hypothesis?
9 How might high skin temperature contribute to fatigue, independent of changes in core temperature?
10 How might different types of hypoxia influence physiology and fatigue?
11 Summarise the primary ways in which acute hypoxia may contribute to fatigue during sport and exercise.

References

1 Casa DJ, Armstrong LE, Hillman SK, et al. National athletic trainers' association position statement: fluid replacement for athletes. *J Athl Train.* 2000;35(2):212–224.
2 American College of Sports M, Sawka MN, Burke LM, et al. American College of Sports Medicine position stand. Exercise and fluid replacement. *Med Sci Sports Exerc.* 2007;39(2):377–390.
3 Logan-Sprenger HM, Heigenhauser GJ, Jones GL, Spriet LL. The effect of dehydration on muscle metabolism and time trial performance during prolonged cycling in males. *Physiol Rep.* 2015;3(8):1–13.
4 Logan-Sprenger HM, Heigenhauser GJ, Killian KJ, Spriet LL. Effects of dehydration during cycling on skeletal muscle metabolism in females. *Med Sci Sports Exerc.* 2012;44(10):1949–1957.
5 Logan-Sprenger HM, Heigenhauser GJ, Jones GL, Spriet LL. Increase in skeletal-muscle glycogenolysis and perceived exertion with progressive dehydration during cycling in hydrated men. *Int J Sport Nutr Exerc Metab.* 2013;23(3):220–229.
6 Ganio MS, Armstrong LE, Casa DJ, et al. Mild dehydration impairs cognitive performance and mood of men. *Br J Nutr.* 2011;106(10):1535–1543.
7 Casa DJ, Clarkson PM, Roberts WO. American college of sports medicine roundtable on hydration and physical activity: consensus statements. *Curr Sports Med Rep.* 2005;4(3):115–127.

8 Cheuvront SN, Carter R, 3rd, Sawka MN. Fluid balance and endurance exercise performance. *Curr Sports Med Rep.* 2003;2(4):202–208.

9 Sawka MN, Noakes TD. Does dehydration impair exercise performance? *Med Sci Sports Exerc.* 2007;39(8):1209–1217.

10 Sawka MN. Physiological consequences of hypohydration: exercise performance and thermoregulation. *Med Sci Sports Exerc.* 1992;24(6):657–670.

11 Dougherty KA, Baker LB, Chow M, Kenney WL. Two percent dehydration impairs and six percent carbohydrate drink improves boys basketball skills. *Med Sci Sports Exerc.* 2006;38(9):1650–1658.

12 Berry CW, Wolf ST, Cottle RM, Kenney WL. Hydration is more important than exogenous carbohydrate intake during push-to-the-finish cycle exercise in the heat. *Front Sports Act Living.* 2021;3:742710.

13 Armstrong LE, Costill DL, Fink WJ. Influence of diuretic-induced dehydration on competitive running performance. *Med Sci Sports Exerc.* 1985;17(4):456–461.

14 James LJ, Funnell MP, James RM, Mears SA. Does hypohydration really impair endurance performance? Methodological considerations for interpreting hydration research. *Sports Med.* 2019;49:103–114.

15 Dugas JP, Oosthuizen V, Tucker R, Noakes TD. Drinking "ad libitum" optimises performance and physiological function during 80 km indoor cycling trials in hot and humid conditions with appropriate convective cooling. *Med Sci Sports Exerc.* 2006;38:S176.

16 Jeukendrup A, Saris WH, Brouns F, Kester AD. A new validated endurance performance test. *Med Sci Sports Exerc.* 1996;28(2):266–270.

17 Mundel T. To drink or not to drink? Explaining "contradictory findings" in fluid replacement and exercise performance: evidence from a more valid model for real-life competition. *Br J Sports Med.* 2011;45(1):2.

18 Dion T, Savoie FA, Asselin A, Gariepy C, Goulet ED. Half-marathon running performance is not improved by a rate of fluid intake above that dictated by thirst sensation in trained distance runners. *Eur J Appl Physiol.* 2013;113(12): 3011–3020.

19 Marino FE, Cannon J, Kay D. Neuromuscular responses to hydration in moderate to warm ambient conditions during self-paced high-intensity exercise. *Br J Sports Med.* 2010;44(13):961–967.

20 Nolte HW, Noakes TD, van Vuuren B. Protection of total body water content and absence of hyperthermia despite 2% body mass loss ('voluntary dehydration') in soldiers drinking ad libitum during prolonged exercise in cool environmental conditions. *Br J Sports Med.* 2011;45(14):1106–1112.

21 Zouhal H, Groussard C, Minter G, et al. Inverse relationship between percentage body weight change and finishing time in 643 forty-two-kilometre marathon runners. *Br J Sports Med.* 2011;45(14):1101–1105.

22 Aragon-Vargas LF, Wilk B, Timmons BW, Bar-Or O. Body weight changes in child and adolescent athletes during a triathlon competition. *Eur J Appl Physiol.* 2013;113(1):233–239.

23 Kao WF, Shyu CL, Yang XW, et al. Athletic performance and serial weight changes during 12- and 24-hour ultra-marathons. *Clin J Sport Med.* 2008;18(2):155–158.

24 Rust CA, Knechtle B, Knechtle P, Wirth A, Rosemann T. Body mass change and ultraendurance performance: a decrease in body mass is associated with an increased running speed in male 100-km ultramarathoners. *J Strength Cond Res.* 2012;26(6):1505–1516.

25 Goulet ED. Effect of exercise-induced dehydration on endurance performance: evaluating the impact of exercise protocols on outcomes using a meta-analytic procedure. *Br J Sports Med.* 2013;47(11):679–686.

26 Maughan RJ, Shirreffs SM, Leiper JB. Errors in the estimation of hydration status from changes in body mass. *J Sports Sci.* 2007;25(7):797–804.

27 Zouhal H, Groussard C, Vincent S, et al. Athletic performance and weight changes during the "Marathon of Sands" in athletes well-trained in endurance. *Int J Sports Med.* 2009;30(7):516–521.

28 Dugas JP, Oosthuizen U, Tucker R, Noakes TD. Rates of fluid ingestion alter pacing but not thermoregulatory responses during prolonged exercise in hot and humid conditions with appropriate convective cooling. *Eur J Appl Physiol.* 2009;105(1):69–80.

29 Gigou PY, Dion T, Asselin A, Berrigan F, Goulet ED. Pre-exercise hyperhydration-induced bodyweight gain does not alter prolonged treadmill running time-trial performance in warm ambient conditions. *Nutrients.* 2012;4(8):949–966.

30 Goulet ED. Effect of exercise-induced dehydration on time-trial exercise performance: a meta-analysis. *Br J Sports Med.* 2011;45(14):1149–1156.

31 Burke LM. Hydration in sport and exercise. In: Periard JD, Racinais S, eds. *Heat Stress in Sport and Exercise: Thermophysiology of Health and Performance.* Switzerland: Springer Nature; 2019:113–138.

32 Kenefick RW. Drinking strategies: planned drinking versus drinking to thirst. *Sports Med.* 2018;48(Suppl 1):31–37.

33 Periard JD, Eijsvogels T, Daanen HAM, Racinais S. Hydration for the Tokyo Olympics: to thirst or not to thirst? *Br J Sports Med.* 2021;55(8):410–411.

34 Goulet EDB. Comment on "Drinking strategies: planned drinking versus drinking to thirst". *Sports Med.* 2019;49(4):631–633.

35 Convertino VA. Heart rate and sweat rate responses associated with exercise-induced hypervolemia. *Med Sci Sports Exerc.* 1983;15(1):77–82.

36 Mischler I, Boirie Y, Gachon P, et al. Human albumin synthesis is increased by an ultra-endurance trial. *Med Sci Sports Exerc.* 2003;35(1):75–81.

37 Leiper JB, McCormick K, Robertson JD, Whiting PH, Maughan RJ. Fluid homoeostasis during prolonged low-intensity walking on consecutive days. *Clin Sci (Lond).* 1988;75(1):63–70.

38 Fellmann N, Ritz P, Ribeyre J, Beaufrere B, Delaitre M, Coudert J. Intracellular hyperhydration induced by a 7-day endurance race. *Eur J Appl Physiol Occup Physiol.* 1999;80(4):353–359.

39 Fellmann N, Sagnol M, Bedu M, et al. Enzymatic and hormonal responses following a 24 h endurance run and a 10 h triathlon race. *Eur J Appl Physiol Occup Physiol.* 1988;57(5):545–553.

40 Skenderi KP, Kavouras SA, Anastasiou CA, Yiannakouris N, Matalas AL. Exertional Rhabdomyolysis during a 246-km continuous running race. *Med Sci Sports Exerc.* 2006;38(6):1054–1057.

41 Knechtle B, Duff B, Schulze I, Kohler G. A Multi-Stage Ultra-Endurance Run over 1,200 KM Leads to a Continuous Accumulation of Total Body Water. *J Sports Sci Med.* 2008;7(3):357–364.

42 Knechtle B, Wirth A, Knechtle P, Rosemann T. Increase of total body water with decrease of body mass while running 100 km nonstop – formation of edema? *Res Q Exerc Sport.* 2009;80(3):593–603.

43 Noakes TD, Sharwood K, Collins M, Perkins DR. The dipsomania of great distance: water intoxication in an Ironman triathlete. *Br J Sports Med.* 2004;38(4):E16.

44 Hew-Butler T, Loi V, Pani A, Rosner MH. Exercise-associated hyponatremia: 2017 update. *Front Med.* 2017;4:21.

45 Rosner MH, Kirven J. Exercise-associated hyponatremia. *Clin J Am Soc Nephrol.* 2007;2(1):151–161.

46 Scheer V, Knechtle B. Exercise associated hyponatremia in endurance sports: a review with practical recommendations. *Arch Med Deporte.* 2020;37(4):260–265.

47 Almond CSD, Shin AY, Fortescue EB, et al. Hyponatraemia among runners in the Boston Marathon. *New Eng J Med.* 2005;352:1550–1556.

48 Knechtle B, Chlibkova D, Papadopoulou S, Mantzorou M, Rosemann T, Nikolaidis PT. Exercise-associated hyponatremia in endurance and ultra-endurance performance-aspects of sex, race location, ambient temperature, sports discipline, and length of performance: a narrative review. *Medicina (Kaunas).* 2019;55(9):1–23.

49 Montain SJ, Cheuvront SN, Sawka MN. Exercise associated hyponatraemia: quantitative analysis to understand the aetiology. *Br J Sports Med.* 2006;40(2):98–105; discussion 98–105.

50 Sharwood KA, Collins M, Goedecke JH, Wilson G, Noakes TD. Weight changes, medical complications, and performance during an Ironman triathlon. *Br J Sports Med.* 2004;38(6):718–724.

51 Noakes TD, Speedy DB. Case proven: exercise associated hyponatraemia is due to overdrinking. So why did it take 20 years before the original evidence was accepted? *Br J Sports Med.* 2006;40(7):567–572.

52 Periard JD, Eijsvogels TMH, Daanen HAM. Exercise under heat stress: thermoregulation, hydration, performance implications, and mitigation strategies. *Physiol Rev.* 2021;101(4):1873–1979.

53 Maughan RJ. Thermoregulatory aspects of performance. *Exp Physiol.* 2012;97(3): 325–326.

54 Nybo L. Hyperthermia and fatigue. *J Appl Physiol (1985).* 2008;104(3):871–878.

55 Nybo L. Brain temperature and exercise performance. *Exp Physiol.* 2012;97(3): 333–339.

56 Gonzalez-Alonso J, Mora-Rodriguez R, Below PR, Coyle EF. Dehydration markedly impairs cardiovascular function in hyperthermic endurance athletes during exercise. *J Appl Physiol (1985).* 1997;82(4):1229–1236.

57 Nybo L, Nielsen B. Hyperthermia and central fatigue during prolonged exercise in humans. *J Appl Physiol (1985).* 2001;91(3):1055–1060.

58 Nielsen B, Strange S, Christensen NJ, Warberg J, Saltin B. Acute and adaptive responses in humans to exercise in a warm, humid environment. *Pflugers Arch.* 1997;434(1):49–56.

59 Shibasaki M, Aoki K, Morimoto K, Johnson JM, Takamata A. Plasma hyperosmolality elevates the internal temperature threshold for active thermoregulatory vasodilation during heat stress in humans. *Am J Physiol Regul Integr Comp Physiol.* 2009;297(6):R1706–R1712.

60 Takamata A, Nagashima K, Nose H, Morimoto T. Osmoregulatory inhibition of thermally induced cutaneous vasodilation in passively heated humans. *Am J Physiol.* 1997;273(1 Pt 2):R197–R204.

61 Sawka MN, Young AJ, Francesconi RP, Muza SR, Pandolf KB. Thermoregulatory and blood responses during exercise at graded hypohydration levels. *J Appl Physiol (1985).* 1985;59(5):1394–1401.

62 Febbraio MA, Carey MF, Snow RJ, Stathis CG, Hargreaves M. Influence of elevated muscle temperature on metabolism during intense, dynamic exercise. *Am J Physiol.* 1996;271(5 Pt 2):R1251–R1255.

63 Febbraio MA, Snow RJ, Stathis CG, Hargreaves M, Carey MF. Effect of heat stress on muscle energy metabolism during exercise. *J Appl Physiol (1985)*. 1994;77(6):2827–2831.

64 Parkin JM, Carey MF, Zhao S, Febbraio MA. Effect of ambient temperature on human skeletal muscle metabolism during fatiguing submaximal exercise. *J Appl Physiol (1985)*. 1999;86(3):902–908.

65 Febbraio MA, Lambert DL, Starkie RL, Proietto J, Hargreaves M. Effect of epinephrine on muscle glycogenolysis during exercise in trained men. *J Appl Physiol (1985)*. 1998;84(2):465–470.

66 Starkie RL, Hargreaves M, Lambert DL, Proietto J, Febbraio MA. Effect of temperature on muscle metabolism during submaximal exercise in humans. *Exp Physiol*. 1999;84(4):775–784.

67 Febbraio MA. Does muscle function and metabolism affect exercise performance in the heat? *Exerc Sport Sci Rev*. 2000;28(4):171–176.

68 Gordon R, Tyler CJ, Castelli F, Diss CE, Tillin NA. Progressive hyperthermia elicits distinct responses in maximum and rapid torque production. *J Sci Med Sport*. 2021;24(8):811–817.

69 Nybo L, Moller K, Volianitis S, Nielsen B, Secher NH. Effects of hyperthermia on cerebral blood flow and metabolism during prolonged exercise in humans. *J Appl Physiol (1985)*. 2002;93(1):58–64.

70 Nybo L, Nielsen B. Middle cerebral artery blood velocity is reduced with hyperthermia during prolonged exercise in humans. *J Physiol*. 2001;534(Pt 1):279–286.

71 Periard JD, Racinais S. Heat stress exacerbates the reduction in middle cerebral artery blood velocity during prolonged self-paced exercise. *Scand J Med Sci Sports*. 2015;25(Suppl 1):135–144.

72 Gonzalez-Alonso J, Dalsgaard MK, Osada T, et al. Brain and central haemodynamics and oxygenation during maximal exercise in humans. *J Physiol*. 2004;557(Pt 1):331–342.

73 Periard JD, De Pauw K, Zanow F, Racinais S. Cerebrocortical activity during self-paced exercise in temperate, hot and hypoxic conditions. *Acta Physiol (Oxf)*. 2018;222(1):1–13.

74 Nielsen B, Nybo L. Cerebral changes during exercise in the heat. *Sports Med*. 2003;33(1):1–11.

75 Nybo L, Nielsen B. Perceived exertion is associated with an altered brain activity during exercise with progressive hyperthermia. *J Appl Physiol (1985)*. 2001;91(5):2017–2023.

76 Caputa SS, McLellan TM. Effect of brain and trunk temperatures on exercise performance in goats. *Pflug Arch Physiol*. 1986;406:184–189.

77 White MD, Greiner JG, McDonald PLL. Point: Humans do demonstrate selective brain cooling during hyperthermia. *J Appl Physiol* 2011;110:569–571.

78 Marino FE. The critical limiting temperature and selective brain cooling: neuroprotection during exercise? *Int J Hyperther*. 2011;27:582–590.

79 Morrison SA, Sleivert GG, Cheung S. Aerobic influence on neuromuscular function and tolerance during passive hyperthermia. *Med Sci Sports Exerc*. 2006;38(10):1754–1761.

80 Periard JD, Christian RJ, Knez WL, Racinais S. Voluntary muscle and motor cortical activation during progressive exercise and passively induced hyperthermia. *Exp Physiol*. 2014;99(1):136–148.

81 Periard JD, Cramer MN, Chapman PG, Caillaud C, Thompson MW. Neuromuscular function following prolonged intense self-paced exercise in hot climatic conditions. *Eur J Appl Physiol.* 2011;111(8):1561–1569.

82 Periard JD, Caillaud C, Thompson MW. Central and peripheral fatigue during passive and exercise-induced hyperthermia. *Med Sci Sports Exerc.* 2011;43(9):1657–1665.

83 Amann M. Central and peripheral fatigue: interaction during cycling exercise in humans. *Med Sci Sports Exerc.* 2011;43(11):2039–2045.

84 Gonzalez-Alonso J, Calbet JA, Nielsen B. Metabolic and thermodynamic responses to dehydration-induced reductions in muscle blood flow in exercising humans. *J Physiol.* 1999;520(Pt 2):577–589.

85 Nielsen B, Hales JR, Strange S, Christensen NJ, Warberg J, Saltin B. Human circulatory and thermoregulatory adaptations with heat acclimation and exercise in a hot, dry environment. *J Physiol.* 1993;460:467–485.

86 Nielsen B, Savard G, Richter EA, Hargreaves M, Saltin B. Muscle blood flow and muscle metabolism during exercise and heat stress. *J Appl Physiol (1985).* 1990;69(3):1040–1046.

87 Ely BR, Ely MR, Cheuvront SN, Kenefick RW, Degroot DW, Montain SJ. Evidence against a 40 degrees C core temperature threshold for fatigue in humans. *J Appl Physiol (1985).* 2009;107(5):1519–1525.

88 Nybo L. Exercise and heat stress: cerebral challenges and consequences. *Prog Brain Res.* 2007;162:29–43.

89 Sawka MN, Cheuvront SN, Kenefick RW. High skin temperature and hypohydration impair aerobic performance. *Exp Physiol.* 2012;97(3):327–332.

90 Chou T, Allen JR, Hahn D, Leary BK, Coyle EF. Cardiovascular responses to exercise when increasing skin temperature with narrowing of the core-to-skin temperature gradient. *J Appl Physiol.* 2018;125:697–705.

91 Thomas MM, Cheung SS, Elder GC, Sleivert GG. Voluntary muscle activation is impaired by core temperature rather than local muscle temperature. *J Appl Physiol (1985).* 2006;100(4):1361–1369.

92 Dubois M, Sato S, Lees DE, et al. Electroencephalographic changes during whole body hyperthermia in humans. *Electroencephalogr Clin Neurophysiol.* 1980;50(5–6):486–495.

93 Montain SJ, Sawka MN, Cadarette BS, Quigley MD, McKay JM. Physiological tolerance to uncompensable heat stress: effects of exercise intensity, protective clothing, and climate. *J Appl Physiol (1985).* 1994;77(1):216–222.

94 Latzka WA, Sawka MN, Montain SJ, et al. Hyperhydration: tolerance and cardiovascular effects during uncompensable exercise-heat stress. *J Appl Physiol (1985).* 1998;84(6):1858–1864.

95 Kenefick RW, Cheuvront SN, Palombo LJ, Ely BR, Sawka MN. Skin temperature modifies the impact of hypohydration on aerobic performance. *J Appl Physiol (1985).* 2010;109(1):79–86.

96 Byrne C, Lee JK, Chew SA, Lim CL, Tan EY. Continuous thermoregulatory responses to mass-participation distance running in heat. *Med Sci Sports Exerc.* 2006;38(5):803–810.

97 Lee JK, Nio AQ, Lim CL, Teo EY, Byrne C. Thermoregulation, pacing and fluid balance during mass participation distance running in a warm and humid environment. *Eur J Appl Physiol.* 2010;109(5):887–898.

98 Burtscher M. Effects of living at higher altitudes on mortality: a narrative review. *Aging Dis.* 2014;5:274–280.

99 Zubieta-Castillo G, Zubieta-Calleja GR, Zubieta-Calleja L, Zubieta-Castillo N. Facts that prove that adaptation to life at extreme altitude (8842m) is possible. *Adapt Biol Med.* 2008;5:348–355.

100 Taylor AT. High-altitude illnesses: physiology, risk factors, prevention, and treatment. *Rambam Maimonides Med J.* 2011;2(1):e0022.

101 Szymczak RK, Marosz M, Grzywacz T, Sawicka M, Naczyk M. Death zone weather extremes mountaineers have experienced in successful ascents. *Front Physiol.* 2021;12:696335.

102 Havenith G. Benchmarking functionality of historical cold weather clothing: Robert F. Scott Roald Amundsen, George Mallory. *J Fiber Bioeng Inform.* 2010;3:121–129.

103 Firth PG, Zheng H, Windsoe JS, et al. Mortality on Mount Everest, 1921–2006: descriptive study. *BMJ.* 2008;337:a2654.

104 Deb SK, Brown DR, Gough LA, et al. Quantifying the effects of acute hypoxic exposure on exercise performance and capacity: A systematic review and meta-regression. *Eur J Sport Sci.* 2018;18(2):243–256.

105 Treml B, Gatterer H, Burtscher J, Kleinsasser A, Burtscher M. A Focused review on the maximal exercise responses in hypo- and normobaric hypoxia: divergent oxygen uptake and ventilation responses. *Int J Environ Res Public Health.* 2020;17(14):1–12.

106 Coppel J, Hennis P, Gilbert-Kawai E, Grocott MP. The physiological effects of hypobaric hypoxia versus normobaric hypoxia: a systematic review of crossover trials. *Extrem Physiol Med.* 2015;4:2.

107 Beidleman BA, Fulco CS, Staab JE, Andrew SP, Muza SR. Cycling performance decrement is greater in hypobaric versus normobaric hypoxia. *Extrem Physiol Med.* 2014;3:8.

108 Saugy JJ, Rupp T, Faiss R, Lamon A, Bourdillon N, Millet GP. Cycling time trial is more altered in hypobaric than normobaric hypoxia. *Med Sci Sports Exerc.* 2016;48(4):680–688.

109 Yan X. Cognitive impairments at high altitudes and adaptation. *High Alt Med Biol.* 2014;15(2):141–145.

110 Roach EB, Bleiberg J, Lathan CE, Wolpert L, Tsao JW, Roach RC. AltitudeOmics: decreased reaction time after high altitude cognitive testing is a sensitive metric of hypoxic impairment. *Neuroreport.* 2014;25(11):814–818.

111 Jung M, Zou L, Yu JJ, et al. Dos exercise have a protective effect on cognitive function under hypoxia? A systematic review with meta-analysis. *J Sport Health Sci.* 2020;9:562–577.

112 Ando S, Komiyama T, Sudo M, et al. The interactive effects of acute exercise and hypoxia on cognitive performance: a narrative review. *Scand J Med Sci Sports.* 2020;30(3):384–398.

113 Grocott MPW, Levett DZH, Ward SA. Exercise physiology: exercise performance at altitude. *Curr Opin Physiol.* 2019;10:210–218.

114 McMorris T, Hale BJ, Barwood M, Costello J, Corbett J. Effect of acute hypoxia on cognition: a systematic review and meta-regression analysis. *Neurosci Biobehav Rev.* 2017;74(Pt A):225–232.

115 Mallet RT, Burtscher J, Richalet JP, Millet GP, Burtscher M. Impact of high altitude on cardiovascular health: current perspectives. *Vasc Health Risk Manag.* 2021;17:317–335.

116 Mourot L. Limitation of maximal heart rate in hypoxia: mechanisms and clinical importance. *Front Physiol.* 2018;9:972.

117 Puthon L, Bouzat P, Robach P, Favre-Juvin A, Doutreleau S, Verges S. Effect of ageing on hypoxic exercise cardiorespiratory, muscle and cerebral oxygenation responses in healthy humans. *Exp Physiol.* 2017;102(4):436–447.

118 Mollard P, Woorons X, Letournel M, et al. Determinant factors of the decrease in aerobic performance in moderate acute hypoxia in women endurance athletes. *Respir Physiol Neurobiol.* 2007;159(2):178–186.

119 Grataloup O, Busso T, Castells J, Denis C, Benoit H. Evidence of decrease in peak heart rate in acute hypoxia: effect of exercise-induced arterial hypoxemia. *Int J Sports Med.* 2007;28(3):181–185.

120 Favret F, Richalet JP. Exercise and hypoxia: the role of the autonomic nervous system. *Respir Physiol Neurobiol.* 2007;158(2–3):280–286.

121 Siebenmann C, Lundby C. Regulation of cardiac output in hypoxia. *Scand J Med Sci Sports.* 2015;25(Suppl 4):53–59.

122 Richalet JP, Hermand E. Cardiovascular response at maximal exercise at high altitude. *J Appl Physiol (1985).* 2023;134(1):147.

123 Lloyd A, Fiala D, Heyde C, Havenith G. A mathematical model for predicting cardiovascular responses at rest and during exercise in demanding environmental conditions. *J Appl Physiol (1985).* 2022;133(2):247–261.

124 Lloyd AB, Havenith G. Reply to Richalet and Hermand. Updating the CVR model for limitations in maximum myocardial contractility at high altitude. *J Appl Physiol (1985).* 2023;134(1):148–149.

125 Williams AM, Levine BD, Stembridge M. A change of heart: mechanisms of cardiac adaptation to acute and chronic hypoxia. *J Physiol.* 2022;600:4089–4104.

126 Wolfel EE, Selland MA, Cymerman A, et al. O2 extraction maintains O2 uptake during submaximal exercise with beta-adrenergic blockade at 4,300 m. *J Appl Physiol (1985).* 1998;85(3):1092–1102.

127 Goebel B, Handrick V, Lauten A, et al. Impact of acute normobaric hypoxia on regional and global myocardial function: a speckle tracking echocardiography study. *Int J Cardiovasc Imaging.* 2013;29(3):561–570.

128 Sengupta PP, Khandheria BK, Narula J. Twist and untwist mechanics of the left ventricle. *Heart Fail Clin.* 2008;4(3):315–324.

129 Calbet JA, Lundby C. Skeletal muscle vasodilatation during maximal exercise in health and disease. *J Physiol.* 2012;590(24):6285–6296.

130 Joyner MJ, Casey DP. Muscle blood flow, hypoxia, and hypoperfusion. *J Appl Physiol (1985).* 2014;116(7):852–857.

131 Calbet JA, Boushel R, Radegran G, Sondergaard H, Wagner PD, Saltin B. Determinants of maximal oxygen uptake in severe acute hypoxia. *Am J Physiol Regul Integr Comp Physiol.* 2003;284(2):R291–R303.

132 Clark SA, Bourdon PC, Schmidt W, et al. The effect of acute simulated moderate altitude on power, performance and pacing strategies in well-trained cyclists. *Eur J Appl Physiol.* 2007;102(1):45–55.

133 Park HY, Kim JW, Nam SS. Metabolic, Cardiac, and Hemorheological Responses to Submaximal Exercise under Light and Moderate Hypobaric Hypoxia in Healthy Men. *Biology (Basel).* 2022;11(1):1–11.

134 Poole DC, Burnley M, Vanhatalo A, Rossiter HB, Jones AM. Critical power: an important fatigue threshold in exercise physiology. *Med Sci Sports Exerc.* 2016;48(11):2320–2334.

135 Richard NA, Koehle MS. Influence and mechanisms of action of environmental stimuli on work near and above the severe domain boundary (critical power). *Sports Med Open.* 2022;8(1):42.

136 Dekerle J, Mucci P, Carter H. Influence of moderate hypoxia on tolerance to high-intensity exercise. *Eur J Appl Physiol.* 2012;112(1):327–335.
137 Sousa AC, Millet GP, Viana J, Milheiro J, Reis V. Effects of normobaric hypoxia on matched-severe exercise and power-duration relationship. *Int J Sports Med.* 2021;42(8):708–715.
138 Townsend NE, Nichols DS, Skiba PF, Racinais S, Periard JD. Prediction of critical power and W' in hypoxia: application to work-balance modelling. *Front Physiol.* 2017;8:180.
139 Craig JC, Vanhatalo A, Burnley M, Jones AM, Poole DC. Critica power: possible the most important fatigue threshold in exercise physiology. In: Zoladz JA, ed. *Muscle and Exercise Physiology.* Academic Press; 2019:159–181.
140 Valli G, Cogo A, Passino C, et al. Exercise intolerance at high altitude (5050 m): critical power and W'. *Respir Physiol Neurobiol.* 2011;177(3):333–341.
141 Ofner M, Wonisch M, Frei M, et al. Influence of acute normobaric hypoxia on physiological variables and lactate turn point determination in trained men. *J Sport Sci Med.* 2014;13:774–781.
142 Maldonado-Rodriguez N, Bentley DJ, Logan-Sprenger HM. Acute physiological response to different sprint training protocols in normobaric hypoxia. *Int J Environ Res Public Health.* 2022;19:1–11.
143 Katayama K, Goto K, Ishida K, Ogita F. Substrate utilization during exercise and recovery at moderate altitude. *Metabolism.* 2010;59(7):959–966.
144 Spriet LL, Watt MJ. Regulatory mechanisms in the interaction between carbohydrate and lipid oxidation during exercise. *Acta Physiol Scand.* 2003;178(4): 443–452.
145 Griffiths A, Shannon OM, Matu J, King R, Deighton K, O'Hara JP. The effects of environmental hypoxia on substrate utilisation during exercise: a meta-analysis. *J Int Soc Sports Nutr.* 2019;16(1):10.
146 McKeown DJ, McNeill CJ, Simmonds MJ, Kavanagh JJ. Time course of neuromuscular responses to acute hypoxia during voluntary contractions. *Exp Physiol.* 2020;105:1855–1868.
147 Liu JZ, Shan ZY, Zhang LD, Sahgal V, Brown RW, Yue GH. Human brain activation during sustained and intermittent submaximal fatigue muscle contractions: an FMRI study. *J Neurophysiol.* 2003;90:300–312.
148 Goodall S, Gonzalez-Alonso J, Ali L, Ross EZ, Romer LM. Supraspinal fatigue after normoxic and hypoxic exercise in humans. *J Physiol.* 2012;590:2767–2782.
149 Goodall S, Twomey R, Amann M. Acute and chronic hypoxia: implications for cerebral function and exercise tolerance. *Fatigue: Biomed, Health Behav.* 2014;2:73–92.
150 Townsend N, Brocherie F, Millet GP, Girard O. Central and peripheral muscle fatigue following repeated-sprint running in moderate and severe hypoxia. *Exp Physiol.* 2020;106:126–138.
151 Amann M, Romer LM, Subudhi AW, Pegelow DF, Dempsey JA. Severity of arterial hypoxaemia affects the relative contributions of peripheral muscle fatigue to exercise performance in healthy humans. *J Physiol.* 2007;581(Pt 1):389–403.
152 Millet GY, Muthalib M, Jubeau M, Laursen PB, Nosaka K. Severe hypoxia affects exercise performance independently of afferent feedback and peripheral fatigue. *J Appl Physiol (1985).* 2012;112(8):1335–1344.

153 Teppema LJ, Dahan A. The ventilatory response to hypoxia in mammals: mechanisms, measurement, and analysis. *Physiol Rev.* 2010;90(2):675–754.

154 Verges S, Bachasson D, Wuyam B. Effect of acute hypoxia on respiratory muscle fatigue in healthy humans. *Respir Res.* 2010;11(1):109.

155 Amann M, Pegelow DF, Jacques AJ, Dempsey JA. Inspiratory muscle work in acute hypoxia influences locomotor muscle fatigue and exercise performance of healthy humans. *Am J Physiol Regul Integr Comp Physiol.* 2007;293(5):R2036–R2045.

5 Potassium, calcium, and inorganic phosphate

5.1 Introduction

Technological advances have enabled the development of more sophisticated human measurement and analysis tools. Magnetic resonance imagery (MRI, see Section 1.4.5), transcranial magnetic stimulation (Section 1.4.6), and a host of other complex technologies usually found in medical and clinical settings are becoming more commonplace within sport and exercise science research.

These technological advances have enabled ever more detailed investigation of the function of the body at a cellular and molecular level during sport and exercise. Consequently, new avenues of knowledge have developed regarding the biochemical processes that control body system functions. Within the context of fatigue during sport and exercise, three substances that have come to light as a result of our improved ability to determine their function are potassium (K), calcium (Ca), and inorganic phosphate (Pi). This chapter will summarise the important functional roles of K, Ca, and Pi before discussing how disturbances in some of these functions during sport and exercise could potentially contribute to fatigue. As with the other chapters in this book, the information provided is a summary of current knowledge; investigations are ongoing.

5.2 Potassium: description and function

The following is a brief description of K and its key functions as related to sport and exercise fatigue. For a more detailed discussion of the nature of K and its roles in performance and health, the interested reader is referred to the excellent article by Lindinger and Cairns.[1]

Potassium is a chemical element that is necessary for the function of all living cells. It is one of the most common elements in the body, representing approximately 0.2% of body mass. Potassium is a mineral, meaning that it is a naturally occurring inorganic solid. Sources of dietary K include orange juice, potatoes, bananas, leafy greens, and salmon.

Potassium is also an electrolyte, meaning that it carries a small electrical charge and enables electricity to be conducted through the solution in which it is

DOI: 10.4324/9781003326137-7

placed (this is very im-
portant for some of the
functional roles that K
plays). The ionic form
of K is abbreviated as
K+. The "+" sign in the
abbreviation indicates a
positively charged ion,
known as a cation. In

Key point 5.1

Potassium is one of the most abundant elements in the body. Dietary sources of K+ include orange juice, potatoes, bananas, leafy greens, and salmon.

fact, K+ is the most abundant cation found within cells. The vast majority of the body's K+ stores (~80%) are located within the nervous system, skeletal muscle, and bone (~60–160 millimoles (mM), depending on cell type) with a small amount (~3.5–5 mM) present in blood plasma.

Potassium plays crucial roles in body function. Firstly, K+, along with another electrolyte, sodium (Na+), helps to regulate intra- and extracellular water content. Water molecules do not have an electrical charge, and cells cannot move water from intra- to extracellular locations directly. However, the components of water, hydrogen and oxygen, do have an electrical charge (hydrogen has a positive charge and oxygen a negative charge). These charges are attracted to the electrical charges of K+ and Na+ ions, meaning that electrolytes "attract" water molecules to them. If a cell membrane is permeable to water, then water will move across the membrane to the side with the highest concentration of electrolytes, as this is the side that is exerting the greatest "pull" on the water molecules. This movement of water will continue until the electrolyte concentration on both sides of the cell membrane is equal.

Movement of K+ and Na+ across cell membranes is achieved via specialised protein-based transport channels. At rest, the inside of a muscle cell has a slightly negative electrical charge compared to the outside of the cell. This negative charge, termed the resting membrane potential, is generated by the relative concentration of Na+ and K+ within and outside the cell. To initiate muscle contraction, an electrical signal moves along a motor neuron, along the surface of a muscle cell, and then inside the cell. The transport, or propagation, of this electrical signal (termed an action potential) is controlled by movement of Na+ and K+ across the cell membrane of the motor neuron and muscle (Figure 5.1). Initial stimulus by the action potential makes the nerve cell membrane permeable to Na+ via the opening of voltage-gated Na+ channels (Figure 5.1). In this situation, Na+ quickly enters the muscle cell, making the interior of the cell positively charged (depolarised) and enabling the action potential to continue. Almost immediately following this, Na+ channels close and voltage-gated K+ channels then open, enabling K+ to quickly leave the cell (Figure 5.1). This process repolarises the cell, making the intracellular charge negative once again (therefore, Na+ movement is excitatory, and K+ movement is inhibitory). The entire process only takes a few milliseconds and occurs during every action potential. Upon repolarisation, the intracellular charge may be slightly

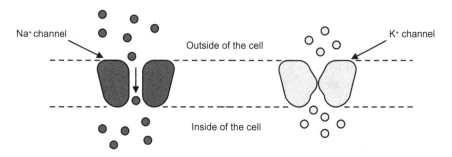

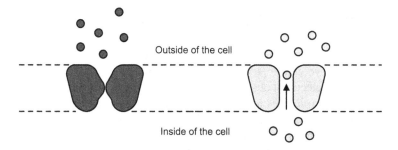

Figure 5.1 At rest, the inside of a nerve or muscle cell has a slightly negative electrical charge compared to the outside of the cell, due in part to the greater concentration of Na^+ outside and greater concentration of K^+ inside the cell. The transport, or propagation, of the electrical signal down a motor neuron and across and into the muscle cell makes the cell membrane permeable to Na^+ via the opening of voltage-gated Na^+ channels. Here, Na^+ quickly enters the muscle cell through ion channels present in the cell membrane, depolarising the cell and enabling the action potential to continue. Almost immediately following this, Na^+ channels close and voltage-gated K^+ channels open, enabling K^+ to quickly leave the cell. This process repolarises the cell, making the intracellular charge negative once again.

more negative than the resting membrane potential (termed hyperpolarisation). In this situation, the Na^+ K^+ pump (integrated specialised channels within the membrane of excitable cells that transport Na^+ and K^+ across the membrane) will regain and maintain resting

Key point 5.2

Potassium has key roles to play in a variety of body functions. Some of the most important of these functions include the regulation of body water content, conduction of action potentials along neurons and muscle cells, and aiding in protein synthesis, carbohydrate metabolism, and glycogenesis.

Outside of the cell

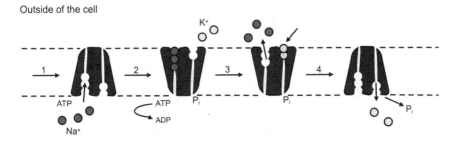

Inside of the cell

Figure 5.2 The Na⁺, K⁺ pump. Specialised channels are present within the membrane of excitable cells such as neurons and muscle. Three Na⁺ molecules and one ATP molecule bind to the channel (step 1). Hydrolysis of ATP drives a conformational change in the channel, causing it to transport Na⁺ across the membrane and out of the cell (step 2). The change also enables two K⁺ molecules to bind to the channel on the outside of the cell membrane (step 3). Removal of inorganic phosphate (Pi) returns the channel to its original shape, in doing so bringing K⁺ across the membrane into the cell and exposing Na⁺ binding sites (step 4). The cycle repeats until resting membrane potential is restored.

membrane potential by actively pumping three Na⁺ ions out of the cell for every two K⁺ ions that move back into the cell (Figure 5.2). A graphical description of action potential propagation is in Figure 5.3.

A lesser known role of K⁺ is in biochemical reactions. Potassium is important in the synthesis of protein, carbohydrate metabolism, and glycogenesis (conversion of glucose to glycogen for storage in the liver and muscles). The roles of K⁺ discussed above highlight the importance of this electrolyte in key processes required for health and function and also for optimal sport and exercise performance.

5.3 Potassium and sport and exercise fatigue

As discussed in Section 5.2, K⁺ plays an important role in conducting the action potential along a motor neuron and muscle fibre. Conduction of this action potential is critical for muscle function, as inadequate electrical stimulation means that insufficient calcium ions (Ca^{2+}) may be released from the sarcoplasmic reticulum (SR), which can prevent the muscle from contracting at its optimum rate and/or force (see Section 2.2.3.2.1). Any interference or breakdown in polarisation (a term for the normal functional processes of depolarisation followed by repolarisation) across a muscle cell membrane could significantly impair cell function. Therefore, alterations in the normal membrane transfer of Na⁺ or K⁺ could contribute to muscle dysfunction and, potentially, fatigue.[2] For example, failure of an action potential can occur due to dysfunction of Na⁺ channels as a result of chronic depolarisation (a continued positive change in cell membrane potential), a reduced Na⁺ concentration gradient (via

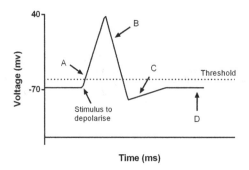

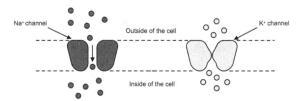

A: Depolarisation

B: Repolarisation and C: Hyperpolarisation

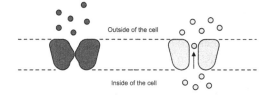

D: Resting potential

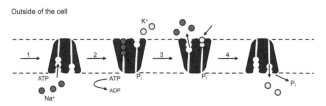

Figure 5.3 A graphical and schematic representation of the depolarisation and repolarisation of a membrane, allowing the propagation of an action potential. The membrane is at a resting potential of −65 to −70 mV. If a depolarising stimulus reaches the required threshold (approximately −50 to −55 mV) then the membrane Na$^+$ channels open and Na$^+$ enters the cell, causing depolarisation (A). At the peak of depolarisation, Na$^+$ channels close and K$^+$ channels open, allowing K$^+$ to leave the muscle, thereby causing repolarisation (B). Potassium channels remain open, causing membrane potential to fall below that of the resting potential (hyperpolarisation, C). Potassium channels then close, and the Na$^+$, K$^+$ pump restores normal resting membrane potential (D).

a decrease in extracellular Na⁺ concentration or an increase in intracellular Na⁺ concentration), or permeability of the cell membrane to K⁺, as an action potential can only progress if the inward Na⁺ current sufficiently exceeds the leak current of K⁺.[2,3]

Dynamic exercise causes a rapid increase in extracellular K⁺ concentration (particularly so in the muscle interstitial space) and a concomitant reduction in intracellular K⁺ concen-

Key point 5.3

Alterations in the membrane transport of K⁺ could interfere with the normal propagation of action potentials, thereby impairing muscle function.

Key point 5.4

Repeated muscle contractions can cause a loss of K⁺ from the muscle cell via the specialised K⁺ transport channels present in the cell membrane.

tration, with this increase greater with more intense/stronger contractions.[1,4] Movement of K⁺ out of the cell likely occurs during action potentials via specific K⁺ transport channels called delayed rectifier K⁺ channels[1,5] and K_{ATP} channels.[6] Haemoconcentration caused by movement of plasma into the interstitial and intracellular compartments also contributes to increased plasma K⁺ concentration.[7] During high-intensity muscle contractions, the capacity of the Na⁺, K⁺ pumps to bring K⁺ back into the muscle may be exceeded,[8] which could also contribute to the net loss of K⁺. Once sport/exercise stops, extracellular K⁺ concentration rapidly falls (half-life ~30 seconds).[9]

A moderate accumulation of K⁺ in the muscle interstitium is actually beneficial to sport and exercise performance as it stimulates muscle blood flow, the exercise pressor reflex, ventilation, and neuromuscular electrical signal transmission (for a summary of the beneficial and detrimental effects of elevated extracellular K⁺ concentration, see Table 5.1).[1] However, the old adage about too much of a good thing applies here. Excessive K⁺ accumulation in the muscle interstitium can impair muscle excitability in two ways. Firstly, increased extracellular K⁺ concentration increases resting K⁺ conductance (movement of charge across the membrane), meaning there is an increase in inhibitory membrane currents.[1,10] Secondly, extracellular K⁺ accumulation can depolarise the membrane potential, slowing the inactivation of voltage-gated Na⁺ channels and consequently reducing the excitatory Na⁺ currents during action potentials.[1,11,12] Together, these processes reduce muscle fibre excitability by tipping the balance between excitatory and inhibitory membrane currents in favour of inhibitory currents.[1] This impact is demonstrated by evidence that exposing muscles to high extracellular K⁺ concentration increases the neural input required to generate an action potential, reduces action potential

Table 5.1 Summary of the beneficial and detrimental effects of extracellular potassium accumulation

Beneficial effects	Detrimental effects
1.Increases muscle blood flow	Increases sensations of pain[a]
Stimulates the exercise pressor reflex	Increases rating of perceived exertion[a]
Increases group III/IV afferent feedback	Increases central fatigue[a]
Increases ventilation	Decreases cardiac muscle contractility
Potentiates neuromuscular transmission	Decreases skeletal muscle force production
Increases skeletal muscle force	
Increases NKA activity	

Source: Adapted from Lindinger and Cairns.[1]

[a] These detrimental effects are likely mediated by stimulation of group III/IV muscle afferents, meaning that afferent neural feedback from extracellular K⁺ accumulation can have positive and/ or negative effects.

amplitude, and can even completely prevent a muscle from being electrically stimulated.[1,10,13–15] Rapid recovery of the action potential and muscle force can be seen when the rate of muscle stimulation (and hence the requirement for action potential propagation) is reduced.[2]

Imbalance in the concentrations of Na^+ and K^+ ions within a muscle cell, in particular K^+ accumulation in the T system (the network of t-tubules that conduct the action potential throughout the fibre so that it can stimulate Ca^{2+} release, see Section 2.2.3.2.1 and Figure 5.4), may prevent the action potential from propagating through the T system, thereby impairing Ca^{2+} release into the muscle.[2] However, despite the suggestion that the largest increases in extracellular K^+ accumulation take place in the T system,[16] there is disagreement as to the role of K^+ accumulation in the T system on Ca^{2+} release, as impairments in Ca^{2+} release may depend on factors including the rate of stimulation and muscle length.[17] All of the potentially negative effects of extracellular

Key point 5.5

Reduced membrane depolarisation, muscle excitation, and force production with muscle K^+ loss have been reported in animals and humans. It appears that the rate of K^+ loss cannot always be compensated for by activity of the Na^+, K^+ pump.

Key point 5.6

Observations of fatigue occurring at the same extracellular K^+ concentration, and high-intensity training reducing the rate of extracellular K^+ accumulation, provide support for a role of extracellular K^+ accumulation in sport and exercise fatigue.

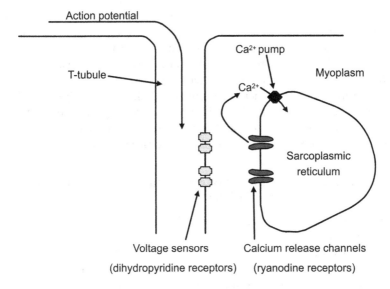

Figure 5.4 The release of Ca^{2+} from the SR. An action potential conducted along the sarcolemma and into the t-tubule stimulates voltage sensors on the t-tubular membrane. These voltage sensors in turn stimulate Ca^{2+} release channels to open, allowing Ca^{2+} to enter the myoplasm. Calcium is sequestered back into the SR via the Ca^{2+} pump.

K^+ accumulation mentioned above can be attributed to inactivation of voltage-gated Na^+ channels in the cell surface and T system membranes.[1,18]

The potential role of extracellular K^+ accu-

Key point 5.7

Extracellular K^+ accumulation may stimulate type III and IV muscle afferents, which could contribute to the development of central fatigue. However, research on this topic is conflicting.

mulation on fatigue is highlighted by observations of reduced time to fatigue when extracellular K^+ accumulation occurs at a faster rate during exercise.[19,20] Fatigue has also been shown to occur at the same extracellular K^+ concentration, despite differences in exercise mode, time to fatigue, and training status[21,22]; however, this has not been consistently found.[19,23] Interestingly, high-intensity training has been shown to reduce the extracellular accumulation of K^+ (likely via increased Na^+, K^+ pump activity) and delay fatigue.[22] This training adaptation may support the suggestion that extracellular K^+ accumulation is involved in fatigue development during sport and exercise.

The influence of extracellular K^+ accumulation on sport and exercise fatigue may not be limited to changes in muscle membrane excitability. Extracellular K^+ accumulation may stimulate group III and IV muscle afferents, which could contribute to the muscle discomfort commonly felt during intense and/

or prolonged exercise (also see Section 3.3.1).[1] Stimulation of these muscle afferents by extracellular K^+ accumulation may also inhibit central motor drive, leading to the development of central fatigue (see Section 6.2.1.1). However, further research is needed to confirm both of these suggestions.

There are also muscle fibre type differences in K^+ dynamics, with fast-twitch fibres releasing more K^+ per action potential than slow-twitch fibres.[24] This fibre type difference indicates that athletes in sports where a higher proportion of fast-twitch fibres is desirable (speed- and power-based sports) may be more affected by performance impairment associated with extracellular K^+ accumulation.

5.4   Modulation of the impact of extracellular K^+ accumulation on sport and exercise fatigue

As discussed in Section 5.3, alterations in K^+ movement across a muscle membrane can reduce muscle cell excitability, and this has been associated with fatigue. As with almost every process in the body, there are associated processes/responses that can attenuate or exacerbate the impact of extracellular K^+ accumulation on fatigue. Some of these will now be discussed.

5.4.1   *Motor unit recruitment*

When a muscle is contracting submaximally, the central nervous system (CNS) is able to vary the specific motor units used to contract the muscle in order to "spread the load" across the different motor units.[2,25,26] Varying the use of motor units to achieve a muscle contraction has the effect of reducing the number of action potentials that a particular muscle fibre has to undergo. As discussed in Section 5.3, K^+ loss from a muscle fibre occurs as a result of the depolarisation of the muscle fibre during an action potential. Reducing the number of action potentials could reduce the amount of K^+ that is lost from that particular muscle fibre, potentially reducing extracellular K^+ accumulation. However, it is unclear what impact that would have on the depressive effect of extracellular K^+ accumulation at the whole muscle level.

5.4.2   *The Na^+, K^+ pump*

The Na^+, K^+ pump is critical for lowering extracellular K^+ concentration, particularly in the T system.[2] When muscle excitability is reduced due to high extracellular K^+ or low extracellular Na^+, stimulation of the Na^+, K^+ pump leads to considerable force recovery.[8,27] Conversely, when the capacity of the Na^+, K^+ pump is reduced, muscle force decline is greater, and force recovery is considerably slower.[8] The Na^+, K^+ pump therefore appears to play a significant role in second-to-second restoration and maintenance of excitability in exercising skeletal muscle across a wider range of extracellular K^+ concentrations than previously thought.[8,28,29] This more involved activity of the Na^+, K^+ pump can provide a degree of resistance to sarcolemmal depolarisation and therefore reduced excitability of muscle during sport and exercise.[1]

5.4.3 Chloride channels

Chloride (Cl⁻) is another negatively charged ion present in skeletal muscle that can significantly influence the potential impact of extracellular K⁺ accumulation on muscle excitability. Recent findings appear to indicate that activity-induced inhibition of CIC-1 chloride channels, one of a family of Cl⁻ selective channels that is almost exclusively present in the outer membrane of skeletal muscles,[30] is one of the most important protective mechanisms against the inhibitory effects of extracellular K⁺ accumulation on muscle excitability.[30] The magnitude of excitatory depolarisation of skeletal muscle caused by the influx of Na⁺ is reduced, or controlled, by outward inhibitory currents carried by K⁺ and Cl⁻, with the degree of excitability a muscle experiences dependent on the balance between these excitatory and inhibitory currents.[30] We have already discussed how extracellular K⁺ accumulation can reduce skeletal muscle excitability. Research has demonstrated that inhibition of CIC-1 channels in a variety of contexts reduces the flow of inhibitory current and helps to restore balance between excitatory and inhibitory currents, thereby restoring excitability and function in contracting muscles with elevated extracellular K⁺ concentrations.[31] Interestingly, lactate appears to be the only compound that can directly inhibit CIC-1 channels under normal physiological conditions and in vivo research.[30,31] This is beneficial for the protective role of CIC-1 inhibition on muscle excitability, as both extracellular K⁺ accumulation and lactate concentration increase with more intense muscle contractions.

There appears to be a "threshold" of benefit regarding inhibition of Cl⁻ conductance. Reductions in Cl⁻ conductance of up to 80% show beneficial effects on muscle excitability, but reductions > 90% lead to impaired muscle function.[32,33] The reasons for this threshold may be that reductions in Cl⁻ conductance > 90% (a) contribute to a loss of resting membrane potential stability, leading to greater loss of excitatory current due to slow inactivation of Na⁺ channels,[1,34] and (b) reduce efficiency of the stabilising effect of Cl⁻ on membrane potential, which leads to an increased accumulation of extracellular K⁺.[1,35] Fortunately, it appears that inhibition of Cl⁻ conductance in exercising muscles does not exceed 80%, meaning that inhibition of Cl⁻ conductance will improve muscle excitability.[35] In summary, regulation of Cl⁻ conductance via CIC-1 channels is regarded as a crucial mechanism in the prevention of extracellular K⁺-induced fatigue.[1] Figure 5.5 summarises the balance between the inhibitory effects of extracellular K⁺ and the counteractive influence of inhibited Cl⁻ conductance on muscle fibre excitability.

5.4.4 Metabolic acidosis

Early work, some of which used animal models, suggested that reduced muscle pH may increase the activity of pH-sensitive K⁺ channels within the muscle membrane, leading to a greater loss of K⁺ from muscle.[36,37] This would imply that any role of extracellular K⁺ accumulation on muscle fatigue would be exacerbated

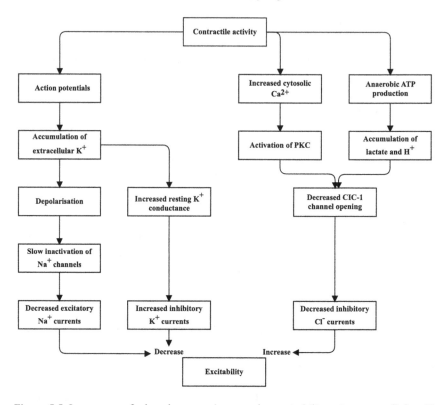

Figure 5.5 Summary of the decrease in muscle excitability via extracellular K⁺ accumulation and the increase in muscle excitability via inhibition of Cl⁻ conductance. The balance between the depressive effects of extracellular K⁺ accumulation and the stimulating effects of inhibition of Cl⁻ conductance is a significant determinant of the extent of muscle excitability during sport and exercise. Re-drawn from Nielsen O, de Paoli FV, Riisager A, Pedersen TH. *Physiology (Bethesda).* 2017;32:425–434.

during high-intensity exercise, where reduced muscle pH is more likely. Several studies have shown an association between reductions in exercising muscle pH and increased K⁺ loss from the muscle.[19,23,36,37] However, this relationship has been questioned by another work

Key point 5.8

The body has many mechanisms that work to prevent losses in muscle excitability. Therefore, these mechanisms can also work to reduce the influence of extracellular K⁺ accumulation on muscle excitability. One of the most crucial "defenders" of muscle excitability is the regulation of chloride conductance.

that appears to show a protective effect of reduced muscle pH on force production in muscles that have lost notable amounts of K⁺.[10,15,38–40]

Increased muscle acidosis can reduce Cl⁻ conductance across the muscle membrane, shifting the balance between inhibitory Cl⁻ currents and excitatory Na⁺ currents in favour of the excitatory current. This shift could potentially counteract the depressive effect of increased extracellular K⁺ levels on membrane excitability (Section 5.4.3). Despite conflicting findings in the literature, the current view is that acidosis may convey some protection for skeletal muscle against the negative effects of elevated K⁺ losses, primarily via inhibition of ClC-1 channels.[1] Interestingly, however, the effects are the opposite for cardiac muscle, where K⁺ loss combined with acidosis is highly detrimental.[1]

5.4.5 External interventions

The above summarises endogenous factors that can modulate the impact of extracellular K⁺ accumulation on sport and exercise fatigue. However, there are also interventions that can be administered which aim to protect against the potentially damaging effects of extracellular K⁺ accumulation on skeletal muscle and cardiac function. These interventions have a more clinical focus, hence why they are not discussed here. However, the interested reader is referred to Lindinger and Cairns[1] for more information.

> **Key point 5.9**
>
> *Acidosis may convey some protection for skeletal muscle against the negative effects of elevated K⁺ losses, primarily via inhibition of ClC-1 channels.*

5.5 Calcium: description and function

Calcium is the most abundant mineral in the body. Milk, yoghurt, and cheese are rich sources of dietary Ca, along with kale, broccoli, sardines, and salmon. Ninety-nine per cent of body Ca stores are located in the skeleton, about 1% is located in intracellular fluid, and about 0.1% in extracellular fluid. The cationic form of calcium (Ca^{2+}) is, like K⁺, an electrolyte that carries a small positive electrical charge.

> **Key point 5.10**
>
> *Calcium is the most abundant mineral in the body. Dietary sources of Ca include milk, yoghurt, cheese, kale, broccoli, sardines, and salmon.*

Calcium plays important roles in a number of physiological and biochemical processes:

- Acting as a second messenger in signal transduction pathways. Signal transduction is a cascade of processes beginning with an extracellular signaller (a hormone or neurotransmitter) interacting with a receptor on a cell surface, which causes a change in the action of an intracellular messenger which in turn alters the function of the cell. For example, the extracellular signal generated by neurotransmission of an action potential into a muscle fibre stimulates the release of Ca^{2+} into the myoplasm where it can then enable the process of muscle contraction to occur.

- Neurotransmitter release from neurons. Neuronal synapses contain Ca^{2+} channels that open when depolarised, allowing Ca^{2+} to flow through the presynaptic membrane and increase internal Ca^{2+} concentration. This activates Ca^{2+}-sensitive proteins attached to vesicles which contain a neurotransmitter. The proteins change shape, allowing the vesicles to open and transfer their neurotransmitter across the synaptic cleft (the narrow space between the pre- and postsynaptic cells).
- A cofactor (a non-protein molecule that assists in biochemical reactions) for enzymes such as those of the blood clotting cascade.
- Cell membrane excitability, particularly in the heart and neurons.

> **Key point 5.11**
>
> *Calcium plays important roles in signal transduction cascades, neurotransmitter release, as a cofactor for enzyme function, in cell membrane excitability, bone formation and density, endothelial tissue vasodilation, and muscle contraction.*

- Bone formation and maintenance of bone mineral density.
- Vasodilation of endothelial tissue (the thin layer of cells coating the inside of blood and lymph vessels).

5.6   Calcium and sport and exercise fatigue

Release of appropriate amounts of Ca^{2+} from its storage site within muscle, the SR, is critical for muscle contraction and appropriate force development (Figure 5.4). If the amount of Ca^{2+} in the SR drops substantially below its normal level, the amount of Ca^{2+} released in each action potential is reduced and muscle force production drops.[41,42] Reduced muscle force will still occur even if the amount of Ca^{2+} in the SR drops but is still sufficient to fully saturate binding sites on troponin C,[41] and increasing SR Ca^{2+} content above that normally found does not increase the amount of Ca^{2+} release during an action potential.[42] Therefore, impairments in SR Ca^{2+} kinetics (the

> **Key point 5.12**
>
> *Release of appropriate amounts of $Ca2^+$ from the SR is crucial for muscle force production. If insufficient $Ca2^+$ is released, muscle force will decline.*

coordinated move-
ment of Ca^{2+} into and
out of the SR and the
myoplasm) can reduce
muscle force and may
contribute to fatigue
development. The ob-
vious question is: what
can cause impaired SR Ca^{2+} kinetics?

> **Key point 5.13**
>
> *Alterations in $Ca2^+$ kinetics can reduce muscle force and may contribute to fatigue development.*

5.6.1 Impaired Ca²⁺ kinetics due to glycogen depletion and acidosis

Chapter 2 discussed how the link between muscle glycogen depletion and muscle force reduction is not fully understood. However, studies have established
an apparent association between muscle glycogen depletion and impaired Ca^{2+}
kinetics.[43-47] Calcium kinetics regulates the amount of free Ca^{2+} that is present
in the myoplasm and is therefore crucial for optimal muscle force production.
Regulation of Ca^{2+} kinetics is controlled by the opening of Ca^{2+} release channels (which control the release of Ca^{2+} from the SR), and by the activity of the
SR Ca^{2+} pump (similar to the Na^+, K^+ pump discussed in Section 5.2) which
moves Ca^{2+} back into the SR (Figure 5.4). Impaired Ca^{2+} release from the SR
could contribute to fatigue by reducing the amount of Ca^{2+} that is available
to bind to troponin C, thereby impairing the excitation-contraction coupling
process, and reduced Ca^{2+} uptake into the SR can slow the rate of relaxation of
a muscle and indirectly cause reduced force production.

There is limited research into the influence of sport and exercise on SR responses in humans. However, existing studies have identified that prolonged
sport/exercise can cause disturbances in Ca^{2+} uptake and release.[44,45,48,49] Interestingly, Ca^{2+} release is impaired in a low-glycogen state, with depletion
of intermyofibrillar and intramyofibrillar glycogen linked to reduced SR Ca^{2+}
release,[50] but this impairment is delayed when sufficient carbohydrate is consumed to modify muscle glycogen stores.[44] There appears to be a critical muscle glycogen threshold of ~250–300 mmol.kg⁻¹ below which SR Ca^{2+} release
rate is impaired.[51]

Despite increasing knowledge of the link between muscle glycogen content
and impaired Ca^{2+} kinetics, the specific mechanisms behind this association are
still under debate.[51] It is plausible that muscles contracting with depleted glycogen stores experience a reduced ability to regenerate adenosine triphosphate
(ATP), leading to ATP depletion in specific areas of the cell that could affect both
SR Ca^{2+} release and uptake (this was also touched upon in Section 2.2.3.2.1).[52,53]
There is also some evidence to suggest the presence of a "complex" of enzymes
associated with glycogen synthesis and breakdown in close association with
the SR.[45,54,55] Depletion of glycogen stores could impair the function of this
enzyme complex, which in turn could impact on energy availability in important areas of the SR (for example, the Ca^{2+} pump and Ca^{2+} release channels).

Therefore, glycogen could impair Ca^{2+} kinetics due to its role as an energy source.

Interestingly, there is some evidence to suggest that the influence of glycogen content on Ca^{2+} kinetics is *not* related to its role as a fuel source. Some studies have shown that the ability of a muscle to respond to depolarisations of the t-tubular system is dependent on muscle glycogen concentration

> **Key point 5.14**
>
> *Calcium release from the SR is delayed in a low muscle glycogen state, which may be related to localised ATP depletion. However, impaired Ca^{2+} kinetics are seen in a low-glycogen state despite the availability of other fuel sources, suggesting the role of glycogen in impaired Ca^{2+} handling may not be related to its role as a fuel source.*

even when other sources of fuel are available, such as ATP and phosphocreatine (PCr). It may be that glycogen depletion locally to the SR could cause structural changes in the SR itself, which may impair SR function.[45,47] Whatever the specific mechanism(s), it does appear that adequate muscle glycogen is important for optimal SR Ca^{2+} kinetics. This further reinforces the potential importance of glycogen in the fatigue process (Chapter 2).

The role of acidosis in SR Ca^{2+} release and binding to troponin C was discussed in Section 3.3.3.1, and the reader is referred to this section. To briefly summarise, it appears that acidosis does not impair

> **Key point 5.15**
>
> *Under normal physiological conditions, acidosis causes little inhibitory effects on Ca^{2+} release from the SR.*

the normal process of Ca^{2+} release from the SR.[56] However, acidosis may negatively influence the interactions between Ca^{2+} and the myofilaments, but this mechanism and its role in fatigue is still being debated.[56,57]

5.6.2　Inorganic phosphate

When energy demand for muscle contraction is high, ATP concentration will remain constant for a very short time but PCr will be broken down to creatine and inorganic phosphate (Pi).[2] As a

> **Key point 5.16**
>
> *Accumulation of Pi can prevent actin-myosin cross-bridges from entering a high-force state, thereby reducing muscle force. This occurs early in the fatigue process, at least in type II fibres.*

result, Pi can accumulate within the muscle (Pi is also produced by the hydrolysis of ATP, as summarised in Equation 2.1). Inorganic phosphate plays very important roles in a number of biochemical and biological processes, including energy metabolism. However, accumulation of Pi outside of normal physiological concentrations can be a problem.

Elevated Pi concentration can directly impair muscle force by inhibiting the ability of the contractile proteins actin and myosin to enter a high-force state.[2] The reduction in muscle force attributed to Pi-induced interference with cross-bridging occurs early on in the fatigue process, at least in type II muscle fibres.

Although the direct influence of Pi on actin-myosin cross-bridging may be comparatively minor, any changes in cross-bridge function can also influence the relationship between intracellular Ca^{2+} concentration and muscle force.[2] Specifically, increased Pi concentration may reduce the contractile response (and hence force production) of the muscle fibre to a given Ca^{2+} concentration.[58-60] This is termed a reduction in Ca^{2+} sensitivity.[58] Interestingly, the reduction in Ca^{2+} sensitivity due to Pi accumulation appears to be greater as muscle temperature gets nearer to normal physiological temperature. This is the opposite response to the inhibition of cross-bridge force by Pi, which decreases as the temperature rises. Therefore, impaired Ca^{2+} sensitivity due to Pi accumulation may play a much more important role than cross-bridge inhibition in muscle fatigue, particularly in the later stages of fatigue when intracellular Ca^{2+} concentration decreases (discussed below).[2]

Continuation of the fatigue process is associated with reduced myoplasmic Ca^{2+}

Key point 5.17

Accumulation of Pi can reduce Ca^{2+} sensitivity (the amount of force produced for a given myoplasmic Ca^{2+} concentration). Therefore, reduced Ca^{2+} sensitivity may be important in the later stages of fatigue when myoplasmic Ca^{2+} concentration decreases.

Key point 5.18

The later stages of the fatigue process are associated with reduced myoplasmic Ca^{2+} concentration. Along with reduced Ca^{2+} sensitivity, this is thought to account largely for the rapid reduction in muscle force that usually precedes exercise termination.

Key point 5.19

Two main ways in which reduced SR Ca^{2+} release may occur are inhibition of the SR Ca^{2+} release channels by Pi, and Ca^{2+} and Pi precipitation in the SR.

concentration which, along with reduced Ca^{2+} sensitivity, is thought to significantly account for the rapid reduction in muscle force that usually precedes exercise termination.[2] Reduced myoplasmic Ca^{2+} concentration suggests that the amount of Ca^{2+} being released from the SR is also reduced. There are two main ways in which Pi-induced reductions in SR Ca^{2+} release may occur: (1) inhibition of the SR Ca^{2+} release channels by Pi and (2) Ca^{2+} and Pi precipitation in the SR.

As summarised in Section 5.6.1 and Figure 5.4, Ca^{2+} leaves the SR via specialised release channels. In the early stages of muscle fatigue, Pi appears to act on the SR Ca^{2+} release channel in such a way that myoplasmic Ca^{2+} concentration increases. However, in the later stages of fatigue, this is reversed, and Pi accumulation contributes to a reduction in myoplasmic Ca^{2+} concentration, probably by affecting the sarcoplasmic Ca^{2+} release mechanism.[2,61] The inhibition of SR Ca^{2+} release by Pi depends on changes in myoplasmic magnesium (Mg^{2+}) concentration (Section 5.6.3), with the inhibitory effect of Pi larger at greater Mg^{2+} concentrations.[62] Magnesium also binds to many of the same intramuscular sites as Ca^{2+}, and it is this competitive binding that allows Mg^{2+} to exert many of its inhibitory effects.

A second way by which Pi may reduce SR Ca^{2+} release is via Ca^{2+}-Pi precipitation in the SR. When Pi accumulates in the myoplasm, some Pi may enter the SR and combine with free Ca^{2+} to form a Ca^{2+}-Pi solid (termed a precipitate). This has the effect of reducing the concentration of free Ca^{2+} in the SR and therefore the amount of Ca^{2+} that is able to be released into the myoplasm with each action potential.

Key point 5.20

In the early stages of fatigue, Pi appears to act on the SR release channel in a way that increases myoplasmic Ca^{2+} concentration. In the later stages of fatigue, this is reversed, and Pi contributes to reduced myoplasmic Ca^{2+} concentration, perhaps by affecting SR Ca^{2+} release.

Key point 5.21

Inhibition of SR Ca^{2+} release by Pi is greater when myoplasmic Mg^{2+} concentration is higher.

Key point 5.22

Accumulation of Pi may cause it to enter the SR and combine with Ca^{2+} to form a Ca^{2+}-Pi precipitate. This would reduce the amount of free Ca^{2+} in the SR, and therefore the amount that is able to be released into the myoplasm.

The existence of a phosphate permeable channel in the SR was discovered in 2001,[63] providing further support for the theory of Ca^{2+}-Pi precipitation in the SR. Subsequent work provided indirect evidence to suggest that precipitation does occur. In vitro studies showed reduced resting myoplasmic Ca^{2+} concentration and faster Ca^{2+} reuptake into the SR following injections of Pi, which points to a reduced SR Ca^{2+} concentration.[64,65] Furthermore, substances that stimulate SR Ca^{2+} release, such as caffeine, stimulated less Ca^{2+} release in fatigued muscle, which is suggestive of a reduced SR Ca^{2+} availability.[66] SR Ca^{2+} concentration was also shown to decrease during fatiguing contractions stimulated by agents such as caffeine or via t-tubular action potentials, with Ca^{2+} leakage/loss from the muscle cells unable to account for this reduction.[67] Finally, the theory of Ca^{2+}-Pi precipitation was strengthened by the fact that reduced myoplasmic Ca^{2+} concentration (suggestive of reduced SR Ca^{2+} concentration/release) was lessened or delayed in mice that did not have the enzyme creatine kinase.[68] This means that the mice are unable to effectively break down PCr, reducing the normal fatigue-induced increase in Pi concentration.

While these studies furthered our understanding of the potential role of Ca^{2+}-Pi precipitation, none of them provided direct evidence for Pi entry into the SR or subsequent precipitation. However, such evidence has now been published. Ferreira et al.[69] provided data demonstrating that Pi does indeed enter the SR of muscle cells (note: this study used an animal model), and this entry is associated with reduced SR Ca^{2+} concentration, indicative of Ca^{2+}-Pi precipitation. The authors were also able to indicate that the method of entry of Pi into the SR appears to be via a Cl– channel, as when this Cl– channel was blocked, the negative impact of Pi on SR Ca^{2+} concentration was not seen. Furthermore, Ferreira et al.[69] provided further evidence that Pi impairs Ca^{2+} kinetics not just by forming a Ca^{2+}-Pi precipitate but also by a direct inhibitory effect on SR Ca^{2+} release channels. Further work by Hureau et al.[70] reinforced the mechanisms evidenced by Ferreira et al.[69] and designed a study that allowed them to separate the effects of H^+ and Pi on fatigue

Key point 5.23

Data has now been published which demonstrates that (1) during sport and exercise, Pi does enter the SR and form a Ca^{2+}-Pi precipitate, and (2) Pi impairs Ca^{2+} kinetics by also exerting a direct inhibitory effect on SR Ca^{2+} release channels.

Key point 5.24

Current evidence suggests that Pi should be considered the primary cause of peripheral fatigue during sport and exercise.

processes. The authors concluded that Pi, via the mechanisms discussed above, should be considered the primary cause of peripheral fatigue during sport and exercise. While further work needs to be done

> **Key point 5.25**
>
> *There is little direct influence of ATP depletion (unless to very low levels) or Mg^{2+} accumulation on the contractile apparatus in muscle. However, high Mg^{2+} levels reduce Ca^{2+} sensitivity.*

to confirm and extend these findings, this is a significant statement within the context of sport and exercise fatigue.

5.6.3   ATP depletion and magnesium accumulation

During intense sport and exercise, ATP concentration may fall (particularly in localised areas), and PCr concentration can be significantly reduced. Adenosine diphosphate (ADP) and Mg^{2+} concentrations can also increase (Mg^{2+} is bound to ATP, and the hydrolysis of ATP releases Mg^{2+} as a byproduct because ADP, adenosine monophosphate (AMP), and inosine monophosphate (IMP), which all can be

> **Key point 5.26**
>
> *ATP depletion at the site of the SR Ca^{2+} pumps can reduce Ca^{2+} reuptake into the SR. Accumulation of ADP also reduces the Ca^{2+} pump rate. Raised Mg^{2+} concentration has little effect on the rate of SR Ca^{2+} uptake.*

produced via ATP hydrolysis, have a lower affinity for Mg^{2+} than does ATP).[1] There is little direct influence of ATP depletion (unless to very low levels) on the contractile apparatus, but reduced ATP concentration and elevated Mg^{2+} can impair SR Ca^{2+} release, and elevated Mg^{2+} can also reduce Ca^{2+} sensitivity.[2,71] There also appears to be an augmentative effect of ATP reduction and Mg^{2+} accumulation on SR Ca^{2+} release.[71]

SR Ca^{2+} pumps play a crucial role in Ca^{2+} kinetics, as they transport Ca^{2+} back into the SR to ensure an appropriate rate of muscle relaxation following contraction (Figure 5.4). If ATP concentration at the sites of the SR pumps is reduced (SR pump activity is ATP dependent) then Ca^{2+} reuptake into the SR is also reduced. Simply put, less Ca^{2+} is pumped into the SR for a given amount of ATP hydrolysis, meaning the process

> **Key point 5.27**
>
> *ATP depletion and Mg^{2+} accumulation both inhibit Ca^{2+} release from the SR, and this reduction is greater when ATP depletion and Mg^{2+} accumulation occur together.*

has become less energy efficient.[2] Increased ADP concentration (which is, of course, associated with greater ATP depletion) also reduces SR Ca^{2+} pump rate and increases leakage of Ca^{2+} back through the pumps into the myoplasm.[2,72] However, this issue appears to be prevalent only in type II muscle fibres.[73] As for the role of Mg^{2+} in SR Ca^{2+} pump activity, raised Mg^{2+} concentration seems to have little to no effect on the rate of SR Ca^{2+} uptake.[74]

The SR Ca^{2+} release channels (Figure 5.4) are stimulated by ATP in a similar way to the SR Ca^{2+} pump. When ATP concentration falls, voltage-sensor-stimulated Ca^{2+} release from the SR is reduced.[2] The presence of Mg^{2+} is a strong inhibitor of SR Ca^{2+} release channels[75] and has been shown to reduce SR Ca^{2+} release by up to 40%.[76] When localised ATP depletion and Mg^{2+} accumulation occur at the same time, the reduction in Ca^{2+} release is even greater.[2] As a result, reduced ATP concentration and increased Mg^{2+} concentration are probably at least partly responsible for the reduced myoplasmic Ca^{2+} concentration that is observed during high-intensity muscle contraction.[2,77] This reduction in myoplasmic Ca^{2+} content may be a protective response from the muscle in the face of reduced ATP concentration. Reduced SR Ca^{2+} release would reduce the amount of Ca^{2+} available to take part in the cross-bridge process and the amount that would be needed to be pumped back into the SR. Both these processes require ATP, so by reducing their activity, the cell is conserving remaining ATP stores, albeit at the expense of muscle force.[2]

5.7 Summary

- Potassium is one of the most common chemical elements in the body and plays important roles in processes such as cellular water balance, many biochemical reactions, and changing of the electrical potential across cell membranes that allows the propagation of action potentials.
- Appropriate action potential propagation is crucial for muscle function, and disturbances could lead to impaired function.
- Repeated muscle contractions cause a net loss of K^+ from the muscle and K^+ accumulation in the extracellular space. This K^+ loss occurs mainly through specialised K^+ channels in the muscle membrane.
- Accumulation of extracellular K^+ has been associated with reduced muscle excitation and force production, perhaps due to the altered electrochemical gradient and reduced membrane depolarisation associated with extracellular K^+ accumulation.
- Recovery of the action potential and muscle force occurs when the rate of muscle stimulation is reduced, which suggests that reduced muscle force is due to reduced muscle cell excitation caused by membrane depolarisation. It also suggests that the influence of extracellular K^+ accumulation is dependent in part on exercise intensity.
- Reduced time to fatigue, and the occurrence of fatigue at the same extracellular K^+ concentration, provides further support for the role of extracellular K^+ accumulation in the fatigue process.

- The body has many mechanisms that work in concert to prevent or minimise losses in membrane excitability, such as alterations to motor unit recruitment, motor neuron firing rate, action potential firing rate, activation of the Na^+, K^+ pump, and the importance of $Cl-$ on the membrane potential and movement of K^+ across the muscle membrane.
- Potassium accumulation may contribute to muscle soreness and discomfort, and the development of central fatigue, via stimulation of type III and IV muscle afferents.
- Calcium is the most abundant mineral in the body and plays important roles in signal transduction, neurotransmitter release, enzyme function, membrane excitability, bone formation and density, endothelial tissue vasodilation, and muscle contraction.
- The release of appropriate amounts of Ca^{2+} into the SR and the adequate reuptake of Ca^{2+} back into the SR is crucial for optimal muscle function.
- If the amount of Ca^{2+} in the SR drops substantially, less Ca^{2+} is released from the SR with each action potential, and muscle force declines.
- Muscle glycogen appears to have a regulatory role in Ca^{2+} release and/or reuptake. This role could relate to glycogen as a source of ATP resynthesis (i.e. a fuel source), or it may be independent of this and instead be due to structural changes in the SR caused by low muscle glycogen content.
- Under normal physiological conditions, acidosis does not appear to impair SR Ca^{2+} release.
- Accumulation of Pi may directly impair the ability of actin and myosin to enter high-force states, reducing muscle force.
- Inorganic phosphate can also reduce the contractile response to a given amount of Ca^{2+} (Ca^{2+} sensitivity) and reduce the amount of Ca^{2+} released from the SR by inhibiting the activity of SR release channels and by precipitating with Ca^{2+} in the SR.
- Calcium-Pi precipitation and Pi-induced impairments in SR Ca^{2+} release are now supported by experimental evidence.
- Inorganic phosphate should be considered a primary cause of peripheral fatigue during sport and exercise.
- Depletion of ATP and accumulation of Mg^{2+} can, individually and in combination, reduce Ca^{2+} release from and reuptake into the SR, although Mg^{2+} does not appear to have much influence on the rate of SR Ca^{2+} uptake.

To think about...

As we develop the ability to study the function of the body in ever more detail, the importance of the complex interplay between so many organ systems, metabolic pathways, hormones, compounds, molecules, and elements and how this influences function and performance becomes more pronounced. Clearly, this benefits our understanding of human exercise physiology. However, it may also open new avenues of human function that could be unfairly exploited in order to gain a competitive advantage in sport.

What are your thoughts on this? What benefits do you see in studying the molecular control of sport and exercise performance? And what are the risks/negatives? Do you think that the benefits outweigh the risks?

Test yourself

Answer the following questions to the best of your ability. Try to understand the information gained from answering these questions before you progress with the book.

1 What are the primary dietary sources of K?
2 What are the main roles that K^+ plays in body function?
3 Describe the process of action potential propagation, with reference to the movement of Na^+ and K^+ across the neuron and muscle membranes.
4 How might the accumulation of extracellular K^+ contribute to muscle dysfunction?
5 List and briefly describe the five mechanisms that can help to minimise the influence of extracellular K^+ accumulation on muscle membrane depolarisation.
6 What are the primary dietary sources of Ca?
7 What are the main roles that Ca plays in body function?
8 What is meant by the term Ca^{2+} kinetics?
9 What are the two ways in which reduced muscle glycogen is thought to impair Ca^{2+} kinetics?
10 List the four ways in which Pi accumulation may impair Ca^{2+} kinetics.
11 What is the main impact of ATP depletion and Mg^{2+} accumulation, alone and in combination, on SR Ca^{2+} release and reuptake?

References

1 Lindinger MI, Cairns SP. Regulation of muscle potassium: exercise performance, fatigue and health implications. *Eur J Appl Physiol.* 2021;121(3):721–748.
2 Allen DG, Lamb GD, Westerblad H. Skeletal muscle fatigue: cellular mechanisms. *Physiol Rev.* 2008;88(1):287–332.
3 Stephenson DG. Tubular system excitability: an essential component of excitation-contraction coupling in fast-twitch fibres of vertebrate skeletal muscle. *J Muscle Res Cell Motil.* 2006;27(5–7):259–274.
4 Gunnarsson TP, Christensen PM, Thomassen M, Nielsen LR, Bangsbo J. Effect of intensified training on muscle ion kinetics, fatigue development, and repeated short-term performance in endurance-trained cyclists. *Am J Physiol Regul Integr Comp Physiol.* 2013;305(7):R811–R821.

5   DiFranco M, Quinonez M, Vergara JL. The delayed rectifier potassium conductance in the sarcolemma and the transverse tubular system membranes of mammalian skeletal muscle fibers. *J Gen Physiol.* 2012;140(2):109–137.

6   Pedersen TH, de Paoli FV, Flatman JA, Nielsen OB. Regulation of ClC-1 and KATP channels in action potential-firing fast-twitch muscle fibers. *J Gen Physiol.* 2009;134(4):309–322.

7   Atanasovska T, Smith R, Graff C, et al. Protection against severe hypokalemia but impaired cardiac repolarization after intense rowing exercise in healthy humans receiving salbutamol. *J Appl Physiol (1985).* 2018;125(2):624–633.

8   Clausen T, Nielsen OB, Harrison AP, Flatman JA, Overgaard K. The Na+,K+ pump and muscle excitability. *Acta Physiol Scand.* 1998;162(3):183–190.

9   Vollestad NK, Hallen J, Sejersted OM. Effect of exercise intensity on potassium balance in muscle and blood of man. *J Physiol.* 1994;475(2):359–368.

10 Pedersen TH, de Paoli F, Nielsen OB. Increased excitability of acidified skeletal muscle: role of chloride conductance. *J Gen Physiol.* 2005;125(2):237–246.

11 Ruff RL, Simoncini L, Stuhmer W. Slow sodium channel inactivation in mammalian muscle: a possible role in regulating excitability. *Muscle Nerve.* 1988;11(5): 502–510.

12 Ruff RL. Sodium channel slow inactivation and the distribution of sodium channels on skeletal muscle fibres enable the performance properties of different skeletal muscle fibre types. *Acta Physiol Scand.* 1996;156(3):159–168.

13 Overgaard K, Nielsen OB. Activity-induced recovery of excitability in K(+)-depressed rat soleus muscle. *Am J Physiol Regul Integr Comp Physiol.* 2001;280(1):R48–R55.

14 Nielsen OB, Ortenblad N, Lamb GD, Stephenson DG. Excitability of the T-tubular system in rat skeletal muscle: roles of K+ and Na+ gradients and Na+-K+ pump activity. *J Physiol.* 2004;557(Pt 1):133–146.

15 Pedersen TH, Nielsen OB, Lamb GD, Stephenson DG. Intracellular acidosis enhances the excitability of working muscle. *Science.* 2004;305(5687):1144–1147.

16 Clausen T. Na+-K+ pump regulation and skeletal muscle contractility. *Physiol Rev.* 2003;83(4):1269–1324.

17 Cairns SP, Dulhunty AF. High-frequency fatigue in rat skeletal muscle: role of extracellular ion concentrations. *Muscle Nerve.* 1995;18(8):890–898.

18 Rich MM, Pinter MJ. Crucial role of sodium channel fast inactivation in muscle fibre inexcitability in a rat model of critical illness myopathy. *J Physiol.* 2003;547(Pt 2):555–566.

19 Nordsborg N, Mohr M, Pedersen LD, Nielsen JJ, Langberg H, Bangsbo J. Muscle interstitial potassium kinetics during intense exhaustive exercise: effect of previous arm exercise. *Am J Physiol Regul Integr Comp Physiol.* 2003;285(1): R143–R148.

20 Bangsbo J, Madsen K, Kiens B, Richter EA. Effect of muscle acidity on muscle metabolism and fatigue during intense exercise in man. *J Physiol.* 1996;495(Pt 2):587–596.

21 Bangsbo J, Graham T, Johansen L, Strange S, Christensen C, Saltin B. Elevated muscle acidity and energy production during exhaustive exercise in humans. *Am J Physiol.* 1992;263(4 Pt 2):R891–R899.

22 Nielsen JJ, Mohr M, Klarskov C, et al. Effects of high-intensity intermittent training on potassium kinetics and performance in human skeletal muscle. *J Physiol.* 2004;554(Pt 3):857–870.

23 Mohr M, Nordsborg N, Nielsen JJ, et al. Potassium kinetics in human muscle interstitium during repeated intense exercise in relation to fatigue. *Pflugers Arch.* 2004;448(4):452–456.

24 Clausen T, Overgaard K, Nilsen OB. Evidence that the Na^+-K^+ leak/pump ratio contributes to the difference in endurance between fast- and slow-twitch muscles. *Acta Physiol Scand.* 2004;180:209–216.

25 Enoka RM, Stuart DG. Neurobiology of muscle fatigue. *J Appl Physiol (1985).* 1992;72(5):1631–1648.

26 Murrant CL, Fletcher NM, Fitzpatrick EJH, Gee KS. Do skeletal muscle motor units and microvascular units align to help match blood flow to metabolic demand? *Eur J Appl Physiol.* 2021;121(5):1241–1254.

27 Nielsen OB, Clausen T. The Na+/K(+)-pump protects muscle excitability and contractility during exercise. *Exerc Sport Sci Rev.* 2000;28(4):159–164.

28 Clausen T. In isolated skeletal muscle, excitation may increase extracellular K+ 10-fold; how can contractility be maintained? *Exp Physiol.* 2011;96(3):356–368.

29 Hakimjavadi H, Stiner CA, Radzyukevich TL, et al. K^+ and Rb^+ affinities of the Na,K-ATPase alpha(1) and alpha(2) isozymes: an application of ICP-MS for quantification of Na(+) pump kinetics in myofibers. *Int J Mol Sci.* 2018;19(9):1–18.

30 Nielsen O, de Paoli FV, Riisager A, Pedersen TH. Chloride channels take center stage in acute regulation of excitability in skeletal muscle: implications for fatigue. *Physiology (Bethesda).* 2017;32(6):425–434.

31 de Paoli FV, Ortenblad N, Pedersen TH, Jorgensen R, Nielsen OB. Lactate per se improves the excitability of depolarized rat skeletal muscle by reducing the Cl– conductance. *J Physiol.* 2010;588(Pt 23):4785–4794.

32 Cairns SP, Ruzhynsky V, Renaud JM. Protective role of extracellular chloride in fatigue of isolated mammalian skeletal muscle. *Am J Physiol Cell Physiol.* 2004;287(3):C762–C770.

33 Dutka TL, Murphy RM, Stephenson DG, Lamb GD. Chloride conductance in the transverse tubular system of rat skeletal muscle fibres: importance in excitation-contraction coupling and fatigue. *J Physiol.* 2008;586(3):875–887.

34 Cairns SP, Lindinger MI. Do multiple ionic interactions contribute to skeletal muscle fatigue? *J Physiol.* 2008;586(17):4039–4054.

35 de Paoli FV, Broch-Lips M, Pedersen TH, Nielsen OB. Relationship between membrane Cl– conductance and contractile endurance in isolated rat muscles. *J Physiol.* 2013;591:531–545.

36 Davies NW, Standen NB, Stanfield PR. The effect of intracellular pH on ATP-dependent potassium channels of frog skeletal muscle. *J Physiol.* 1992;445:549–568.

37 Davis NW, Standen NB, Stanfield PR. ATP-dependent potassium channels of muscle cells: their properties, regulation, and possible functions. *J Bioenerg Biomembr.* 1991;23(4):509–535.

38 Hansen AK, Clausen T, Nielsen OB. Effects of lactic acid and catecholamines on contractility in fast-twitch muscles exposed to hyperkalemia. *Am J Physiol Cell Physiol.* 2005;289(1):C104–C112.

39 Kristensen M, Albertsen J, Rentsch M, Juel C. Lactate and force production in skeletal muscle. *J Physiol.* 2005;562(Pt 2):521–526.

40 Overgaard K, Hojfeldt GW, Nielsen OB. Effects of acidification and increased extracellular potassium on dynamic muscle contractions in isolated rat muscles. *J Physiol.* 2010;588(Pt 24):5065–5076.

41 Dutka TL, Cole L, Lamb GD. Calcium phosphate precipitation in the sarcoplasmic reticulum reduces action potential-mediated Ca2+ release in mammalian skeletal muscle. *Am J Physiol Cell Physiol*. 2005;289(6):C1502–C1512.

42 Posterino GS, Lamb GD. Effect of sarcoplasmic reticulum Ca2+ content on action potential-induced Ca2+ release in rat skeletal muscle fibres. *J Physiol*. 2003;551 (Pt 1):219–237.

43 Chin ER, Allen DG. Effects of reduced muscle glycogen concentration on force, Ca2+ release and contractile protein function in intact mouse skeletal muscle. *J Physiol*. 1997;498(Pt 1):17–29.

44 Duhamel TA, Perco JG, Green HJ. Manipulation of dietary carbohydrates after prolonged effort modifies muscle sarcoplasmic reticulum responses in exercising males. *Am J Physiol Regul Integr Comp Physiol*. 2006;291(4):R1100–R1110.

45 Duhamel TA, Green HJ, Stewart RD, Foley KP, Smith IC, Ouyang J. Muscle metabolic, SR Ca(2+) -cycling responses to prolonged cycling, with and without glucose supplementation. *J Appl Physiol (1985)*. 2007;103(6):1986–1998.

46 Helander I, Westerblad H, Katz A. Effects of glucose on contractile function, [Ca2+]i, and glycogen in isolated mouse skeletal muscle. *Am J Physiol Cell Physiol*. 2002;282(6):C1306–C1312.

47 Lees SJ, Franks PD, Spangenburg EE, Williams JH. Glycogen and glycogen phosphorylase associated with sarcoplasmic reticulum: effects of fatiguing activity. *J Appl Physiol (1985)*. 2001;91(4):1638–1644.

48 Duhamel TA, Green HJ, Perco JG, Sandiford SD, Ouyang J. Human muscle sarcoplasmic reticulum function during submaximal exercise in normoxia and hypoxia. *J Appl Physiol (1985)*. 2004;97(1):180–187.

49 Duhamel TA, Green HJ, Sandiford SD, Perco JG, Ouyang J. Effects of progressive exercise and hypoxia on human muscle sarcoplasmic reticulum function. *J Appl Physiol (1985)*. 2004;97(1):188–196.

50 Nielsen J, Cheng AJ, Ortenblad N, Westerblad H. Subcellular distribution of glycogen and decreased tetanic Ca2+ in fatigued single intact mouse muscle fibres. *J Physiol*. 2014;592(9):2003–2012.

51 Ortenblad N, Nielsen J, Morton JP, Areta JL. Exercise and muscle glycogen metabolism. In: McConell G, ed. *Exercise Metabolism: Physiology in Health and Disease*. Switzerland: Springer Nature; 2022:71–114.

52 Favero TG. Sarcoplasmic reticulum Ca^{2+} release and muscle fatigue. *J Appl Physiol*. 1999;87:471–483.

53 Korge P. Factors limiting ATPase activity in skeletal muscle. In: Hargreaves M, Thompson M, eds. *Biochemistry of Exercise X*. Champaign, IL: Human Kinetics; 1998:125–134.

54. Ortenblad N, Westerblad H, Nielsen J. Muscle glycogen stores and fatigue. *J Physiol*. 2013;591(18):4405–4413.

55 Xu K, Zweier J, Becker L. Functional coupling between glycolysis and sarcoplasmic reticulum Ca^{2+} transport. *Circ Res*. 1995;77:88–97.

56 Place N, Westerblad H. Metabolic factors in skeletal muscle fatigue. In: McConell G, ed. *Exercise Metabolism: Physiology in Health and Disease*. Switzerland: Springer Nature; 2022:377–399.

57 Sundberg CW, Fitts RH. Bioenergetic basis of skeletal muscle fatigue. *Curr Opin Physiol*. 2019;10:118–127.

58 Varian KD, Raman S, Janssen PM. Measurement of myofilament calcium sensitivity at physiological temperature in intact cardiac trabeculae. *Am J Physiol Heart Circ Physiol*. 2006;290(5):H2092–H2097.

59 Martyn DA, Gordon AM. Force and stiffness in glycerinated rabbit psoas fibers. Effects of calcium and elevated phosphate. *J Gen Physiol.* 1992;99(5):795–816.

60 Millar NC, Homsher E. The effect of phosphate and calcium on force generation in glycerinated rabbit skeletal muscle fibers. A steady-state and transient kinetic study. *J Biol Chem.* 1990;265(33):20234–20240.

61 Steele DS, Duke AM. Metabolic factors contributing to altered Ca2+ regulation in skeletal muscle fatigue. *Acta Physiol Scand.* 2003;179(1):39–48.

62 Jahnen-Dechent W, Ketteler M. Magnesium basics. *Clin Kidney J.* 2012;5:3–14.

63 Laver DR, Lenz GK, Dulhunty AF. Phosphate ion channels in sarcoplasmic reticulum of rabbit skeletal muscle. *J Physiol.* 2001;535(Pt 3):715–728.

64 Allen DG, Clugston E, Petersen Y, Roder IV, Chapman B, Rudolf R. Interactions between intracellular calcium and phosphate in intact mouse muscle during fatigue. *J Appl Physiol (1985).* 2011;111(2):358–366.

65 Westerblad H, Allen DG. The effects of intracellular injections of phosphate on intracellular calcium and force in single fibres of mouse skeletal muscle. *Pflugers Arch.* 1996;431(6):964–970.

66 Westerblad H, Allen DG. Changes of myoplasmic calcium concentration during fatigue in single mouse muscle fibers. *J Gen Physiol.* 1991;98(3):615–635.

67 Kabbara AA, Allen DG. The use of the indicator fluo-5N to measure sarcoplasmic reticulum calcium in single muscle fibres of the cane toad. *J Physiol.* 2001;534(Pt 1):87–97.

68 Dahlstedt AJ, Westerblad H. Inhibition of creatine kinase reduces the rate of fatigue-induced decrease in tetanic [Ca(2+)](i) in mouse skeletal muscle. *J Physiol.* 2001;533(Pt 3):639–649.

69 Ferreira JJ, Pequera G, Launikonis BS, Rios E, Brum G. A chloride channel blocker prevents the suppression by inorganic phosphate of the cytosolic calcium signals that control muscle contraction. *J Physiol.* 2021;599(1):157–170.

70 Hureau TJ, Broxterman RM, Weavil JC, Lewis MT, Layec G, Amann M. On the role of skeletal muscle acidosis and inorganic phosphates as determinants of central and peripheral fatigue: a (31) P-MRS study. *J Physiol.* 2022;600(13):3069–3081.

71 Blazev R, Lamb GD. Low [ATP] and elevated [Mg^{2+}] reduce depolarization-induced Ca^{2+} release in mammalian skeletal muscle. *J Physiol.* 1999;520:203–215.

72 Macdonald WA, Stephenson DG. Effects of ADP on sarcoplasmic reticulum function in mechanically skinned skeletal muscle fibres of the rat. *J Physiol.* 2001;532(Pt 2):499–508.

73 Macdonald WA, Stephenson DG. Effect of ADP on slow-twitch muscle fibres of the rat: implications for muscle fatigue. *J Physiol.* 2006;573(Pt 1):187–198.

74 Kabbara AA, Stephenson DG. Effects of Mg2+ on Ca2+ handling by the sarcoplasmic reticulum in skinned skeletal and cardiac muscle fibres. *Pflugers Arch.* 1994;428(3–4):331–339.

75 Laver DR, O'Neill ER, Lamb GD. Luminal Ca^{2+}-regulated Mg^{2+} inhibition of skeletal RyRs reconstituted as isolated channels or coupled clusters. *J Gen Physiol.* 2004;124:741–758.

76 Dutka TL, Lamb GD. Effect of low cytoplasmic [ATP] on excitation-contraction coupling in fast-twitch muscle fibres of the rat. *J Physiol.* 2004;560(Pt 2):451–468.

77 A.J. D, Katz A, Wieringa B, Westerblad H. Is creatine kinase responsible for fatigue? Studies of isolated skeletal muscle deficient in creatine kinase. *FASEB J.* 2000;14:982–989.

6 Central fatigue, and central regulation of performance

6.1 Introduction

In Chapter 1, the two most prevalent fatigue theories were introduced: peripheral fatigue and central fatigue (Section 1.2). Briefly, peripheral fatigue refers to causes of fatigue that are outside of the central nervous system (CNS), through processes distal to the neuromuscular junction. Central fatigue refers to causes of fatigue located within the CNS, proximal to the neuromuscular junction (within the brain, spinal nerves, and motor neurons). In addition, the more recent argument that we should conceptualise fatigue less as a specific "type", such as central or peripheral fatigue, and more like a global symptom was also discussed (Section 1.2.4). This recent suggestion about the re-conceptualisation of fatigue perhaps questions the worth/appropriateness of having a chapter called "central fatigue". However, there is a large body of research that has been published under the traditional definition of central fatigue, and it is important to be aware of this work both for its standalone significance but also to better understand how it informs contemporary fatigue research and understanding.

This chapter will begin by discussing some of the classic and contemporary potential "causes" of central fatigue (or perhaps what Enoka and Duchateau[1] would call perceived fatiguability) during sport and exercise before addressing a related concept – the central regulation of sport and exercise performance. As we proceed through the chapter, the findings will be discussed in light of the classical and more contemporary conceptualisations of fatigue, as appropriate.

6.2 Central fatigue

6.2.1 Potential "causes" of central fatigue

Reduced CNS drive to the motor neurons can be caused by a reduction in corticospinal impulses reaching the motor neuron (descending) and/or neurally mediated afferent feedback from muscle (ascending). The development of central fatigue was addressed in Chapter 4 with regard to hyperthermia. However, there are other hypotheses of how central fatigue may develop, and these are discussed in the following sections.

DOI: 10.4324/9781003326137-8

6.2.1.1 Sensory feedback from muscle afferents

There is evidence to suggest that the extent of peripheral muscle fatigue during whole-body sport and exercise does not exceed a level specific to the exercising individual and the task being completed,[2-5] a concept known as the "critical threshold of peripheral fatigue". This consistent level of peripheral fatigue has been demonstrated despite altering parameters such as inspired oxygen availability,[6] activity intensity,[7] and work:rest ratios.[8] Such evidence indicates that our performance during sport and exercise is carefully regulated to prevent excessive peripheral fatigue. This regulation occurs primarily via sensory feedback provided by group III (mechanosensitive) and IV (metabosensitive) afferent fibres, which relay information about the intra- and extra-muscular environment back to the CNS. Greater muscle contraction-induced changes in mechanical stress and metabolic/molecular products (particularly adenosine triphosphate (ATP), hydrogen (H^+), and potassium (K^+)) cause these sensory afferents to fire to a greater extent, resulting in reduced corticospinal excitability and hence reduced muscle activation in an attempt to limit the extent of peripheral fatigue.[9] Put another way, peripheral fatigue is attenuated via an increase in central fatigue. Research employing a variety of methodologies to reduce or completely block afferent feedback from group III and IV afferents, including pharmacological blocking via spinal administration of anaesthetic and opioid drugs such as lidocaine and fentanyl, have reported significant increases in peripheral fatigue during sport and exercise.[10-12] Interestingly, the studies also report suboptimal cardiovascular and ventilatory responses to exercise.[9] These findings serve to highlight the importance of group III/IV afferents in optimising the exercise pressor reflex. Interested readers are referred to Teixeira and Vianna[13] for more information on the exercise pressor reflex and the role of group III/IV afferents.

Consideration of the role of group III/IV afferents in the pressor reflex emphasises one of the primary challenges of investigating the impact of these afferents on fatigue, namely their dual role in reducing peripheral fatigue and increasing central fatigue. The first study to robustly investigate the central impact of group III/IV afferents by controlling for the reduction in muscle oxygenation with afferent blockade provided clear evidence that group III/IV afferents limit sport and exercise performance by reducing neural activation of skeletal muscle (i.e. generating central fatigue).[9,12]

There is also evidence that counters the critical threshold of peripheral fatigue hypothesis. Several studies

Key point 6.1

Stimulation of group III and IV muscle afferents by mechanical and chemical stimuli during sport and exercise can inhibit central motor drive, reducing muscle activation and generating a central fatigue response.

have shown that the extent of peripheral fatigue is dependent on the intensity and duration of the activity, suggesting that the extent of peripheral fatigue is task-specific and varied. These findings may indicate that the critical threshold hypothesis does not hold true when comparing fatigue across different exercise modes, intensities, durations, and in different environmental conditions.[2] A second hypothesis, termed the sensory tolerance limit, was originally proposed in 2001 and is still forming part of the conceptual framework for contemporary fatigue investigations.[2,14]

6.2.1.2 Brain neurotransmitters

Newsholme *et al*.[15] developed the first hypothesis to implicate changes in central neurotransmission with the development of fatigue, termed the "central fatigue hypothesis". These authors suggested that during prolonged sport and exercise the production and metabolism of key monoamines (compounds with a single amine group, in particular neurotransmitters) was altered, and that this influenced central function. Of particular interest was the neurotransmitter serotonin. The serotinergic system is an important modulator of mood, sleep, emotion and appetite.[16] Simply put, increased production of serotonin increases feelings of lethargy and tiredness. Serotonin is synthesised within the brain, as it is unable to cross the blood-brain barrier (BBB). A key precursor for the synthesis of serotonin is the essential amino acid tryptophan (TRP). TRP transport across the BBB is the rate-limiting step in serotonin synthesis within the brain,[16] meaning that the more TRP that crosses the BBB into the brain, the more brain serotonin is synthesised. At rest, most (80%–90%) available TRP is transported in the blood bound to a binding protein called albumin, with the rest circulating freely in plasma (free TRP, or f-TRP). However, during sport and exercise an increase in blood free fatty acid (FFA) concentration occurs. These FFAs compete with TRP for binding to albumin, meaning that during prolonged sport and exercise (when blood FFA may increase the most due to lower glycogen availability), a significant increase in f-TRP can occur. A strong positive relationship has been found between the proportion of f-TRP in blood and brain TRP concentrations,[17] suggesting that TRP crosses the BBB more easily when it is present in its free form. As increased concentrations of brain TRP lead to increased brain serotonin production, it is this sport and exercise-induced brain TRP uptake that was originally proposed to cause the sensations of tiredness, lethargy, and lack of motivation characteristic of central fatigue.[15]

TRP utilises the same BBB transport proteins as the amino acids leucine, isoleucine, and valine. These three amino acids are known as branched chain amino acids (BCAAs) as their structures contain side-chains composed of carbon atoms. The greater the plasma concentration of BCAAs, the more competition there will be between TRP and BCAAs for entry into the brain, and less TRP will make it to the brain. During prolonged sport and exercise, plasma BCAA concentration remains stable or falls.[18] This, combined with the exercise-induced increase in plasma f-TRP concentration, would further increase brain TRP uptake and, therefore, serotonin synthesis. A logical assumption is that reducing the plasma concentration ratio of f-TRP to BCAA via ingestion of BCAA during prolonged sport and exercise would reduce brain TRP uptake, serotonin production, and, hence, central fatigue.[16] While initial field-based research did find support for the use of BCAAs in improving physical and mental performance during prolonged sport and exercise,[19] much subsequent laboratory work has not corroborated these findings.[20-25] As with most topics in sport and exercise science, there are individual research studies that find a benefit of BCAAs on central fatigue and those that find no benefit; however, the most recent consensus from systematic reviews is that BCAA supplementation does not attenuate central fatigue during sport and exercise.[26] Furthermore, there is some evidence that BCAA supplementation during sport and exercise may lead to increased blood ammonia concentrations, which could impair muscle performance and contribute to central fatigue (see Section 6.2.1.3), although more work is required here.[27]

The complexity of brain function makes it unlikely that a single neurotransmitter would be responsible for central fatigue, and this is further supported by the contradictory and largely negative results from studies that have manipulated only serotonergic activity.[16] Dopamine and noradrenaline are catecholaminergic neurotransmitters that have been implicated in enhancing prolonged sport and exercise performance,[28,29] potentially via inhibition of serotonin synthesis and direct activation of central motor pathways.[22] Dopamine has been implicated in increased arousal, motivation and cognition, and the control of motor behaviour.[30] However, in humans exercising in mild ambient temperatures, supplementation with dopamine precursors (substances that are required for the synthesis of dopamine) and reuptake inhibitors (substances that block the removal of dopamine from its synaptic targets and its return to its presynaptic neuron) consistently fails to improve prolonged sport and exercise performance.[31-33] This may be because the influence of dopamine is not strong enough in normal environmental temperatures.[34] During sport and exercise in the heat, inhibition of dopamine reuptake allowed participants to maintain a higher intensity and a higher body temperature, with no changes in their perception of exertion.[35] This effect was also present when both dopamine and noradrenaline reuptake inhibitors were used (see below).[35] Clearly, dopamine can influence our sport and exercise performance through central means.[36] However, the presence of moderating factors (specifically ambient temperature) suggests again that any involvement of brain neurotransmitters in central fatigue is complex. Regarding dopamine, this complexity may not have been appreciated due to early work taking place using animal models, the findings of which we now know do not translate to humans.

Similarly to dopamine, noradrenaline is involved in the regulation of arousal, consciousness, and brain reward centres. Less well researched than dopamine, the use of noradrenaline reuptake inhibitors has failed to find significant improvements in endurance sport and exercise performance.[37] In fact, noradrenaline reuptake inhibitors are associated with reduced endurance performance of ~5%–10%. This may be due to the stimulatory effect of noradrenaline neurons on the serotinergic system.[38] Interestingly, the use of a dopamine reuptake inhibitor that also inhibits the reuptake of noradrenaline has been demonstrated to improve prolonged sport and exercise only when performed in the heat.[33] Both dopamine and noradrenaline have been linked to thermoregulation, and this may explain why manipulations that increase their concentration seem to improve performance during sport and exercise in the heat, as they may work to extend the "safe" limits of hyperthermia.[35]

The influence of brain neurotransmitters on central fatigue during prolonged sport and exercise in humans is still being investigated. While it does appear that serotonin and dopamine are involved in central fatigue, they do not seem able to significantly influence fatigue individually.[38] Noradrenaline negatively affects sport and exercise performance in a temperate environment. During sport and exercise in the heat, dopamine and noradrenaline appear to have a greater effect on performance than serotonin. The apparent difficulty in altering sport and exercise performance in thermoneutral environments by manipulation of neurotransmitters suggests other potential causes of central fatigue should be investigated.

> **Key point 6.2**
>
> *Any potential role of central neurotransmitters on fatigue is likely to involve a combination of the key neurotransmitters serotonin, dopamine, and noradrenaline. The exact influence, if any, may also depend on activity duration and environmental temperature.*

6.2.1.3 Brain ammonia accumulation

Ammonia is a natural by-product of the metabolism of nitrogenous compounds such as proteins and amino acids. It is crucial that ammonia is metabolised as excess accumulation can result in significant cellular and organ dysfunction which can be life threatening. In humans, ammonia is metabolised to urea via the urea cycle in the liver. This urea is then excreted in urine.

Ammonia is produced in the body in several ways. At rest, most ammonia is produced from the gastrointestinal tract via the breakdown of the amino acid glutamine and urea.[39] Ammonia is also produced in the brain, kidneys, and skeletal muscle. Within skeletal muscle, ammonia is produced via the deamination (removal of an amine group) of adenosine monophosphate (AMP) as part of the purine nucleotide cycle (Figure 6.1). This indicates that skeletal muscle ammonia production will increase during intense muscle contraction. Indeed, at intensities below 50%–60% $\dot{V}O_2$max, very little ammonia accumulation occurs, but accumulation rapidly increases as intensity rises above this level.[40] During

1. $AMP + H_2O + H^+ \xrightarrow{\text{AMPD}} IMP + NH_4^+$

2. $IMP + GTP + Aspartate \xrightarrow{\text{AS}} Adenylosuccinate + GDP + P_i$

3. $Adenylosuccinate \xrightarrow{\text{AL}} AMP + Fumarate$

Figure 6.1 The three interlinked reactions that compose the purine nucleotide cycle. This metabolic pathway acts to increase the concentration of Krebs cycle metabolites via the production of fumarate, an intermediate of the Krebs cycle. Note the production of ammonium ($NH4^+$, protonated ammonia) as a result of the deamination of AMP (reaction 1). During intense sport and exercise, accumulation of IMP inhibits reactions 2 and 3 of the cycle. This prevents the reamination of AMP, promoting the accumulation of IMP and ammonia. AMP = adenosine monophosphate; AMPD = AMP deaminase, IMP = inosine monophosphate; GTP = Guanosine-5'-triphosphate; AS = adenylosuccinate synthetase, GDP = Guanosine diphosphate; AL = adenylosuccinate lyase.

sport and exercise, skeletal muscle oxidation of BCAAs can increase ~four-fold over resting rates. If activity is prolonged, BCAA oxidation increases further due to the depletion of glycogen stores.[41]

Key point 6.3

During sport and exercise, ammonia is produced in muscle through the breakdown, in separate reactions, of AMP and branched chain amino acids.

Greater oxidation of BCAAs can also significantly increase ammonia production. Anything from 75% to 90% of the ammonia produced in muscle during sport and exercise is retained in the muscle until completion of exercise, where it is gradually released and metabolised.[42] This is beneficial, as rapid release from muscle could raise blood ammonia concentrations to levels that could cause significant health risks.

Ammonia influences brain function positively at low concentrations by providing substrate for neuron metabolism and neurotransmission and negatively at high concentrations by impairing normal cellular function.[43] These negative influences manifest in symptoms including impaired brain mitochondrial function[44] and inhibition of locomotor activity via ammonia-stimulated glutamate production in brain regions controlling motor activity.[43] Performing fatiguing, intense sport and exercise has been shown to produce systemic ammonia concentrations similar to those observed in patients with liver disorders. The influence of ammonia accumulation in the periphery, even during severe sport and exercise, appears inconsequential with regard to fatigue development,[45] and as a result the role of ammonia in sport and exercise-induced fatigue fell somewhat out of favour as a research topic.[43] However, research investigating the influence of ammonia production on central function during sport and exercise has revealed some interesting findings. It appears that peripheral ammonia production, as occurs during hard and/or exhaustive sport and exercise, may lead to an increase in ammonia transport across the BBB and into the cerebral tissues.[43] Once in the brain ammonia may act negatively on central function. Indeed, research has now demonstrated a significant uptake and accumulation of ammonia in the cerebral tissue during long duration (2–3 hours cycling)[44] and shorter exhaustive exercise (arm and leg, 9–16 minutes duration).[46] However, it is not yet clear whether this accumulation is significant enough to contribute to cellular and neurotransmitter dysfunction.[43]

Ammonia appears to accumulate and exert effects mainly in brain areas associated with learning, memory, and motor activity.[47] It is unlikely that this accumulation will exert any negative effects during short duration sport and exercise, regardless of the intensity.[46] During prolonged sport and exercise, uptake of ammonia across the BBB can exceed its rate of detoxification, leading to an accumulation that could have negative consequences.[44] Therefore, any contribution of ammonia to fatigue is likely to occur during prolonged sport and exercise, and manifest as negative alterations in cognitive function. However, more research is required that directly tests and evidences this theory.[43]

> **Key point 6.4**
>
> *The influence of ammonia accumulation on fatigue development during sport and exercise would probably be limited to cognitive disturbances during prolonged sport and exercise only.*

6.2.1.4 Cytokines

Cytokines are intercellular signalling proteins produced by numerous cells including skeletal muscle. They play a key role in intercellular communication and are intimately involved in the immune system response to illness. For example, pro-inflammatory cytokines (those involved in generating a systemic inflammatory response) are thought to induce the feelings of fatigue, lethargy, and sluggishness characteristic of many common transient and more chronic illnesses.

It is this fatigue-inducing role of cytokines during illness that led to the hypothesis that cytokine production elicits sensations of fatigue during and after sport and exercise.[48] During sport and exercise, skeletal muscle production of the cytokine interleukin 6 (IL-6) can reach 50 times that at rest.[48] This is likely stimulated by an energy crisis in the working muscles (Figure 6.2),[49] suggesting IL-6 production is greater during prolonged sport and exercise. Interleukin-6 may also be produced post sport and exercise in the inflammatory response to contraction-induced muscle damage (IL-6 can have both

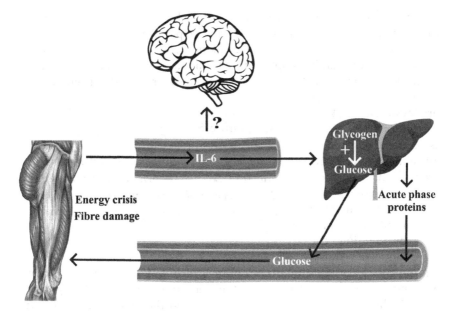

Figure 6.2 Energy crisis within working skeletal muscle, most likely glycogen depletion, increases the skeletal muscle production of interleukin 6 (IL-6). This
increases the systemic concentration of IL-6, which acts to promote liver
glycogenolysis, lipolysis, and production of acute-phase proteins. Interleukin 6 may also influence the development of central fatigue, individually
and in combination with interleukin 1 (IL-1) and tumour necrosis factor
(TNF), both of which are produced partly as a result of IL-6 production.
Redrawn from Gleeson M. *J Physiol.* 2000;529:1.

pro- and anti-inflammatory actions).[50] Importantly, IL-6 produced in skeletal muscle can cross the BBB as well as being produced directly within the
CNS.[51,52] Both IL-6 and interleukin-1, which is produced during intense
sport and exercise, induce sleep promoting effects on the CNS and have py-
rogenic (fever-inducing) capabilities.[53,54] Therefore, they may produce sensations of fatigue during sport and exercise. This is reinforced by research
demonstrating correlations between cytokine concentrations and alterations
in brain activity during sport and exercise and with self-reported perceptions
of fatigue, stress, and mood during intense training periods,[52,55] and increased
sensations of fatigue and reduced exercise performance with acute administration of IL-6.[56]

Related to the above is an idea termed the selfish immune system theory.[57]
This theory posits that high rates of cytokine production indicates high immune cell turnover. Such activation of the immune system is a very energy in-
tensive process, and as a result, immune cells receive energetic "priority" over
other tissues including neurons.[58] Decreased energy availability to neurons

would likely cause reduced neuronal activity, which in the case of motor neurons would lead to reduced sport and exercise performance.[58,59]

Further evidence for a role of cytokine production on central fatigue comes from research in people with chronic diseases that have a strong inflammatory component, such as rheumatoid arthritis and cancer. In these conditions, lethargy, tiredness, and lack of motivation have been associated with pro-inflammatory cytokine production.[56] Furthermore, cytokine production can influence central neurotransmission by altering the availability of amino acid precursors of brain neurotransmitters including dopamine and serotonin, and the function of the neurotransmitters themselves (highlighting a potential link between cytokine production and the brain neurotransmitter hypothesis discussed in Section 6.2.1.2).[56] However, the relevance of this in an acute sport and exercise situation has not been studied. While cytokine production may correlate with loss of muscle function, or at least reduced performance,[60] the causal relationship between their production and fatigue still needs to be clearly demonstrated.[61]

> **Key point 6.5**
>
> *Cytokines are small intercellular signalling proteins. Skeletal muscle produces cytokines during sport and exercise that may be involved in generating fatigue-inducing sensations in the CNS.*

As with almost every physiological process in the body, the production of cytokines during sport and exercise is far from a negative occurrence. Yes, increased cytokine production may contribute to central fatigue and therefore limit sport and exercise performance. However, this increased central fatigue may be an evolutionary mechanism to prevent excessive disruptions to homeostasis and therefore preserve health and function.[62] Furthermore, cytokine production is associated with promotion of an anti-inflammatory environment within the body, meaning cytokines are involved in key sport- and exercise-associated health benefits with regard to chronic inflammatory diseases related to physical inactivity.[62]

6.2.1.5 Summary

Central fatigue has multiple hypotheses for its development. Each hypothesis has research that both supports and refutes it, in a similar vein to the peripheral fatigue hypotheses discussed in earlier chapters. The difficulty in identifying a specific cause(s) for the onset of central fatigue probably relates to the complexity behind the central control of sport and exercise performance, the multitude of factors that can influence this control, and the difficulty in establishing experimental designs that can accurately and reliably measure parameters associated with central fatigue hypotheses.

6.3   Central regulation of sport and exercise performance

The historical inability of peripheral and central fatigue processes to conclusively explain sport and exercise fatigue required scientists to widen their view in an attempt to solve the fatigue "riddle". An interesting perspective that has arisen, or more accurately been revived, over the last 20 years or so is the concept of the brain acting as a central "master regulator" of sport and exercise performance.

6.3.1   Origins of the role of the brain in sport and exercise regulation

Figure 6.3 is an overview of the cardiovascular/anaerobic/catastrophic model of sport and exercise performance, originally proposed by Hill and colleagues in the 1920s. In the top left corner of the figure is an image of the brain with the words "*governor in the brain or heart causing a*

> **Key point 6.6**
>
> *The peripheral catastrophe model of exercise fatigue described by Hill and colleagues in the 1920s is traditionally considered a purely peripheral model of fatigue. However, the original model actually referred to a "central governor" that was hypothesised to protect the heart from ischaemic damage.*

'slowing of the circulation'". Hill suggested the presence of a "governor" either in the heart or brain that was responsible for reducing the pumping capacity of the heart, thereby protecting it from damage due to the myocardial ischaemia that, it was thought at the time, was the cause of fatigue during sport and exercise (Section 1.2.1).[63] Therefore, Hill and colleagues model of fatigue, traditionally thought of as a purely peripheral model, actually included a central component which was also alluded to in the even earlier work of Mosso[64] (Chapter 1, Section 1).

As discussed by Noakes,[65] the "governor" component of Hill's peripheral model of sport and exercise fatigue was omitted in subsequent generations of academic teaching. This may be at least partly because research established that the healthy heart does not become ischaemic during even maximal sport and exercise, thereby discrediting the role of this "governor" as proposed by Hill *et al*. Rather than using the absence of myocardial ischaemia as stimulus to challenge Hill's

> **Key point 6.7**
>
> *The "central governor" component of Hill's peripheral fatigue model was omitted in subsequent generations of teaching, perhaps due to the finding that the healthy heart does not become ischaemic during even the most severe sport and exercise.*

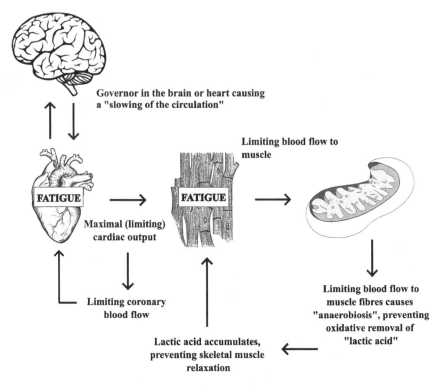

Figure 6.3 Overview of the cardiovascular/anaerobic/catastrophic model of exercise performance originally proposed by Hill and colleagues in the 1920s. Redrawn From Noakes TD. *Front Physiol.* 2012;3:82.

model, it appears that the "governor" component was ignored/forgotten, and the peripheral catastrophe model of sport and exercise fatigue went on to dominate teaching and research (Section 1.2.1).

6.3.2 *Reintroduction of the role of the brain in sport and exercise regulation*

Ulmer[66] reintroduced the concept of a central programmer or governor that regulates muscle metabolic activity and performance through afferent peripheral feedback. Ulmer[66] suggested that this central programmer takes into account the finishing point of a sport or exercise bout by using previous experience and training and knowledge of the current bout and regulates metabolic demand from the onset of sport/exercise to achieve successful completion without catastrophic physiological failure. This maintenance of an "appropriate" metabolic demand by the brain is termed teleoanticipation.

In a series of articles, the central governor was developed further,[67-71] culminating in a full description of a model termed the "anticipatory feedback model" of exercise regulation by Tucker.[72] The model is summarised in Figure 6.4, and a more detailed description of each phase of the model is in Table 6.1. Briefly, the model states that self-paced sport and exercise is regulated from the outset by previous sport and exercise experience, knowledge of the expected distance or duration of the current bout, and afferent physiological feedback regarding variables such as muscle glycogen levels and skin and core temperatures. The synthesis of this information allows the brain to "predict" the most appropriate intensity that will enable optimal performance without causing severe homeostatic disruption. This prediction

> **Key point 6.8**
>
> *The concept of a central governor that regulates sport and exercise performance was reintroduced in the 1990s. Subsequent research developed the model into the anticipatory regulation model of sport and exercise performance.*

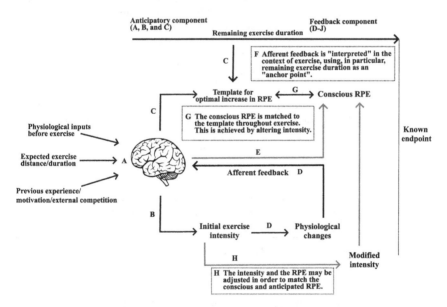

Figure 6.4 The anticipatory feedback model of sport and exercise regulation. This proposes that afferent information from a variety of sources allows the brain to develop an ideal template RPE and, therefore, intensity for a given sport/exercise bout that will enable optimal performance while preventing significant homeostatic disruption. From the onset of activity, actual RPE is measured against this template, and intensity is modulated to ensure that the actual intensity does not deviate significantly from the template. Continued regulation is enabled by afferent monitoring of physiological changes and knowledge of the remaining duration of the bout. Redrawn from Tucker R. *Br J Sports Med.* 2009;43:392–400.

Table 6.1 Summary of each phase of the proposed anticipatory feedback model of exercise regulation. The descriptions in the table should be read with continued reference to Figure 6.1 to aid clarity

Phase of Model (See Figure 6.1)	Description
A	Afferent information from physiological variables, knowledge of the expected exercise duration, previous experience, and level of motivation/competition enables the brain to forecast the most appropriate exercise intensity (and RPE) for the upcoming exercise bout
B	Using the information derived from phase A, the athlete selects the most appropriate exercise intensity at the onset of exercise
C	In conjunction with phase B, a template for optimal rate of rise in RPE is developed, with the goal of reaching maximal RPE at exercise termination and not before. Conscious (i.e. actual) RPE is continually compared to this "ideal" RPE throughout exercise
D	Changes in physiological variables that occur during exercise are constantly relayed back to the brain
E	These signals are interpreted by the brain, and conscious RPE is developed and modulated depending on the nature of these afferent physiological signals
F	The remaining exercise duration is a key anchor that afferent physiological data is compared against, and thereby influences conscious RPE
G	Conscious RPE is continually compared with the anticipated ideal rate of rise in RPE, to determine if the current, conscious RPE is acceptable based on the brains initial projections made in phases A and B
H	Exercising workrate is adjusted, if necessary, to ensure that the conscious RPE and the template RPE remain closely matched
I	Workrate is continually adjusted until conscious RPE returns to an acceptable level that the brain interprets can be sustained until the end of the exercise bout

Source: Information in the table is based on the descriptions of Tucker.[72]

manifests as a rating of perceived exertion (RPE) "template" whereby RPE will progressively rise from the beginning of sport and exercise and reach its maximum at the predicted termination of the bout. Physical, mechanical, and biochemical variables are continuously monitored by the brain, and this afferent feedback is used to generate the conscious RPE which is continually compared to the "template" RPE. Intensity is modulated if actual RPE deviates too much (either lower or higher) from the template RPE. Modulation of intensity continues until the conscious RPE returns to a level that the brain interprets can be tolerated. The anticipatory feedback model therefore holds that fatigue, rather than a physical state, is in-fact a conscious sensation generated from interpretation of subconscious regulatory processes (perhaps now would be a good time to revisit Section 1.2 to see how the anticipatory feedback model may sit within classical and contemporary conceptualisations of fatigue).[70,73] It also suggests that RPE, rather than simply a direct manifestation of afferent physiological feedback, plays a significant role in preventing excessive sport and exercise duration/intensity by acting as the motivator behind an athlete's decision to stop or to adjust intensity to ensure completion without significant physical damage.[72] In essence, the model states that the brain protects us from ourselves.

It is important to note that the anticipatory feedback model described in Figure 6.4 and Table 6.1 relates to self-paced sport and exercise, where the athlete is able to voluntarily alter intensity. During fixed-intensity exercise to exhaustion, it is proposed that RPE is set by the brain at the onset of exercise as described above, and that the rate of rise of RPE is influenced by afferent feedback and the duration of exercise completed. However, the expected duration/distance cannot be used to modify RPE as there is no known duration/distance. Also, the athlete is unable to modify intensity based on changes in RPE. As a result, time to fatigue is determined by the rate at which RPE rises to the maximal level that can be tolerated.[72] A slower rate of rise in RPE would facilitate a longer time to fatigue; a higher rate of rise would mean a shorter time to fatigue.

> **Key point 6.9**
>
> *The anticipatory regulation model of sport and exercise performance states that the brain "predicts" the appropriate intensity based on prior experience, knowledge of the duration/distance, and physiological status. During sport and exercise, continual afferent feedback and knowledge of remaining duration/distance generates the conscious perception of effort (RPE) which is compared to the template RPE, and intensity is modified to keep the template and conscious RPE as similar as possible.*

6.4 Support for the anticipatory regulation model of sport and exercise performance

6.4.1 Anecdotal support

Anecdotal support for a hypothesis or theory (particularly one as complex as the anticipatory regulation model) is of course the weakest type of support. However, it is still worth touching on. Sport or exercise, regardless of the type, intensity, or duration, is almost always voluntarily ended by the individual before they encounter serious physical damage to any body systems (physical damage through sport and exercise as a result of underlying health problems or acute injury is not considered here). Absence of physical damage regardless of how motivated a person may be to push themselves to their "maximum" is interesting. If sport/exercise termina-

Key point 6.10

Regardless of type, duration, or intensity, sport and exercise is almost always voluntarily ended without serious physical damage, regardless of the motivation of the individual to push themselves to their "maximum". If termination is due to the occurrences predicted in the peripheral catastrophe model of fatigue, the prevalence of physical damage and health consequences could be expected to be greater.

tion were due to the peripheral catastrophe suggested by Hill and colleagues, whereby the intensity immediately preceding termination represented maximal recruitment of all available motor units and an exertion on the heart so great that the heart was near failure, then it would be reasonable to expect a greater prevalence of negative health consequences during hard/maximal sport and exercise.

6.4.2 The end-spurt phenomenon

Look back at the "to think about" case study at the end of Chapter 1. The case study discussed the great Ethiopian runner Kenenisa Bekele setting the word record for the 10,000 metres of 26 minutes 17 seconds. Bekele ran the first 9 km of the race at an average pace of 2:38 per km, yet ran the final km in 2:32, 6 seconds faster than the average speed for 90% of the race. You could of course suggest that Bekele made a pacing error; suddenly realising that he had taken the first 9 km too easy and having to pick up his pace over the final km – highly unlikely for an athlete of his calibre during a world record run! More likely is that Bekele displayed an end-spurt – a phenomenon that is quite commonplace in endurance sport and exercise. The end-spurt phenomenon is characterised by a significant increase in intensity near the end of a race, almost regardless of how hard the athlete was pushing throughout the event. Impor-

tant questions are: (1) What causes, or more accurately enables, the end-spurt phenomenon to occur? And (2) How does the existence of an end-spurt fit with current theories of sport and exercise fatigue?

Key point 6.11

The end-spurt phenomenon is characterised by a significant increase in intensity near the end of a race, almost regardless of how hard the athlete was pushing during the activity.

The anticipatory regulation model states that sport and exercise demand is continually monitored by the brain through afferent feedback, and this monitoring is used to allow the athlete to achieve the optimal rate of rise in RPE that maximises performance. Logically, the model states that knowledge of the end-point of exercise (both expected duration from the onset of the bout and the duration remaining at any point during the bout) is a crucial part of the calculations made by the brain in determining the appropriate intensity to maintain (Figure 6.4 and phase A in Table 1). However, during sport and exercise, there is often a degree of uncertainty about the precise end-point and the type of effort that will need to be expended (particularly with longer duration activity). This would be particularly true of competition events, where the completion time and the required intensity throughout the event would be partly dependent on the tactics and pace employed by an athlete's competitors. These factors would influence the pace of the athlete at any given time and could necessitate alterations to pace that could not be anticipated prior to the bout. As the proposed purpose of the anticipatory regulatory role of the brain is to prevent the occurrence of catastrophic changes in homeostasis,[72] this uncertainty may result in the maintenance of a motor unit and metabolic "reserve".[72] Simply put, the athlete cannot be certain of what may occur in the remainder of the bout, so they (subconsciously) hold something back to enable them to respond to any potential physical challenges and to complete the bout without significant homeostatic disruption. As the end-point draws nearer, the athlete's uncertainty may decrease to the point where this "reserve" is no longer required and the athlete is "allowed" to significantly increase metabolic demand and speed/power output.[72] Hence, the occurrence of the end-spurt. An alternative but related view is that the end-spurt occurs as a result of an athlete's belief that their actions will have a large impact on their performance (termed perceived impact).[74] For example, a track runner with two laps remaining knows that completion of a single lap represents 50% of the remaining race distance; as a result, the perceived impact of completing that lap is greater than the perceived impact of completing a single lap when there are five laps remaining (the single lap here represents only 20% of the remaining distance).[74] Motivation to complete the "50% lap" will be greater than that for the "20% lap", giving rise to a greater increase in intensity manifesting as an end-spurt.[74]

Key point 6.12

Uncertainty regarding the end-point of sport/exercise may cause a subconscious maintenance of a motor unit/metabolic "reserve" to allow the athlete to respond to any potential physical challenges and finish without significant homeostatic disruption. As the end of the activity draws nearer, uncertainty may decrease to the point where this "reserve" is no longer required, and the athlete is "allowed" to increase speed/power output.

The end-spurt phenomenon is not just anecdotal. Schabort *et al.*[75] asked participants to complete a 100-km cycle time trial (TT) comprising four 1-km and four 4-km maximal sprints at regular intervals, to be completed as quickly as possible. Power output decreased in each successive 1 km and 4 km sprint. However, power output increased signifi-

> **Key point 6.13**
>
> *Research has shown reductions in power output and EMG activity from the early stages of prolonged sport and exercise, followed by an increase in these measures to levels similar to those at the beginning of sport and exercise. This provides support for the suggestion that a metabolic and neuromuscular reserve is maintained, which the athlete is subsequently able to access near the end of the bout.*

cantly in the last 5 km of the TT compared to the first 5 km. Put another way, the participants were cycling harder from 95 to 100 km than they were from 0 to 5 km. Similarly, Kay *et al.*[76] asked participants to complete a 60 minutes self-paced cycle TT in warm, humid conditions with six 1 minute sprints interspersed throughout the TT. The authors reported that average power output, as a percentage of initial sprint power output, and quadriceps electromyography (EMG; Section 1.4.2) during the sprints fell from sprints 2–5. However, during the final sprint, power output and quadriceps EMG recovered to 94% and 90% of sprint one values, respectively. These findings demonstrate that neuromuscular activity declines early in sport and exercise despite a conscious effort by participants to maintain maximal power output.[77] The EMG data suggests that the CNS reduces the amount of muscle mass recruited, even in the presence of a large muscle reserve, perhaps in order to prevent a significant metabolic crisis from occurring.[71] This metabolic/neuromuscular reserve is emphasised by St Clair Gibson *et al.*[77] who found that muscle force production during a 100-km TT declines from very early on in the TT, despite recruitment of only about 20% of available muscle mass.

It also appears that the end-spurt phenomenon is not limited to prolonged sport and exercise. Marcora and Staiano[78] measured peak power output during a 5-second cycle sprint. On a separate occasion, participants cycled at a resistance equal to 80% of their peak aerobic power until they could no longer maintain that power output (i.e. they became "fatigued"). At this time, participants immediately completed another 5-second cycle sprint. While peak power in the sprint following the exhaustive exercise was lower than that in the isolated sprint, it was still on average three times greater than power output at 80% of peak aerobic power which the participants had been unable to maintain just a few seconds earlier. Therefore, participants must have been physiologically able to continue exercise at 80% of peak aerobic power for longer than they did. So why did they stop? Marcora and Staiano[78] suggest that the known short duration of the peak power test (5 seconds) motivated the participants to exert a greater effort compared with the submaximal cycle to exhaustion, which had an unknown duration. The authors also stated their findings

as evidence that fatigue (at least during the type of exercise used in their study) is not caused by an inability of the muscle to produce force. The findings also agree to some extent with the anticipatory feedback model; if sport/exercise duration is unknown then the brain cannot accurately reconcile the physiological status of the body with the remaining duration, and exercise may be stopped with a notable physiological and neuromuscular reserve. Further support comes from research that shows people only exert their true peak power if the expected sport/exercise duration is less than 30 seconds.[79]

The end-spurt phenomenon has been characterised by an increase in EMG activity to working muscle.[76] This suggests that the end-spurt is central in origin as EMG is a measure of the electrical signal arriving at the muscle from the motor neurons. The presence of an end-spurt ability refutes the peripheral catastrophe model of fatigue on at least two counts. Firstly, the linear catastrophe model states that fatigue is a catastrophic failure of muscle force production that occurs when all motor units, and hence, muscle fibres have been fully activated. However, it has been clearly demonstrated that all motor units are not simultaneously recruited during sport and exercise (in fact, far from it), even when people are required to perform maximally.[77] Secondly,

the catastrophic nature of the peripheral fatigue model implies complete failure of force production due to factors including intramuscular substrate depletion or metabolite accumulation. If this were the case then an athlete would be unable to increase muscle force towards the end of sport/exercise when they would be most "fatigued", as energy depletion/metabolite accumulation would not allow it.[9] Simply put, according to the peripheral fatigue model an end-spurt response is impossible.[80] Indeed, most of our current definitions of fatigue (Table 1.1) quantify it as an inability to maintain the required intensity. However, the display of an end-spurt at the point when an athlete should be most tired means that the athlete cannot be fatigued according to these prevalent definitions. A contrast between sport and exercise regulation according to the peripheral catastrophe and the anticipatory regulation model is in Figure 6.5.

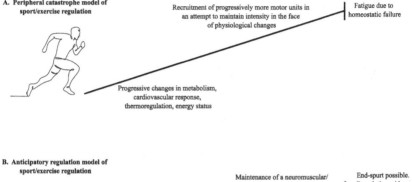

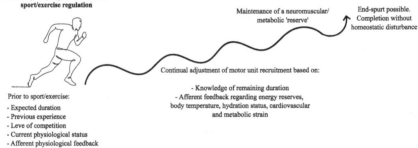

Figure 6.5 A summary of sport and exercise regulation as explained by the peripheral catastrophe model (A) and the anticipatory regulation model (B). The peripheral catastrophe model describes a linear, progressive change in various cardiovascular, metabolic, and thermoregulatory parameters that would increasingly challenge the athlete's ability to maintain intensity. In response to these changes, more motor units are recruitment in an effort to maintain intensity until all motor units are fully recruited and fatigue occurs due to a failure in homeostasis. In contrast, the anticipatory regulation model states that an initial intensity is set prior to activity based on knowledge of exercise duration, experience, and afferent physiological feedback. During activity, continual afferent feedback and awareness of remaining duration allows a continued adjustment of motor unit recruitment and intensity, allowing the athlete to maintain a neuromuscular and/or metabolic reserve that can be accessed in the final stages. Access to this reserve enables the end-spurt phenomenon to occur and allows the athlete to complete the bout without significant homeostatic failure.

6.4.3 Pacing strategies

The concept of pacing strategies is not exclusive to sport and exercise; it applies to all situations where effort must be distributed in some fashion to accomplish a task.[81] With regard to sport and exercise, pacing has been defined as "*the goal directed distribution and management of effort across the duration of an exercise bout*".[81] As has been discussed previously in this book, during sport and exercise in healthy people, no physiological system demonstrates catastrophic failure[77] and no single physiological variable accurately predicts performance or the development of fatigue in all situations.[65,82] Therefore, the concept of pacing in sport and exercise cannot be investigated from a purely physiological perspective.[81] Consequently, the role of central processes must be considered in the development of a pacing strategy and how this strategy is carried out.

Five common pacing strategies used in sport and exercise are shown in Figure 6.6. The presence of pacing strategies such as these during self-paced sport and exercise is important from the perspective of the proposed anticipatory regulation model of sport and exercise performance. People perform sport and exercise less well when the sport/exercise is unfamiliar to them and the demands are unclear.[83] Furthermore, people voluntarily reduce their intensity when confronted with factors such as high ambient temperature or humidity but this reduction in intensity is often in advance of any actual physical need to do so (e.g. before significant increases in body heat storage), and before impairment of performance occurs as a result of any physiological system failure.[84-86] These findings all suggest that the modification of intensity (i.e. pacing) during self-paced sport and exercise is conducted in anticipation of, rather than as a result of, physiological system stress/failure.[81,87]

> **Key point 6.16**
>
> *Research shows that people voluntarily reduce intensity in challenging environments and situations before there is a physical need to do so, indicating an anticipatory aspect to pacing.*

As discussed in Section 6.3.2, Figure 6.4, and Table 6.1, the athlete's prior knowledge/experience of the sport/exercise that is about to be completed may be important information that the brain uses to select an appropriate initial intensity. Research into pacing strategies in sport and exercise has confirmed that the ability to pace accurately is improved

> **Key point 6.17**
>
> *Prior experience improves the ability to pace effectively during sport and exercise. This validates one aspect of the anticipatory regulation model of performance.*

with training and experience.[88,89] As Edwards and Polman[81] state, if pacing strategies are used as a way of enabling successful completion without physical damage then previous experience along with accurate knowledge of exercise demands is critical (see Section 6.4.4).

The above paragraphs demonstrate how the use of pacing strategies in sport and exercise may provide support for aspects of the anticipatory feedback model. However, use of pacing strategies also refutes aspects of the peripheral linear catastrophe model. For example, during sport and exercise that begins in hot conditions, athletes will initiate pacing almost from the onset of exercise,[90,91] demonstrating a lower intensity than would be seen at the onset of the same bout in a thermoneutral environment. This pacing strategy is implemented despite fully functioning thermoregulatory systems.[90] If this scenario were described by the peripheral linear catastrophe model, then fatigue would occur gradually and inexorably due to a failing physiological system (in this case, thermoregulation) which would culminate in complete thermoregulatory failure.[81] However, this scenario does not occur when an athlete can self-regulate their own performance (of course some people do suffer heat exhaustion during sport and exercise in severe environments; however, the peripheral fatigue model states that everyone taking part in sport and exercise in the heat would experience this. Clearly, that is not the case). Instead, during self-paced sport and exercise, a pacing strategy is observed that is dependent on the environment, exercise demands and goals, and afferent physiological feedback, which is in line with the anticipatory regulation model.[81]

If an athlete's pacing strategy is determined by the accumulation of metabolic by-products or depletion of energy stores, as predicted by the peripheral linear catastrophe model, then athletes would always begin sport and exercise at an unsustainable pace and then gradually slow as the negative effect of the particular peripheral variable(s) took hold.[65] In other words, the peripheral linear catastrophe model states that the only pacing

> **Key point 6.18**
>
> *The peripheral linear catastrophe model predicts that an exercising person would show a gradual and inexorable decline in pace due to a failing physiological system, before total failure of that system renders the athlete exhausted. However, this is rarely seen in a person who is free to self-regulate their performance.*

> **Key point 6.19**
>
> *The peripheral linear catastrophe model does not allow for the existence of the varied pacing strategies that have been clearly documented in the sport and exercise literature.*

strategy it is possible to follow in sport and exercise is akin to the positive strategy depicted in Figure 6.6A. The model simply does not allow for the existence of the other strategies in Figure 6.6. Yet, evidence for these other strategies is plentiful.

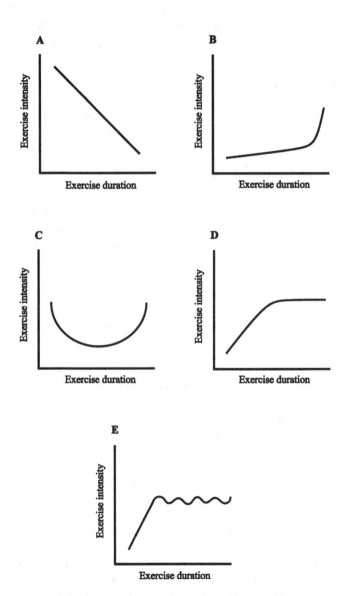

Figure 6.6 Five pacing strategies commonly employed in sport and exercise. A = positive strategy; B = negative strategy; C = parabolic strategy; D = even strategy; E = variable strategy.

6.4.4   Deception studies

The importance of knowledge of sport and exercise duration as a regulator of performance is perhaps most clear when deception is employed in research studies. Commonly, participants in these studies believe they are

> **Key point 6.20**
>
> *When people are asked to continue exercising for longer than they anticipated, RPE can increase and affect decrease despite no difference in intensity or physiological responses to exercise.*

exercising for a given time, but almost at completion of this time are asked to continue exercising for longer. A good example of this research model is the study of Baden *et al.*[92] These authors asked participants to run on a treadmill at 75% of their peak speed. On one occasion, they were asked to run for 20 minutes and were stopped at 20 minutes. On a second occasion, they were asked to run for 10 minutes, but at 10 minutes were asked to run for a further 10 minutes. On a third occasion, they were asked to run but were not told for how long (they were stopped after 20 minutes). The important thing to remember is that all trials were conducted at the same running speed, and all lasted for 20 minutes. However, participants' RPE increased significantly between 10 and 11 minutes in the 10-minute deception trial, which was immediately after the deception was revealed. Correspondingly, participants affect score (a measure of how pleasurable exercise is) decreased significantly at the same time point. These changes to the perception of effort and pleasure occurred despite no changes in running speed or physiological responses to the exercise bout. The significant increase in RPE when participants are required to exercise for longer than originally thought has also been found by other researchers using very similar protocols.[93] In the study of Eston *et al.*,[93] affect also increased in the last few minutes of exercise, perhaps due to the participants being aware that the exercise was almost over. This finding relates back to the end-spurt phenomenon discussed in Section 6.4.2; an increase in pleasurable feelings towards the end of sport/exercise may play a role in "allowing" the end-spurt to occur. Perhaps unsurprisingly, Eston *et al.*[93] found no increase in affect in the trial where participants did not know how long they were to exercise for; in fact, affect continued to decrease throughout this trial. It therefore seems that knowledge of sport and exercise duration is crucial for appropriate regulation of performance, as suggested in the anticipatory feedback model (Figure 6.4). The increase in RPE when deception is revealed may reflect a disruption to the feed-forward/feedback mechanism (of which RPE is crucial) also suggested by the model (Figure 6.4 and Table 6.1).

An interesting point is that Eston *et al.*[93] reported a significant increase in RPE immediately following participants being asked to continue running for longer than they thought they would have to, but this increase in RPE was not seen when participants were asked to continue cycling for longer than they thought. This finding suggests that activity mode may influence the perceptual regulation of sport and exercise. Eston *et al.*[93] suggested that the absence of an increase in RPE during deceived cycling may be due to the lower relative intensity used in the cycling compared with running trials, or related to the way in which RPE was collected. Eston *et al.*[93] asked participants to rate their overall (whole body) RPE; however, during cycling, the perceptual signals arising from the leg muscles are greater than the overall perception of exertion.[94] Therefore, overall RPE may not have been sensitive enough to reflect sudden changes in RPE arising from the legs as a result of the deception of cycling duration.[93]

As well as a significant increase in RPE accompanying deception of sport and exercise duration, it has also been shown that both RPE and physiological responses ($\dot{V}O_2$, heart rate) are lower during sport and exercise with an unknown duration compared to a known duration, despite no difference in the intensity.[92,93] These responses may reflect a subconscious improvement in economy of effort to conserve energy due to the unknown duration of the activity. This again highlights that knowledge of the end point of sport and exercise plays a large role in

> **Key point 6.21**
>
> *When people are required to exercise for an unknown duration, both RPE and physiological responses such as $\dot{V}O_2$ and heart rate may be lower compared to exercise at the same intensity for a known duration. This may reflect a subconscious improvement in economy in order to conserve energy due to the unknown exercise duration.*

the perceptual and physiological responses to that activity.[95] This is further evidenced by the observation that RPE responses to exercise are robust when the exercise duration is known, even when no information is provided to the participant about how much distance has been covered or duration is remaining.[96]

Some research has also investigated the influence of deception during repeated sprint exercise. Billaut *et al.*[97] asked participants to perform 10 × 6-second cycle sprints interspersed with 24 seconds of recovery. On a second occasion, they told the participants that they would be performing 5 × 6-second sprints, but immediately after the fifth sprint, participants were asked to complete a further five sprints. In a third trial, participants were asked to perform repeated 6-second sprints, but were not told how many they were going to do (they did 10). Interestingly, while RPE was not different between the three trials, more work was done in the first five sprints of the deception trial compared to the control and unknown trials. Also, the work completed in all sprints in the unknown trial was significantly lower than in the other two trials. This suggests that participants were "holding something back" in the control and unknown trials, despite being asked to perform the sprints maximally. These findings show that pacing also occurs during short, repeated sprint exercise, and that this pacing is related to the anticipated number of sprints to be completed.

Interestingly, deception used in the "opposite" way appears able to improve sport and exercise performance. For example, Ansdell et al.[98] asked participants to complete a 4-km cycling TT on a laboratory ergometer in the shortest possible time. Subsequently, they completed another two 4-km TTs where they raced against a virtual avatar that they believed was moving at the average power output they produced in their first TT. In reality, in one trial, the average power output was equal to their first TT, and in the other, the average power was 102% of their first TT. Participants were able to improve their performance when racing

Key point 6.22

Pacing in anticipation of sport and exercise duration also occurs during short, repeated sprints. It appears that the pacing during this type of exercise is related to anticipation of the number of sprints to be performed.

the 102% vs. the 100% avatar and demonstrated no significant increase in neuromuscular fatigue compared to the other trials (the improvement was attributed to a change in pacing strategy).

Research findings from deception studies provide further evidence for some process by which people can hold back a physiological reserve during sport and exercise of an uncertain duration. These findings also provide support for a key role of the CNS in the regulation of sport and exercise performance,[93] perhaps to ensure the maintenance of homeostasis and the presence of an emergency "reserve" of energy/physical ability.[93,99]

6.4.4.1   The relationship between rate of rise in RPE and performance

During constant-intensity exercise that continues until exhaustion, RPE increases linearly across a variety of intensities and environmental conditions,[73] and time to fatigue is inversely related to the rate of rise in RPE.[73,100] These findings indicate that time to fatigue can essentially be "predicted" within the first few moments of exercise.[73] Crewe et al.[73] suggested that the subconscious brain predicts exercise duration (perhaps

Key point 6.23

During constant load exercise to exhaustion, RPE increases linearly across a range of intensities and environmental conditions, and time to fatigue is inversely related to the rate of rise in RPE. Therefore, the rate of rise in RPE can be used to predict exercise duration.

through feedback from the information suggested in Figure 6.4 and Table 6.1) and sets both the early-exercise RPE and its rate of increase. This was evident in the fact that the rate of rise in RPE was set at a faster rate from the start of exercise when cycling at higher intensities and in higher ambient temperatures. The findings suggest that the brain can sense both the increased intensity and hotter conditions, and rapidly factor these variables into its prediction of how exercise should best be regulated.

Tucker *et al.*[101] conducted a novel study in which they asked participants to cycle at a pre-determined RPE. Participants were free to vary the intensity they were cycling at in order to maintain this RPE. A protocol such as this enables investigation of the influence of physiological changes on RPE and performance. Participants cycled in three different ambient temperatures (15°C, 25°C, and 35°C). The authors found that after only a few minutes of exercise in the hot trial (35°C), cycling power output began to decrease more rapidly than in the other two temperatures. In other words, participants were having to reduce their intensity to maintain the pre-determined RPE. Importantly, this lowering of intensity (i.e. alteration in pacing strategy) occurred despite the absence of a higher core temperature or heart rate in the hot trial compared with the other two trials. By lowering the intensity, participants slowed their rate of body heat storage so that heat storage was similar between all three trials after 20 min and remained so for the rest of the exercise. Tucker *et al.*[101] concluded that intensity in the heat is regulated by afferent feedback related to the rate of body heat storage in the first few minutes of exercise, and that this is used to regulate intensity and, hence, rate of heat storage for the remainder of the activity. The observation of a change in intensity within the first few minutes of exercise in the heat, no difference in body heat storage between ambient temperatures, and that a critically high core temperature was not reached in any trial, suggests that the alteration in intensity was made in an anticipatory fashion, driven through changes in RPE, to prevent the occurrence of a homeostatic crisis (in this case, an excessively high core body temperature).

Studies showing a relationship between changes in RPE during exercise and exercise duration shed further light on the anticipatory regulation model as they suggest that RPE is a crucial regulator of performance. Also, the suggestion that RPE can be modified from the onset of exercise by changes in ambient

> **Key point 6.24**
>
> *It appears that RPE changes during sport and exercise in anticipation of physiological changes occurring, not as a result of those physiological changes. This provides support for the importance of RPE in the anticipatory regulation of sport and exercise. It also poses the suggestion that fatigue may be an emotion rather than an actual physical process.*

temperature and intensity, in advance of actual physiological changes, and that this change in RPE also alters intensity, provides support for a role of RPE in the *anticipatory* regulation of sport and exercise. This also leads to the suggestion that RPE may not be a direct reflection of an exercising person's physiological state, but may instead be an anticipatory sensory regulator of performance. Put another way, RPE may change in anticipation of physiological changes occurring, not as a result of those physiological changes. This suggestion also requires us to consider the nature of fatigue itself. As Baden *et al.*[92] states, fatigue may be an emotional construct as opposed to a physical process, and this emotion may be driven by expectations about the nature of the exercise that is to be completed.

6.4.5   Support from other research areas

Further indirect support for the anticipatory feedback model can be found by looking at the wider base of sport and exercise fatigue research such as that reviewed in earlier chapters. As we have already discussed, the peripheral linear catastrophe model of performance states that homeostatic failure will occur at the point of fatigue. This perspective implies that fatigue is a developing characteristic of exercising to a point of exhaustion where it becomes of critical physiological importance to stop exercising immediately.[81] However, skeletal muscle is never fully recruited, even during maximal intensity sport and exercise,[77,102] as discussed earlier in this chapter. Secondly, muscle ATP concentration is not fully depleted during sport and exercise (Section 2.2.1). Therefore, the presence of an "energy crisis" in working muscle cannot be the homeostatic failure that the peripheral linear catastrophe model states has to occur in order to "cause" fatigue. In line with this, the intramuscular fuel sources phosphocreatine (PCr) and glycogen can be significantly depleted during prolonged and/or intense sport and exercise, but they are not fully depleted in all muscle fibres (Sections 2.2.2 and 2.2.3). Along with the use of fat, this means that ATP resynthesis is always possible. Finally, exercise termination can occur without significant accumulation of metabolites such as lactate, H^+, or extracellular K^+, without disturbances to muscle calcium (Ca^{2+}) kinetics,[68,81] and without attainment of an abnormally high core temperature or significant hypohydration

> **Key point 6.25**
>
> *Indirect support for the anticipatory regulation model comes from the wider base of sport and exercise fatigue research discussed in previous chapters. This includes the absence of full skeletal muscle recruitment, lack of complete ATP, PCr, and muscle glycogen depletion, and termination of exercise in the absence of metabolite accumulation, a critically high core temperature, or hypohydration.*

(Chapters 3–5). All these observations contradict the prediction of the peripheral linear catastrophe model that some form of homeostatic failure has to occur in order to "cause" fatigue. While these observations may contradict the peripheral linear catastrophe model, and thereby provide indirect support for alternative models of fatigue, they do not provide focussed support for the anticipatory feedback model, hence why the support is indirect.

6.5   Criticism of the anticipatory feedback model

The above findings seem to confirm that fatigue during self-paced sport and exercise is mediated by central alterations in perception of effort and neuromuscular activation, not peripheral failure of the contractile mechanism. However, there is criticism of the anticipatory feedback model that should be presented to provide a balanced perspective.

Some authors have argued that the anticipatory feedback model is unnecessarily complicated. For example, Marcora[103] speculated that the model is *"internally inconsistent, unnecessarily complex, and biologically implausible"*. Some of the reasons given for this suggestion are as follows. The anticipatory feedback model states that a central regulator in the brain holds subconscious control over skeletal muscle recruitment during sport and exercise to prevent the recruitment of sufficient muscle mass that would allow the individual to exercise to the point of physical damage. However, the presence of a single region of the brain that is dedicated to regulating sport and exercise performance is highly unlikely as the suggestion goes against all we know of how the brain functions, namely as an incredibly complex integrated organ where each region contributes to overall brain function.[81] This may also explain why the specific brain region thought to be the central regulator has not been located.

The model also states that the perception of effort is crucial in deterring the individual from continuing to dangerous levels of exercise. However, Marcora[103] points out that if a subconscious central regulator has control over skeletal muscle recruitment then the conscious perception of effort is, in theory, redundant, as the subconscious regulator will stop the individual regardless of how much motivation there is to continue. The argument, essentially, is that the anticipatory feedback model could exist without inclusion of effort perception (hence the issues with consistency and complexity).

It has also been suggested that the progressive increase in RPE over time and at different rates in response to changes in intensity and ambient temperature (Section 6.4.4.1) can be explained by factors other than a central regulator that uses effort perception as a "safety brake". The anticipatory feedback model states that afferent feedback from different physiological and metabolic systems during exercise is interpreted by the brain and used to generate the conscious RPE (Figure 6.4; Table 6.1). However, other authors claim that RPE actually arises from *efferent* sensory signals.[103,104] This claim has partly arisen from research that has attempted to quantify RPE while controlling for or removing afferent feedback that is commonly thought to regulate RPE. For example, studies using drugs that induce muscle weakness have shown significant increases in RPE during exercise without a corresponding increase in measures of metabolic stress.[105] Similar studies have examined RPE responses to exercise with spinal blockade, which greatly reduces sensory afferent feedback from skeletal muscles.[106,107] If afferent feedback from skeletal muscle is important for perception of effort during sport and exercise, it would be expected that RPE would be reduced when exercising with spinal blockade. However, these studies have found that RPE is either unchanged or actually increases with spinal blockade.[104]

Similar findings have been reported regarding the influence of afferent feedback from the heart and lungs on RPE. In experiments where heart rate is reduced by methods such as blocking the stimulating effect of adrenaline, the RPE response to exercise is unchanged.[108] It also appears that people who have had a heart transplant and do not have the same afferent sensory links between the heart and CNS show a normal effort perception during exercise.[109] Similarly, the sensations of difficult or laboured breathing experienced during exercise are due to central motor commands being sent to the respiratory muscles, as opposed to afferent feedback from those muscles.[104,110]

If sensory afferent feedback to the CNS is not responsible for generating RPE, what is? Marcora[103] contends that it is moment-to-moment increases in central motor command to working muscles (both skeletal and respiratory) that are needed to compensate for reductions in motor neuron and muscle responsiveness during prolonged submaximal sport and exercise that explains the increase in RPE over time. The fundamental suggestion is that RPE is generated via signals leaving the CNS, rather than by signals arriving at the CNS. However, in this explanation, Marcora[103] specifically referred to *"prolonged submaximal exercise at a constant workload"*. What about other forms of sport and exercise, such as the self-paced, variable intensity exercise commonly seen in team games or many other forms of competitive sport? This is highlighted in a rebuttal to the paper of Marcora[103] by Noakes and Tucker.[111] Noakes and Tucker[111] discuss that RPE has been shown to alter almost from the onset of sport and exercise as a result of differences in intensity and ambient temperature,[73] and that this finding is not well explained by the suggestion of Marcora[103] that RPE increases due to requirement for a

Key point 6.26

Some authors have suggested that RPE during sport and exercise is generated by increased efferent signals from the CNS, rather than peripheral afferent feedback. Support for this comes from observation of a normal RPE response when various afferent signals are blocked. However, counter arguments suggest that some afferent feedback must still be required to stimulate the increased efferent signals from the CNS.

progressive increase in CNS discharge. Also, Noakes and Tucker[111] argue that if the CNS is being required to increase its motor commands to the working muscles, and this is responsible for the increase in RPE, then the CNS must be receiving some afferent information from the working muscles which "tells" it that these increased motor commands are needed. The argument is that the model proposed by Marcora[103] cannot work without afferent sensory feedback, which makes it conceptually similar to the anticipatory feedback model.[111]

The above discussion highlights the difficulties and debates surrounding the anticipatory feedback model of sport and exercise performance. Whether to accept or reject this model is hampered by the fact that the nature of perceived exertion, primarily how it is generated during sport and exercise, is still unknown. This uncertainty was highlighted in a review[112] where the author suggested that generation of effort perception during sport and exercise is likely centrally generated, with peripheral feedback playing an unimportant role (agreeing with Marcora[103]). However, it was also stated that ultimately, regulation of performance is likely due to sense of effort (centrally generated) and specific sensations such as temperature, pain, and other muscular sensations (from afferent sensory feedback).[112] As

> **Key point 6.27**
>
> *There is ongoing debate surrounding the origins of RPE during sport and exercise. As RPE is a central tenet of the anticipatory feedback model, it is likely that the validity of this model will continue to be argued until exercising RPE is better understood.*

RPE is a central tenet of the anticipatory feedback model, it is likely that the model will remain a source of debate until the mechanisms behind the sensation of effort during sport and exercise are better understood. One of the ways in which understanding of RPE in sport and exercise has been clouded, and therefore a way in which it can also be better understood, is the use of multiple definitions and measurement tools related to the concept of perceived effort.[113] Clarifying and reducing the number of definitions and measurement tools, and measuring other perceptions and emotions alongside perceived effort, will improve our understanding of the concept of perceived effort and therefore of any models that include perceived effort.[113]

Shephard[114] published an article commenting on many components of the anticipatory feedback model. The author argued that the presence of a central governor that regulates physical performance was from an evolutionary perspective unnecessary and unlikely to have developed in humans. The ability of the anticipatory regulator to protect the body from critical damage during sport and exercise was also questioned. Shephard[114] supported this argument with data on the prevalence of death from heat stroke in American Football Players, and the approximate 50-fold increase in the risk of sudden cardiac death as a result of vigorous exercise. However, these arguments were followed by statements that reduced their strength. For example, discussion of the increase in the risk of sudden cardiac death during vigorous exercise was qualified by the statement that many of those contributing to the statistic might have had existing cardiac or vascular disease. Shephard[114] also argues that technical issues associated with measuring equipment could be responsible for some of the data that supports the central governor/anticipatory feedback model. However, no specific examples of such technical issues were provided.

The fundamental argument of Shephard[114] is that the anticipatory feedback model should be treated with scepticism as there is a lack of experimental evidence for its existence. However, the model is exceedingly complex and poses significant challenges to researchers who attempt to investigate it experimentally.[115] Furthermore, much of the evidence that argues against the model comes from studies on isolated component physiological systems. Caution should be used when interpreting this research as evidence against the model, as investigating isolated component systems disregards the complex physiological, psychological, and neurological interplay proposed by the anticipatory feedback model.[115]

This complexity may be one of the key reasons behind much of the criticism of the central governor/anticipatory feedback model. The available research supporting the model, while generally well conducted, cannot conclusively state that the observations made are a result of the existence of an anticipatory regulating system that "oversees" in real time the balance between exercise demand and athlete ability. The combined integration of numerous physiological, metabolic, neurological, psychological, and environmental factors (as well as the self-regulation of most of these factors in isolation) means that fully controlling and accounting for the influence of all within a centrally governed network has not yet been achieved within a research design. Indeed, this may not be possible. Furthermore, arguing for the existence of the model is hampered by the inability to clearly identify the "location" of the central governor/regulator, or which specific central/brain processes are involved, or comprise, the governor or the development of RPE. More extensive research focussing on, amongst other things, the relationships and influences between physiological/metabolic factors, central brain and motor function, and the conscious perception of effort, is required to more clearly address whether the anticipatory feedback model exists in its proposed form.

While the central governor/anticipatory feedback models of sport and exercise performance were admirable attempts to universally describe what is a highly complex process, they do fall short of this goal. Some of the reasons why are discussed above, and the need to continue searching for better ways to explain regulation of sport and exercise performance is evidenced by the original proponents of these earlier models acknowledging their limitations and continuing to propose alternative theories. One such theory is the integrative governor theory, first published in 2018.[116] Integrative governor theory proposes that considering potential regulatory mechanisms as "central" or "peripheral" is limiting; rather, it is competition between psychological and physiological drives/requirements and the associated regulation of each via dynamic negative feedback that regulates performance.[116] Continued interplay between these psychological and physiological drives means that activity in all related systems will constantly "oscillate", and this oscillation provides information that can be compared with prior information/experience, the current activity, or activity "templates" and generate subsequent efferent responses to alter performance as deemed appropriate.[116] While this proposed model has alterations from the anticipatory regulation model, it clearly also has similarities, namely the existence of a central "organiser" that makes sense of system oscillations and elicits appropriate responses. Therefore, the integrative governor model may suffer from some of the issues aimed at the anticipatory regulation model.

Probably the most successful alternative theory of performance regulation is the psychobiological model of sport and exercise regulation, first described in 2008.[103] The psychobiological model combines physiology with motivational psychology research and contends that the conscious brain makes the decision to modulate intensity or terminate exercise when (A) the effort required to continue is equal to the maximum effort the athlete is willing to exert or (B) when the athlete believes they have exerted their true maximal effort and continuation is therefore perceived to be impossible. Part B can be considered an upper limit (although one that can be increased by training), and increasing part A (essentially facilitating greater motivation from the athlete) will improve sport and exercise tolerance/performance.

Through a series of publications, proponents of the psychobiological model have provided evidence and made arguments claiming that the model explains sport and exercise performance regulation effectively and in a simpler and more plausible manner than the

> **Key point 6.28**
>
> *Rival theories of sport and exercise regulation continue to be developed. One of the most recent theories is the integrated governor theory, but probably the most researched is the psychobiological model of sport and exercise regulation.*

> **Key point 6.29**
>
> *The existence of the anticipatory feedback model is refuted by some based on a lack of experimental evidence. However, the complex nature of the model hampers the ability to experimentally test it. Also, some experimental research used to refute the model does not reflect the complexity of the model to be a sufficiently valid test of its existence.*

anticipatory regulation model.[78,117–121] This work appears to show that the psychobiological model is valid in explaining the effects of psychological and physiological manipulations on constant-load and self-paced endurance sport and exercise performance.[119] However, as is only right in science, debate goes on and alternative/extension theories continue to be published (e.g. Venhorst *et al.*[122]) in an effort to develop the most valid, encompassing explanation of the highly complex regulation of sport and exercise performance.

6.6   Summary

- Stimulation of group III and IV muscle afferents by mechanical and chemical stimuli during sport and exercise can inhibit central motor drive and may contribute to increased effort perception by increasing sensations of muscular pain/discomfort.
- Alterations in central neurotransmitters, particularly serotonin, dopamine, and noradrenaline, are likely involved in central fatigue in a synergistic fashion. The relative influence of central neurotransmitters is probably influenced by factors including exercise duration and environmental temperature. The exact role of central neurotransmitter disturbances on central fatigue is still being investigated.
- Ammonia produced during sport and exercise can cross the BBB and accumulate in the cerebral tissues, impairing cognitive function and potentially motor activity. Any contribution of ammonia to fatigue during sport and exercise is likely to occur during prolonged sport/exercise.
- Pro-inflammatory cytokines may induce feelings of fatigue, lethargy, and sluggishness characteristic of many illnesses and increased cytokine production during sport and exercise could encourage similar sensations. Cytokine production can also influence central neurotransmitter production and function. The causal relationship between cytokine production and fatigue still needs to be better demonstrated.
- Central regulation of sport and exercise performance is not a new concept. Some form of central regulation of performance has been speculated upon for over 100 years.
- Central regulation of sport and exercise was reintroduced in the mid-1990s with the concept of a central programmer or governor that uses information about the finishing point of a sport/exercise bout and regulates metabolic demand to achieve this end-point without catastrophic physiological failure (teleoanticipation).
- This concept was developed further, culminating in the anticipatory feedback model of sport and exercise performance.
- The anticipatory feedback model states that sport/exercise is regulated from the outset by previous experience, knowledge of the expected distance or duration of the current bout, and afferent physiological feedback. The synthesis of this information allows the brain to "predict" the most appropriate intensity that will enable optimal performance without causing severe homeostatic disruption.

- Central to the anticipatory feedback model is the RPE. The model states that a "template" RPE is developed that will enable RPE to reach its maximum at the predicted termination of sport/exercise. Afferent physiological feedback is continuously monitored by the brain and used to generate conscious RPE. If the conscious RPE and "template" RPE deviate too much, intensity is altered as appropriate to correct the imbalance.

- The anticipatory feedback model holds that fatigue is a conscious sensation rather than a physical state, and that RPE plays a crucial role in preventing excessive duration/intensity by acting as the motivator to stop or adjust intensity to ensure exercise is completed at an intensity that allows optimal performance without significant physical damage.

- Support for the anticipatory feedback model is anecdotal (sport and exercise is almost always voluntarily ended before serious physical damage occurs) and evidence-based (the end-spurt phenomenon, the use of varied pacing strategies, the physiological and psychological responses to deception of intensity or duration, the relationship between RPE and exercise at different durations, intensities, and conditions, and the frequent occurrence of fatigue despite the absence of a direct physiological or metabolic cause).

- Criticism of the anticipatory feedback model includes the questioning of whether a central regulator in the brain is necessary for central sport and exercise regulation to occur, the requirement for conscious RPE to be such a significant part of the model, and the nature of RPE generation during exercise (whether it is generated from afferent feedback of efferent signals).

- One of the consistent criticisms of the model is that it has not been sufficiently tested experimentally. However, the complexity of the model, along with the separate debate concerning components of the model such as RPE, makes its integrated testing extremely difficult, perhaps even impossible.

- Alternative models of sport and exercise regulation continue to be developed, such as the integrative governor theory and psychobiological model.

- Integrative governor theory posits that competition between psychological and physiological drives/requirements and the associated regulation of each, via dynamic negative feedback, regulates performance. Similar to the anticipatory regulation model, integrative governor theory implicates prior information/experience, the nature of the current activity, and activity "templates" in the regulatory process.

- The psychobiological model contends that the conscious brain makes the decision to modulate intensity or terminate exercise when the effort required to continue is equal to the maximum effort the athlete is willing to exert or when the athlete believes they exerted their true maximal effort and continuation is therefore perceived to be impossible.

- Proponents of the psychobiological model argue that it explains sport and exercise performance regulation effectively and in a simpler and more plausible manner than the central governor/anticipatory regulation models.

- Debate is ongoing, and alternative models of sport and exercise regulation continue to be published.

To think about...

It is becoming ever clearer that the brain plays a very important role in sport and exercise performance. This role can be related to our fundamental desire to exercise (or not!), the will to keep going when things get difficult, and more complex potential roles such as the potential regulation of sport and exercise discussed in this chapter. Also mentioned in this chapter is the difficulty in investigating and determining the exact roles of the brain during sport and exercise. Due to these difficulties, most research infers the role of the brain by collecting measures that allow exclusion of the role of peripheral factors, by asking participants about their thoughts and feelings during sport and exercise, and designing studies that may show alterations in these thought processes and emotions. The lack of objective measures focussed on brain function itself is clearly a hindrance to this form of research.

Consider the information in Chapters 2–6 of this book. Based on this information, do you feel that the body of knowledge is sufficient to state that a brain-regulated model of sport and exercise performance is the most logical explanation for sport and exercise regulation? Or do we still need to wait for that one study that finally gives us the conclusive "proof" of this? Is it ever sufficient to use a process of elimination and anecdotal support to accept a hypothesis or model? When you are considering these questions, look for some literature outside of the sport and exercise sciences that discusses how the brain regulates things such as our emotions and motivation. This information may shed more light on the above questions.

Test yourself

Answer the following questions to the best of your ability. Try to understand the information gained from answering these questions before you progress with the book.

1 Summarise the key proposed mechanisms behind the development of central fatigue during sport and exercise.
2 In your own words, briefly explain the central governor model of sport and exercise regulation.
3 In your own words, briefly explain the anticipatory feedback model of sport and exercise regulation. Highlight differences between the anticipatory feedback model and the central governor model.
4 Explain the proposed importance of RPE in the anticipatory feedback model.
5 What are the five main areas of support for the anticipatory feedback model?

6 Briefly explain how each of the areas you noted in question 5 supports the existence of the anticipatory feedback model.

7 What are the main arguments that have been put forwards against the anticipatory feedback model?

8 Summarise the main difference(s) between the anticipatory feedback model and the psychobiological model of sport and exercise regulation.

9 What are the main research findings that indicate RPE may be generated due to efferent signals rather than afferent peripheral feedback?

10 What are the key factors that make it extremely difficult for the anticipatory feedback model to be appropriately tested in a research setting?

References

1 Enoka RM, Duchateau J. Translating fatigue to human performance. *Med Sci Sports Exerc.* 2016;48(11):2228–2238.

2 Hureau TJ, Romer LM, Amann M. The 'sensory tolerance limit': a hypothetical construct determining exercise performance? *Eur J Sport Sci.* 2018;18(1):13–24.

3 Amann M, Dempsey JA. Locomotor muscle fatigue modifies central motor drive in healthy humans and imposes a limitation to exercise performance. *J Physiol.* 2008;586(1):161–173.

4 Hureau TJ, Ducrocq GP, Blain GM. Peripheral and central fatigue development during all-out repeated cycling sprints. *Med Sci Sports Exerc.* 2016;48(3):391–401.

5 Hureau TJ, Olivier N, Millet GY, Meste O, Blain GM. Exercise performance is regulated during repeated sprints to limit the development of peripheral fatigue beyond a critical threshold. *Exp Physiol.* 2014;99(7):951–963.

6 Hogan MC, Richardson RS, Haseler LJ. Human muscle performance and PCr hydrolysis with varied inspired oxygen fractions: a 31P-MRS study. *J Appl Physiol (1985).* 1999;86(4):1367–1373.

7 Burnley M, Vanhatalo A, Fulford J, Jones AM. Similar metabolic perturbations during all-out and constant force exhaustive exercise in humans: a (31)P magnetic resonance spectroscopy study. *Exp Physiol.* 2010;95(7):798–807.

8 Chidnok W, DiMenna FJ, Fulford J, et al. Muscle metabolic responses during high-intensity intermittent exercise measured by (31)P-MRS: relationship to the critical power concept. *Am J Physiol Regul Integr Comp Physiol.* 2013;305(9): R1085–R1092.

9 Amann M, Wan HY, Thurston TS, Georgescu VP, Weavil JC. On the influence of group III/IV muscle afferent feedback on endurance exercise performance. *Exerc Sport Sci Rev.* 2020;48(4):209–216.

10 Amann M, Proctor LT, Sebranek JJ, Pegelow DF, Dempsey JA. Opioid-mediated muscle afferents inhibit central motor drive and limit peripheral muscle fatigue development in humans. *J Physiol.* 2009;587(1):271–283.

11 Blain GM, Mangum TS, Sidhu SK, et al. Group III/IV muscle afferents limit the intramuscular metabolic perturbation during whole body exercise in humans. *J Physiol.* 2016;594(18):5303–5315.

12 Hureau TJ, Weavil JC, Thurston TS, et al. Pharmacological attenuation of group III/IV muscle afferents improves endurance performance when oxygen delivery to locomotor muscles is preserved. *J Appl Physiol (1985).* 2019;127(5):1257–1266.

13 Teixeira AL, Vianna LC. The exercise pressor reflex: an update. *Clin Auton Res.* 2022;32(4):271–290.

14 Azevedo RA, Silva-Cavalcante MD, Cruz R, Couto P, Lima-Silva AE, Bertuzzi R. Distinct pacing profiles result in similar perceptual responses and neuromuscular fatigue development: why different "roads" finish at the same line? *Eur J Sport Sci.* 2022;22(7):1046–1056.

15 Newsholme EA, Acworth I, Blomstrand E. Amino acids, brain neurotransmitters and a function link between muscle and brain that is important in sustained exercise. In: Benzi G, ed. *Advances in Myochemistry.* London: John Libbey Eurotext; 1987:127–133.

16 Meeusen R, Watson P, Hasegawa H, Roelands B, Piacentini MF. Central fatigue: the serotonin hypothesis and beyond. *Sports Med.* 2006;36(10):881–909.

17 Chaouloff F, Kennett GA, Serrurrier B, Merino D, Curzon G. Amino acid analysis demonstrates that increased plasma free tryptophan causes the increase of brain tryptophan during exercise in the rat. *J Neurochem.* 1986;46(5):1647–1650.

18 MacLean DA, Graham TE, Saltin B. Branched-chain amino acids augment ammonia metabolism while attenuating protein breakdown during exercise. *Am J Physiol.* 1994;267(6 Pt 1):E1010–E1022.

19 Blomstrand E, Hassmen P, Ekblom B, Newsholme EA. Administration of branched-chain amino acids during sustained exercise – effects on performance and on plasma concentration of some amino acids. *Eur J Appl Physiol Occup Physiol.* 1991;63(2):83–88.

20 Blomstrand E, Andersson S, Hassmen P, Ekblom B, Newsholme EA. Effect of branched-chain amino acid and carbohydrate supplementation on the exercise-induced change in plasma and muscle concentration of amino acids in human subjects. *Acta Physiol Scand.* 1995;153(2):87–96.

21 Blomstrand E, Hassmen P, Ek S, Ekblom B, Newsholme EA. Influence of ingesting a solution of branched-chain amino acids on perceived exertion during exercise. *Acta Physiol Scand.* 1997;159(1):41–49.

22 Davis JM, Welsh RS, De Volve KL, Alderson NA. Effects of branched-chain amino acids and carbohydrate on fatigue during intermittent, high-intensity running. *Int J Sports Med.* 1999;20(5):309–314.

23 Greer BK, White JP, Arguello EM, Haymes EM. Branched-chain amino acid supplementation lowers perceived exertion but does not affect performance in untrained males. *J Strength Cond Res.* 2011;25(2):539–544.

24 Madsen K, MacLean DA, Kiens B, Christensen D. Effects of glucose, glucose plus branched-chain amino acids, or placebo on bike performance over 100 km. *J Appl Physiol (1985).* 1996;81(6):2644–2650.

25 Struder HK, Hollmann W, Platen P, Donike M, Gotzmann A, Weber K. Influence of paroxetine, branched-chain amino acids and tyrosine on neuroendocrine system responses and fatigue in humans. *Horm Metab Res.* 1998;30(4):188–194.

26 Hormoznejad R, Z. JA, Mansoori A. Effect of BCAA supplementation on central fatigue, energy metabolism substrate and muscle damage to the exercise: a systematic review with meta-analysis. *Sport Sci Health.* 2019;15:265–279.

27 Holecek M. Branched-chain amino acids in health and disease: metabolism, alterations in blood plasma, and as supplements. *Nutr Metab (Lond).* 2018;15:33.

28 Heyes MP, Garnett ES, Coates G. Central dopaminergic activity influences rats ability to exercise. *Life Sci.* 1985;36(7):671–677.

29 Gerald MC. Effects of (+)-amphetamine on the treadmill endurance performance of rats. *Neuropharmacology.* 1978;17(9):703–704.

30 Nestler EJ, Hyman SE, Malenka RC. *Molecular Neuro-Pharmacology: A Foundation for Clinical Neuroscience.* New York: McGraw-Hill; 2001.

31 Meeusen R, Roeykens J, Magnus L, Keizer H, De Meirleir K. Endurance performance in humans: the effect of a dopamine precursor or a specific serotonin (5-HT2A/2C) antagonist. *Int J Sports Med.* 1997;18(8):571–577.

32 Piacentini MF, Meeusen R, Buyse L, De Schutter G, De Meirleir K. Hormonal responses during prolonged exercise are influenced by a selective DA/NA reuptake inhibitor. *Br J Sports Med.* 2004;38(2):129–133.

33 Watson P, Hasegawa H, Roelands B, Piacentini MF, Looverie R, Meeusen R. Acute dopamine/noradrenaline reuptake inhibition enhances human exercise performance in warm, but not temperate conditions. *J Physiol.* 2005;565(Pt 3):873–883.

34 Roelands B, Watson P, Cordery P, et al. A dopamine/noradrenaline reuptake inhibitor improves performance in the heat, but only at the maximum therapeutic dose. *Scand J Med Sci Sports.* 2012;22(5):e93–e98.

35 Meeusen R, Roelands B. Fatigue: is it all neurochemistry? *Eur J Sport Sci.* 2018;18:37–46.

36 Flack K, Pankey C, Ufholz K, Johnson L, Roemmich JN. Genetic variations in the dopamine reward system influence exercise reinforcement and tolerance for exercise intensity. *Behav Brain Res.* 2019;375:112148.

37 Piacentini MF, Meeusen R, Buyse L, et al. No effect of a noradrenergic reuptake inhibitor on performance in trained cyclists. *Med Sci Sports Exerc.* 2002;34(7):1189–1193.

38 Roelands B, Meeusen R. Alterations in central fatigue by pharmacological manipulations of neurotransmitters in normal and high ambient temperature. *Sports Med.* 2010;40(3):229–246.

39 Romero-Gomez M, Jover M, Galan JJ, Ruiz A. Gut ammonia production and its modulation. *Metab Brain Dis.* 2009;24(1):147–157.

40 Buono MJ, Clancy TR, Cook JR. Blood lactate and ammonium ion accumulation during graded exercise in humans. *J Appl Physiol Respir Environ Exerc Physiol.* 1984;57(1):135–139.

41 Wagenmakers AJ, Coakley JH, Edwards RH. Metabolism of branched-chain amino acids and ammonia during exercise: clues from McArdle's disease. *Int J Sports Med.* 1990;11(Suppl 2):S101–S113.

42 Graham TE, MacLean DA. Ammonia and amino acid metabolism in human skeletal muscle during exercise. *Can J Physiol Pharmacol.* 1992;70:132–141.

43 Wilkinson DJ, Smeeton NJ, Watt PW. Ammonia metabolism, the brain and fatigue; revisiting the link. *Prog Neurobiol.* 2010;91(3):200–219.

44 Nybo L, Dalsgaard MK, Steensberg A, Moller K, Secher NH. Cerebral ammonia uptake and accumulation during prolonged exercise in humans. *J Physiol.* 2005;563(Pt 1):285–290.

45 Shanely RA, Coast JR. Effect of ammonia on in vitro diaphragmatic contractility, fatigue and recovery. *Respiration.* 2002;69(6):534–541.

46 Dalsgaard MK, Ott P, Dela F, et al. The CSF and arterial to internal jugular venous hormonal differences during exercise in humans. *Exp Physiol.* 2004;89(3):271–277.

47 Monfort P, Cauli O, Montoliu C, et al. Mechanisms of cognitive alterations in hyperammonemia and hepatic encephalopathy: therapeutical implications. *Neurochem Int.* 2009;55(1–3):106–112.

48 Pedersen BK, Hoffman-Goetz L. Exercise and the immune system: regulation, integration, and adaptation. *Physiol Rev.* 2000;80(3):1055–1081.

49 Gleeson M. Interleukins and exercise. *J Physiol.* 2000;529(Pt 1):1.

50 Clarkson PM, Hubal MJ. Exercise-induced muscle damage in humans. *Am J Phys Med Rehabil.* 2002;81(11 Suppl):S52–S69.

51 Banks WA, Kastin AJ, Gutierrez EG. Penetration of interleukin-6 across the murine blood-brain barrier. *Neurosci Lett.* 1994;179(1–2):53–56.

52 Vargas NT, Marino F. A neuroinflammatory model for acute fatigue during exercise. *Sports Med.* 2014;44(11):1479–1487.

53 Kapsimalis F, Richardson G, Opp MR, Kryger M. Cytokines and normal sleep. *Curr Opin Pulm Med.* 2005;11(6):481–484.

54 Cerqueira E, Marinho DA, Neiva HP, Lourenco O. inflammatory effects of high and moderate intensity exercise-a systematic review. *Front Physiol.* 2019;10:1550.

55 Cullen T, Thomas AW, Webb R, Phillips T, Hughes MG. sIL-6R is related to weekly training mileage and psychological well-being in athletes. *Med Sci Sports Exerc.* 2017;49(6):1176–1183.

56 Dantzer R, Heijnen CJ, Kavelaars A, Laye S, Capuron L. The neuroimmune basis of fatigue. *Trends Neurosci.* 2014;37(1):39–46.

57 Straub RH. Insulin resistance, selfish brain, and selfish immune system: an evolutionarily positively selected program used in chronic inflammatory diseases. *Arthritis Res Ther.* 2014;16(Suppl 2):S4.

58 Proschinger S, Freese J. Neuroimmunological and neuroenergetic aspects in exercise-induced fatigue. *Exerc Immunol Rev.* 2019;25:8–19.

59 Matsui T, Omuro H, Liu YF, et al. Astrocytic glycogen-derived lactate fuels the brain during exhaustive exercise to maintain endurance capacity. *Proc Natl Acad Sci U S A.* 2017;114(24):6358–6363.

60 Robson-Ansley PJ, de Milander L, Collins M, Noakes TD. Acute interleukin-6 administration impairs athletic performance in healthy, trained male runners. *Can J Appl Physiol.* 2004;29(4):411–418.

61 Finsterer J. Biomarkers of peripheral muscle fatigue during exercise. *BMC Musculoskelet Disord.* 2012;13:218.

62 Nash D, Hughes MG, Butcher L, et al. IL-6 signaling in acute exercise and chronic training: potential consequences for health and athletic performance. *Scand J Med Sci Sports.* 2023;33(1):4–19.

63 Hill AV, Long CHN, Lupton H. Muscular exercise, lactic acid and the supply and utilisation of oxygen: parts VII-VIII. *Prog Royal Soc.* 1924;97:155–176.

64 Mosso A. *Fatigue.* London: Allen and Unwin Ltd; 1915.

65 Noakes TD. Fatigue is a brain-derived emotion that regulates the exercise behavior to ensure the protection of whole body homeostasis. *Front Physiol.* 2012;3:82.

66 Ulmer HV. Concept of an extracellular regulation of muscular metabolic rate during heavy exercise in humans by psychophysiological feedback. *Experientia.* 1996;52(5):416–420.

67 Lambert EV, St Clair Gibson A, Noakes TD. Complex systems model of fatigue: integrative homoeostatic control of peripheral physiological systems during exercise in humans. *Br J Sports Med.* 2005;39(1):52–62.

68 Noakes TD. Physiological models to understand exercise fatigue and the adaptations that predict or enhance athletic performance. *Scand J Med Sci Sports.* 2000;10(3):123–145.

69 Noakes TD, Peltonen JE, Rusko HK. Evidence that a central governor regulates exercise performance during acute hypoxia and hyperoxia. *J Exp Biol.* 2001;204(Pt 18):3225–3234.

70 Noakes TD, St Clair Gibson A, Lambert EV. From catastrophe to complexity: a novel model of integrative central neural regulation of effort and

fatigue during exercise in humans: summary and conclusions. *Br J Sports Med.* 2005;39(2):120–124.

71 St Clair Gibson A, Noakes TD. Evidence for complex system integration and dynamic neural regulation of skeletal muscle recruitment during exercise in humans. *Br J Sports Med.* 2004;38(6):797–806.

72 Tucker R. The anticipatory regulation of performance: the physiological basis for pacing strategies and the development of a perception-based model for exercise performance. *Br J Sports Med.* 2009;43(6):392–400.

73 Crewe H, Tucker R, Noakes TD. The rate of increase in rating of perceived exertion predicts the duration of exercise to fatigue at a fixed power output in different environmental conditions. *Eur J Appl Physiol.* 2008;103(5):569–577.

74 Emanuel A. Perceived impact as the underpinning mechanism of the end-spurt and U-shape pacing patterns. *Front Psychol.* 2019;10:1082.

75 Schabort EJ, Hawley JA, Hopkins WG, Mujika I, Noakes TD. A new reliable laboratory test of endurance performance for road cyclists. *Med Sci Sports Exerc.* 1998;30(12):1744–1750.

76 Kay D, Marino FE, Cannon J, St Clair Gibson A, Lambert MI, Noakes TD. Evidence for neuromuscular fatigue during high-intensity cycling in warm, humid conditions. *Eur J Appl Physiol.* 2001;84(1–2):115–121.

77 St Clair Gibson A, Schabort EJ, Noakes TD. Reduced neuromuscular activity and force generation during prolonged cycling. *Am J Physiol Regul Integr Comp Physiol.* 2001;281(1):R187–R196.

78 Marcora SM, Staiano W. The limit to exercise tolerance in humans: mind over muscle? *Eur J Appl Physiol.* 2010;109(4):763–770.

79 Wittekind AL, Micklewright D, Beneke R. Teleoanticipation in all-out short duration cycling. *Br J Sports Med.* 2011;45:114–119.

80 Amann M, Blain GM, Proctor LT, Sebranek JJ, Pegelow DF, Dempsey JA. Implications of group III and IV muscle afferents for high-intensity endurance exercise performance in humans. *J Physiol.* 2011;589(Pt 21):5299–5309.

81 Edwards AM, Polman RC. Pacing and awareness: brain regulation of physical activity. *Sports Med.* 2013;43(11):1057–1064.

82 Noakes TD. Time to move beyond a brainless exercise physiology: the evidence for complex regulation of human exercise performance. *Appl Physiol Nutr Metab.* 2011;36(1):23–35.

83 Paterson S, Marino FE. Effect of deception of distance on prolonged cycling performance. *Percept Mot Skills.* 2004;98(3 Pt 1):1017–1026.

84 Dugas JP, Oosthuizen U, Tucker R, Noakes TD. Rates of fluid ingestion alter pacing but not thermoregulatory responses during prolonged exercise in hot and humid conditions with appropriate convective cooling. *Eur J Appl Physiol.* 2009;105(1):69–80.

85 Marcora SM, Staiano W, Manning V. Mental fatigue impairs physical performance in humans. *J Appl Physiol (1985).* 2009;106(3):857–864.

86 Rauch HG, St Clair Gibson A, Lambert EV, Noakes TD. A signalling role for muscle glycogen in the regulation of pace during prolonged exercise. *Br J Sports Med.* 2005;39(1):34–38.

87 Marino FE. Anticipatory regulation and avoidance of catastrophe during exercise-induced hyperthermia. *Comp Biochem Physiol B Biochem Mol Biol.* 2004;139(4):561–569.

88 Mauger AR, Jones AM, Williams CA. Influence of feedback and prior experience on pacing during a 4-km cycle time trial. *Med Sci Sports Exerc.* 2009;41(2):451–458.

89 Micklewright D, Papadopoulou E, Swart J, Noakes T. Previous experience influences pacing during 20 km time trial cycling. *Br J Sports Med.* 2010;44(13): 952–960.

90 Saunders AG, Dugas JP, Tucker R, Lambert MI, Noakes TD. The effects of different air velocities on heat storage and body temperature in humans cycling in a hot, humid environment. *Acta Physiol Scand.* 2005;183(3):241–255.

91 Tucker R, Bester A, Lambert EV, Noakes TD, Vaughan CL, St Clair Gibson A. Non-random fluctuations in power output during self-paced exercise. *Br J Sports Med.* 2006;40(11):912–917; discussion 917.

92 Baden DA, McLean TL, Tucker R, Noakes TD, St Clair Gibson A. Effect of anticipation during unknown or unexpected exercise duration on rating of perceived exertion, affect, and physiological function. *Br J Sports Med.* 2005;39(10):742–746; discussion 742–746.

93 Eston R, Stansfield R, Westoby P, Parfitt G. Effect of deception and expected exercise duration on psychological and physiological variables during treadmill running and cycling. *Psychophysiology.* 2012;49(4):462–469.

94 Bolgar MR, Baker CE, Goss FL, Nagle E, Robertson RJ. Effect of exercise intensity on differentiated and undifferentiated ratings of perceived exertion during cycle and treadmill exercise in recreationally active and trained women. *J Sports Sci Med.* 2010;9(4):557–563.

95 Morton RH. Deception by manipulating the clock calibration influences cycle ergometer endurance time in males. *J Sci Med Sport.* 2009;12(2):332–337.

96 Faulkner J, Arnold T, Eston R. Effect of accurate and inaccurate distance feedback on performance markers and pacing strategies during running. *Scand J Med Sci Sports.* 2011;21(6):e176–183.

97 Billaut F, Bishop DJ, Schaerz S, Noakes TD. Influence of knowledge of sprint number on pacing during repeated-sprint exercise. *Med Sci Sports Exerc.* 2011;43(4):665–672.

98 Ansdell P, Thomas K, Howatson G, Amann M, Goodall S. Deception improves time trial performance in well-trained cyclists without augmented fatigue. *Med Sci Sports Exerc.* 2018;50(4):809–816.

99 Swart J, Lindsay TR, Lambert MI, Brown JC, Noakes TD. Perceptual cues in the regulation of exercise performance – physical sensations of exercise and awareness of effort interact as separate cues. *Br J Sports Med.* 2012;46(1):42–48.

100 Presland JD, Dowson MN, Cairns SP. Changes of motor drive, cortical arousal and perceived exertion following prolonged cycling to exhaustion. *Eur J Appl Physiol.* 2005;95(1):42–51.

101 Tucker R, Marle T, Lambert EV, Noakes TD. The rate of heat storage mediates an anticipatory reduction in exercise intensity during cycling at a fixed rating of perceived exertion. *J Physiol.* 2006;574(Pt 3):905–915.

102 Noakes TD. Testing for maximum oxygen consumption has produced a brainless model of human exercise performance. *Br J Sports Med.* 2008;42(7): 551–555.

103 Marcora SM. Do we really need a central governor to explain brain regulation of exercise performance? *Eur J Appl Physiol.* 2008;104(5):929–931; author reply 933–925.

104 Marcora S. Perception of effort during exercise is independent of afferent feedback from skeletal muscles, heart, and lungs. *J Appl Physiol (1985).* 2009;106(6): 2060–2062.

105 Gallagher KM, Fadel PJ, Stromstad M, et al. Effects of partial neuromuscular blockade on carotid baroreflex function during exercise in humans. *J Physiol.* 2001;533(Pt 3):861–870.

106 Kjaer M, Hanel B, Worm L, et al. Cardiovascular and neuroendocrine responses to exercise in hypoxia during impaired neural feedback from muscle. *Am J Physiol.* 1999;277(1):R76–R85.

107 Smith SA, Querry RG, Fadel PJ, et al. Partial blockade of skeletal muscle somatosensory afferents attenuates baroreflex resetting during exercise in humans. *J Physiol.* 2003;551(Pt 3):1013–1021.

108 Myers J, Atwood JE, Sullivan M, et al. Perceived exertion and gas exchange after calcium and beta-blockade in atrial fibrillation. *J Appl Physiol (1985).* 1987; 63(1):97–104.

109 Braith RW, Wood CE, Limacher MC, et al. Abnormal neuroendocrine responses during exercise in heart transplant recipients. *Circulation.* 1992;86(5):1453–1463.

110 Grazzini M, Stendardi L, Gigliotti F, Scano G. Pathophysiology of exercise dyspnea in healthy subjects and in patients with chronic obstructive pulmonary disease (COPD). *Respir Med.* 2005;99(11):1403–1412.

111 Noakes TD, Tucker R. Do we really need a central governor to explain brain regulation of exercise performance? A response to the letter of Dr Marcora. *Eur J Appl Physiol.* 2008;104:933–935.

112 Smirmaul Bde P. Sense of effort and other unpleasant sensations during exercise: clarifying concepts and mechanisms. *Br J Sports Med.* 2012;46(5):308–311.

113 Halperin I, Emanuel A. Rating of perceived effort: methodological concerns and future directions. *Sports Med.* 2020;50(4):679–687.

114 Shephard RJ. Is it time to retire the 'central governor'? *Sports Med.* 2009;39: 709–721.

115 Micklewright D, Parry D. The central governor model cannot be adequately tested by observing its components in isolation. *Sports Med.* 2010;40(1):91–92; author reply 92–94.

116 St Clair Gibson A, Swart J, Tucker R. The interaction of psychological and physiological homeostatic drives and role of general control principles in the regulation of physiological systems, exercise and the fatigue process – the integrative governor theory. *Eur J Sport Sci.* 2018;18(1):25–36.

117 Pageaux B, Lepers R, Dietz KC, Marcora SM. Response inhibition impairs subsequent self-paced endurance performance. *Eur J Appl Physiol.* 2014;114(5): 1095–1105.

118 Salam H, Marcora SM, Hopker JG. The effect of mental fatigue on critical power during cycling exercise. *Eur J Appl Physiol.* 2018;118(1):85–92.

119 Pageaux B. The psychobiological model of endurance performance: an effort-based decision-making theory to explain self-paced endurance performance. *Sports Med.* 2014;44(9):1319–1320.

120 Dallaway N, Lucas S, Marks J, Ring C. Prior brain endurance training improves endurance exercise performance. *Eur J Sport Sci.* 2023;23(7):1–10.

121 Gattoni C, O'Neill V, Tarperi C, Schena F, Marcora SM. The effect of mental fatigue on half-marathon performance: a pragmatic trial. *Sport Sci Health.* 2021;17:807–816.

122 Venhorst A, Micklewright D, Noakes TD. Towards a three-dimensional framework of centrally regulated and goal-directed exercise behaviour: a narrative review. *Br J Sports Med.* 2018;52(15):957–966.

7 Mental fatigue

Dr Suzanna Russell, Sports, Performance, Recovery, Injury and New Technology (SPRINT) Research Centre, Australian Catholic University, in partnership with the Australian Institute of Sport and Queensland Academy of Sport

7.1 Introduction

The understanding of mental fatigue and its relationship with physical performance can be traced back to work by Angelo Mosso in 1891. Mosso proposed that feelings of brain fatigue could have implications on attentiveness, reaction time, and the perceived effort individuals are willing to invest.[1] Although the pioneering work of Mosso took place over a century ago, research investigating mental fatigue and its impact on sport and exercise performance has gained momentum in more recent years. A key publication by Marcora, Staiano and Manning[2] investigated cycling performance under mental fatigue, with the findings sparking increased scientific interest in the area. Subsequently, the area gained rapid scientific attention leading to a systematic review by Van Cutsem, Marcora, De Pauw, Bailey, Meeusen and Roelands,[3] which evidenced a decrease in physical performance as a result of mental fatigue. The findings also revealed duration, intensity, and higher perceived exertion as important factors in the relationships between mental fatigue and physical performance. Since 2017, several research groups have focused their attention towards undertaking fundamental research investigating mental fatigue and aspects of physical performance. More recently, an intensification of research into the impact of mental fatigue on sporting performance has occurred. The growing body of evidence has situated mental fatigue as a current 'hot topic' in sports and exercise science. Mental fatigue is now positioned as an aspect of fatigue that all researchers or practitioners who are working in sport and exercise performance contexts should be cognisant of. Despite the substantial growth in the field of research, the body of high-quality evidence remains in its infancy and numerous questions regarding the impact, assessment, and management of mental fatigue in relation to sport and exercise performance are yet to be answered.

7.2 Defining mental fatigue

Consistent with the topics covered in other chapters of this book, it is crucial to recognise that mental fatigue is positioned as one of many aspects of fatigue that hold relevance to sport and exercise performance. Whilst mental fatigue possesses

DOI: 10.4324/9781003326137-9

its own distinct characteristics that differentiate it from other related concepts, it is important to acknowledge that fatigue is a multifaceted phenomenon with the numerous aspects, e.g., mental, physical, and neuromuscular, often interacting and presenting concurrently. To illustrate this concept, consider the example of deliberately intensifying team sporting drills by overloading defenders compared to attackers. In this scenario, physical fatigue would occur from physical demands including acceleration, deceleration, change of direction, and vertical elevation. Concurrently, mental fatigue may also emerge due to cognitive demands such as information processing, attentional demands, response-inhibition, and sustained attention.

> **Key point 7.1**
>
> *The growing body of evidence highlighting the impact of mental fatigue on sport and exercise performance demonstrates its relevance to both research and practice.*

Mental fatigue is also commonly known as cognitive fatigue, but for the purpose of this chapter, it will be referred to as mental fatigue and discussed in the context of the following definition. Mental fatigue can be defined as the exertion experienced as a result of prolonged demanding cognitive activity that requires sustained mental efficiency.[4] While mental fatigue is commonly named as a psychobiological state, it is typically indicated by a change in subjective, behavioural, or neuro-physiological markers.[5] In other domains, such as cognitive science, the definition of mental fatigue expands to include reduced motivation to sustain attention as required for task performance,[6] lack of energy,[7] and feelings of exhaustion.[8] However, this chapter explores the exercise-related and sports-specific symptoms, which are discussed in Section 7.5.1. Whilst not extensively covered, mental recovery is also addressed in this chapter. Mental recovery is defined as the process of regaining allostatic balance and replenishment of one's cognitive resource and capability through restorative processes.[9]

> **Key point 7.2**
>
> *Mental fatigue is typically defined as a psycho-biological state which is indicated by changes in subjective, behavioural, or neurophysiological markers. Mental recovery refers to the regaining of allostatic balance and replenishment of cognitive resource and capability.*

7.3 Proposed mechanisms of mental fatigue

The precise mechanisms responsible for performance impairments seen with the inducement of mental fatigue remain elusive.[10] The challenge in direct measurement of neurotransmitter changes in humans, particularly during sport and exercise, has hindered our ability to draw definitive conclusions about the specific nature of these neuro-physiological changes. However, various researchers have proposed mechanisms that offer valuable perspectives on the potential mechanisms underlying the performance impairments associated with mental fatigue. The following paragraphs will briefly introduce some of these proposed mechanisms.

7.3.1 Adenosine accumulation

Martin, Meeusen, Thompson, Keegan and Rattray[11] propose a theoretical framework that suggests the accumulation of extracerebral adenosine serves as the primary mechanism responsible for the metal-fatigue-related impairments observed in endurance performance (Figure 7.1). It is widely recognised that the observed reductions in endurance performance are primarily mediated by an increased perception of effort, resulting in a greater rating of perceived exertion (RPE) while other physiological variables such as heart rate, lactate, and neuromuscular function remain largely unaffected by mental fatigue. Martin, Meeusen, Thompson, Keegan and Rattray[11] discuss how demanding cognitive activity leads to the accumulation of extracerebral adenosine, which subsequently impacts endurance performance in two ways. Firstly, adenosine accumulation increases the perception of effort experienced during effortful tasks. Secondly, it impairs motivation, or willingness to exert effort via an interaction with dopamine in the anterior cingulate cortex. Although this proposed mechanism has not yet been quantified through fundamental research, the observed effectiveness of caffeine as an ergogenic aid to counter fatigue provides empirical support for the proposition. Adenosine accumulates in the brain during periods of wakefulness and effortful cognitive activity can accelerate this accumulation, augmenting its role as a modulator of neural activity. This includes inhibiting the release of dopamine and potentially altering the

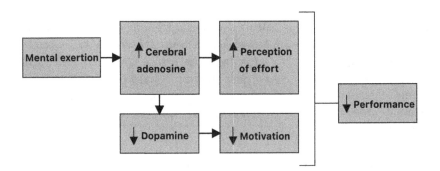

Figure 7.1 Schematic representation of the proposed mechanism.

Source: Re-drawn from Martin K, Meeusen R, Thompson KG, Keegan R, Rattray B. *Sports medicine (Auckland, NZ).* 2018;48(9):2041–2051.

affinity of dopamine receptor binding, with subsequent impacts on regulation of effort-based decision making. While the exploration of adenosine and dopamine antagonism pathways in humans is still pending, findings from ergogenic aids and animal research provide support for the proposed theoretical model. The model highlights the significance of these neuromodulators on adenosine (A1, A2A) and dopamine (D1) receptors in relation to mental fatigue, and subsequent sport and exercise performance.

7.3.2 *Phosphocreatine concentration*

The positive impact of creatine supplementation on cognitive performance also suggests a potential role of the brain concentration of phosphocreatine (PCr) in mental fatigue. Van Cutsem, Roelands, Pluym, Tassigno, Verschueren, De Pauw and Meeusen[12] proposed this theory and investigated the use of creatine supplementation as a potential strategy to counter mental fatigue. Direct measurement of the relationship between PCr availability in the brain, and the consequence of mental fatigue on sport and exercise performance, is currently lacking. However, the study reported improvements in strength, endurance, and cognitive Stroop task performance. Interestingly, these improvements were not attributed to changes in the assessed perceptual or physiological outcomes.[12] Accordingly, the authors suggest that the observed cognitive performance enhancement may involve factors beyond the assessed perceptual and physiological parameters. This model proposes that the localised drop in PCr could mediate neuronal excitability to counteract adenosine release and accumulation, thereby reducing the perception of effort and its behavioural consequences as discussed above. While further investigation is required, the mechanistic role of PCr in mental fatigue and its subsequent effects is plausible.

7.3.3 *Role of Interoception*

The interoceptive mechanism theory, proposed by McMorris,[13] offers insights into the role of motivation and perception of effort costs in explaining the impact of mental fatigue on sport and exercise performance. The theory encompasses multiple brain regions and complex processes, involving interactions between top-down predictions of effort and bottom-up feedback. According to McMorris,[13] the theory suggests that the differential predications of expected sensory consequences of undertaking exercise, as compared to the actual cost experienced during the exercise, may moderate performance output. Motivation is therefore closely tied to this theory, as evidence suggests that using psychological strategies to manipulate motivation can aid in mitigating the impairments on exercise performance that are induced by mental fatigue (Figure 7.2).

The influence of mental fatigue on sport and exercise performance outcomes is likely a result of a complex interaction among neurobiological, physiological, psychological, and behavioural processes. Accordingly, it is reasonable that the

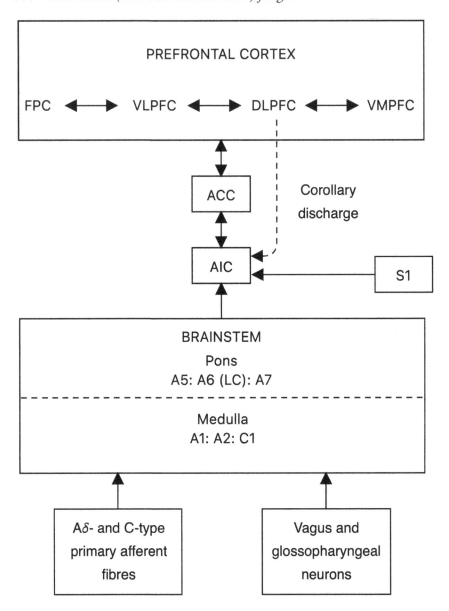

Figure 7.2 Schematic of afferent activation in the interoceptive system. *ACC* anterior
cingulate cortex, *AIC* anterior insula cortex, *DLPFC* dorsolateral prefrontal cortex, *FPC* frontopolar cortex, *VLPFC* ventrolateral prefrontal cortex,
VMPFC ventromedial prefrontal cortex, *S1* somatosensory cortex.

Source: Re-drawn from McMorris T. *Sports Medicine.* 2020:1–6.

mechanisms discussed above all contribute to a degree to the observed performance impairments resulting from mental fatigue. Continued advancements in imaging techniques for direct measurement of neuro-physiological changes, adherences to methodological research guidelines for reporting, and the implementation of countermeasures will significantly contribute to the expansion of knowledge concerning the proposed mechanisms underlying the impact of mental fatigue on exercise performance.

> **Key point 7.3**
>
> *Various researchers have proposed mechanisms that offer valuable perspectives on the potential mechanisms underlying the performance impairments associated with mental fatigue. Whilst the relationship likely involves a complex interaction among neurobiological, physiological, psychological, and behavioural processes, adenosine accumulation, brain concentration of phosphocreatine, and a role of interception are hypothesised mechanisms.*

7.4 Impact of mental fatigue on sport and exercise performance

Prior systematic reviews and meta-analyses have provided comprehensive evaluations of the effects of mental fatigue on physical performance[3,14] and sports-specific psychomotor performance.[15] This evidence supports the potential for mental fatigue to impact the everyday exerciser or those participating in recreational sport. More recently, systematic and scoping reviews focused on aspects such as athlete skilled performance,[16] team sport athletes,[17,18] soccer,[19,20] and basketball performance[21] have been published. In addition, narrative reviews and perspective articles have synthesised the evidence and provided contextual discussion of mental fatigue in elite team sports[22] and specifically in soccer.[23] Collectively, these publications synthesise the growing body of literature which highlights the potential adverse effects of mental fatigue on sport and exercise performance. It is important to note that the intention of this section is not to provide detail or critical analysis of individual studies investigating this impact, and such information can be found in the original research manuscripts or relevant reviews. Individual studies may however be referenced as examples to illustrate how mental fatigue has been shown to negatively influence different aspects of sport and exercise performance.

7.4.1 Physical performance

From a physical performance standpoint, the evidence convincingly supports the notion that mental fatigue has a negative impact on endurance performance. However, the findings regarding its impact on strength, power, and anaerobic-type tasks are mixed.

7.4.1.1   Endurance performance

Extensive research has investigated mental fatigue and its subsequent impairment on endurance performance. Various task types, such as time to exhaustion, time trial (completion time), and standardised endurance ramp-based protocols have been employed to demonstrate the negative impacts following inducement of mental fatigue. These effects have been observed across different whole-body exercise modalities including cycling, running, and swimming.[3]

Marcora, Staiano and Manning[2] investigated the influence of mental fatigue on cycling time to exhaustion at 80% of peak power output, using a 90-minute cognitively demanding task (AX-continuous performance test) or a 90-minute control condition (watching emotionally neutral documentaries). Time to exhaustion was significantly reduced compared with the control condition, and perception of effort was significantly higher, following the inducement of mental fatigue. These findings provide evidence that mental fatigue reduces the duration of endurance exercise an individual can perform and reinforces the mediating role of higher perception of effort.

Mental fatigue has also been shown to impair performance in time trials. Pires, Silva-Júnior, Brietzke, Franco-Alvarenga, Pinheiro, de França, Teixeira and Meireles Santos[24] demonstrated mental fatigue to impair 20km time-trial cycling performance by ~2.7%. Following a 30-minute cognitively demanding task (rapid visual information processing), compared to a 30-minute control of seated rest, lower wattage and a steeper increase in RPE were also observed. In the context of running, mental fatigue was found to increase completion time in a 3,000 m time trial on an indoor track. Completion time increased significantly following a 90-minute cognitively demanding task (AX-continuous performance test), compared to a 90-minute emotionally neutral documentary.[25] Similarly, Pageaux, Lepers, Dietz and Marcora[26] reported a greater impairment in 5,000 m running time-trial performance following 30 minutes of a cognitively demanding response-inhibition task, compared to a control task requiring no response-inhibition. These findings highlight the negative impact of demanding cognitive tasks on average running speed and consequent performance outputs during a self-paced set distance. Penna, Wanner, Campos, Quinan, Filho, Mendes, Smith and Prado[27] investigated the effect of mental fatigue on the completion time of a 1,500 m swim. Completion time increased by 1.2% following a 30-minute cognitively demanding task (Stroop task), compared to the control of watching an emotionally neutral video.

Mental fatigue has also been shown to negatively impact incremental ramp-based protocols commonly used in laboratory and field settings. For instance, Brietzke, Franco-Alvarenga, Canestri, Goethel, Vínicius, Painelli, Santos, Hettinga and Pires[28] investigated the effect of mental fatigue on cycling performance during a maximal incremental test. Following a 40-minute cognitive task (rapid visual information processing test), a reduction in cycling performance during the maximal incremental test was found, compared to when no cognitive task was completed prior. The Yo-Yo intermittent recovery test is commonly used as an indicator of fitness in team sports and requires the repeated performance of high-intensity aerobic work. A 30-minute cognitive task (Stroop) resulted in a significantly reduced running distance covered by soccer players in the Yo-Yo intermittent recovery test, compared to the 30-minute control of reading emotionally neutral magazines.[29] The same 30-minute cognitively demanding and control protocols have been replicated with elite cricketers. Again, a significant reduction in distance covered was observed following the inducement of mental fatigue.[30] Together, the findings provide support for a negative impact of mental fatigue on performance during the Yo-Yo intermittent recovery test across team sports.

> **Key point 7.4**
>
> *The large majority of the evidence to date has investigated the impact of mental fatigue on subsequent endurance performance. The findings consistently indicate a negative impact on both whole-body and isolated endurance protocols, across a range of different exercise modalities.*

In addition to its impact on whole-body endurance tasks, mental fatigue has been shown to have a negative impact on local muscle or isolated endurance protocols. Dallaway, Lucas and Ring[31] found a 20-minute cognitively demanding task (Stroop or N-back) to result in impairment of performance on a rhythmic handgrip exercise, which was not impaired by the control condition (watching an emotionally neutral documentary).

7.4.1.2 *Strength, power, and anaerobic performance*

Research conducted on the impact of mental fatigue on physical performance has primarily focused on endurance tasks, revealing consistent impairments in performance. However, some research has been directed towards the impact of mental fatigue on strength, power, and anaerobic performance tasks, which has yielded less consistent results. Due to the limited available evidence, and the greater variability in outcomes, it is important to interpret such findings with caution until a more robust and extensive evidence base is established. Nonetheless, several individual studies have provided insight into the detrimental effects of mental fatigue on these specific tasks.

In a study by Gantois, Lima-Júnior, Fortes, Batista, Nakamura and Fonseca,[32] social networking application use was employed as a 30-minute cognitive demanding task. Following this, when participating in a strength training session consisting of a half-back squat exercise to failure at 80% of 15 repetition max, a lower volume load during the session was observed. Additionally, Staiano, Bonet, Romagnoli and Ring[33] investigated a 90-minute cognitively demanding task (AX-continuous performance test) compared to a 90-minute control of watching emotionally neutral videos, on subsequent resistance training performance. The findings indicated a greater RPE resulting from lifting with the inducement of mental fatigue. Evidence further demonstrates that mental fatigue can impact performance during a high-intensity, body weight, resistance task involving repetition of 5 pull ups, 10 push ups, and 15 unweighted squats. A 52-minute cognitively demanding intervention (vigilance task of Low Go/High No-Go) was shown to decrease the percentage of time-on-task during the workout, compared to the control of an emotionally neutral video.[34]

It is important to consider the nature of the performance task and associated demands when assessing the impact of mental fatigue on non-endurance-based tasks. Although high-intensity exercise is typically renowned for being largely unaffected by mental fatigue, overall distance covered during a 45-minute intermittent running protocol has been reduced with the presence of mental fatigue.[35] Accordingly, while individuals may be able to maintain performance during an all-out bout of high-intensity activity, this may have consequences on recovery, or overall task performance. When considering the impact on non-endurance-based physical tasks, it is important to reflect on the demands of how the task is usually performed in practice, i.e., as a one-off isolated effort or in a repeated manner.

7.4.2   Technical performance

Early research largely focused on the potential consequences of mental fatigue on physical aspects of performance. However, attention has been increasingly directed beyond physical performance towards psychomotor performance, including technical and skill aspects.[15] The vast majority of this research has been focused on soccer, however the impact of mental fatigue on racquet sports, cricket, and sprinting technique have also been investigated.

Smith, Zeuwts, Lenoir, Hens, De Jong and Coutts[36] reported soccer passing response time and accuracy to be impaired during small-sided games following a 30-minute cognitively demanding task (Stroop) compared to a 30-minute control of reading emotionally neutral magazines. In a different study, Smith, Coutts, Merlini, Deprez, Lenoir and Marcora[29] again employed the same 30-minute cognitively demanding and 30-minute control protocol and found mentally fatigued players committed more passing and ball control errors and had reduced shot accuracy and speed. Together, these findings demonstrate how mental fatigue may impair speed and accuracy of soccer-specific skill execution and decision making.

A negative impact of mental fatigue has also been demonstrated on racquet sports including tennis and table tennis. Filipas, Rossi, Codella and Bonato[37] assessed tennis serve accuracy following a 30-minute cognitively demanding task (Stroop) or control of an easy cognitive task. Whilst no differences in serve speed were detected between conditions, the percentage of failed services from the deuce (right) side of the court was greater following the cognitively demanding task. Le Mansec, Pageaux, Nordez, Dorel and Jubeau[38] also reported a negative impact of a 90-minute cognitively demanding task (AX-continuous performance test), on technical aspects of table tennis performance, when compared to a 90-minute control of watching an emotionally neutral movie. Mental fatigue significantly decreased the ball speed and shot accuracy and increased the number of faults committed. Collectively, these findings indicate mental fatigue can have a negative impact on technical execution in racquet sports.

Sprinting is a physically demanding task, yet the technical components of sprinting (e.g., reaction time) are also important to the overall performance outcome of the task. Englert and Bertrams[39] used a 6-minute cognitively demanding transcription task and a non-depletion (fatiguing) condition followed by 10 m maximal sprints. A slower reaction time was found following the fatiguing condition. Englert, Persaud, Oudejans and Bertrams[40] used the same cognitively demanding and control tasks with results showing an increased number of false starts following the cognitively demanding task. Coupled together, these studies demonstrate an increase in the reaction time to start the task and in the number of false starts, demonstrating prior cognitive demand to impair technical components of sprinting performance.

In addition to the observed impairments in simple reaction time, Van Cutsem, De Pauw, Vandervaeren, Marcora, Meeusen and Roelands[41] demonstrated a negative effect of a 90-minute cognitively demanding task (Stroop) on response time during a more complex visuomotor task. Following the cognitively demanding condition, a significantly slower response time to the complex stimuli task was found, compared to the 90-minute control of watching an emotionally neutral documentary. The visuomotor task required participants to respond to the random appearance of specific-coloured light stimuli with differing physical movements required, depending on the colour that appeared. Veness, Patterson, Jeffries and Waldron[30] employed the study protocol as described above, and also demonstrated an increase in the cricket run-two test, an English Cricket Board standardised test. This task also assesses response time and technical execution, by timing the total duration it takes an invididual to sprint the equivalent to one length of a cricket pitch (17.68 m), touch their cricket bat over the crease line, and turn 180° to sprint back. Mental fatigue was found to statistically increase the run-two completion time. Mental fatigue can therefore not only impair simple response time but also execution of more complex technical skills.

7.4.3 *Tactical performance*

The impact of mental fatigue on tactical performance has again not been extensively researched. However, there is some evidence to support that mental fatigue may alter tactical execution. Coutinho, Gonçalves, Travassos, Wong, Coutts and Sampaio[42] demonstrated an impact on tactical performance using a 20-minute whole-body coordination task to induce mental fatigue and compared to a control condition involving light physical activity without the cognitive demand. Following the cognitively demanding task, a decrease in the level of dyadic synchronisation was found, demonstrating tactical behaviour to be negatively impacted. Kunrath, Nakamura, Roca, Tessitore and Teoldo Da Costa[43] found a 30-minute mentally fatiguing task (Stroop) to impact tactical execution in comparison to the 30-minute control task of watching an emotionally neutral documentary. Following the cognitively demanding task, alternations in several tactical behaviours were observed. Mental fatigue appeared to constrain players to more frequently perform penetration, depth mobility, and defensive unity. Further, players less frequently performed the actions of defensive coverage and balance. This had a con-

> **Key point 7.5**
>
> *Recent studies have revealed mental fatigue can impact not only physical performance, but also technical and tactical aspects of performance. In simple terms, mental fatigue can influence the speed or accuracy when executing skills, in addition to how players interact and move in relation to each other.*

sequence on physical work done, with greater distances covered overall at a moderate speed with mental fatigue, demonstrating that the impact of mental fatigue on tactical performance can result in an overall reduction in players' movement efficiency.

7.4.4 Psychological performance

Several studies, from both within the sport and exercise domain and other areas including transport and mining research, demonstrate a negative impact of mental fatigue on reaction time. Often an increase in response time and a decrease in response accuracy are used as a behavioural manipulation check to determine the inducement of mental fatigue. Habay, Van Cutsem, Verschueren, De Bock, Proost, De Wachter, Tassignon, Meeusen and Roelands[15] summarise this in their systematic review, where several examples of this impact are referenced. As briefly discussed in the section of this chapter summarising the proposed mechanisms behind the performance impairments seen with mental fatigue, RPE is believed to be a major mediator. Again, multiple examples of studies demonstrating a greater RPE with the inducement of mental fatigue can be found in the systematic review by Van Cutsem, Marcora, De Pauw, Bailey, Meeusen and Roelands.[3] The relationship between mental fatigue and motivation is complex, in that the effect of mental fatigue appears to be potentially counteracted by increased motivation.[3] Accordingly, effects on motivational processes need to be considered as a psychological consequence of mental fatigue. However, further research is needed to explore this notion and understand the intricacies of the relationship.[15]

> **Key point 7.6**
>
> *In line with the psychobiological nature of mental fatigue, psychological impacts, including increased perception of effort and reduced exercise intention, are also found with mental fatigue. This can impact the way the everyday exerciser may engage with physical activity and exercise.*

Further, Brown and Bray[44] have demonstrated that 50 minutes of high cognitive load can reduce the subsequent intended RPE and reduce the amount of total work performed by individuals. The findings evidence that mental fatigue reduces the amount of effort individuals are willing to invest in a workout, resulting in a reduction in the work they do and their ability to adhere to current physical activity guidelines. In line with this, Harris and Bray[45] demonstrated that higher cognitive demand and the subsequent mental fatigue are linked to higher perceived costs of engaging in exercise, rather than sedentary alternatives. Combined these studies indicate that mental fatigue can reduce both exercise performance and an individual's motivation to engage in physical activity.

7.5   Athlete experiences of mental fatigue

7.5.1   *Athlete perceptions of mental fatigue*

The above impacts of mental fatigue on sport and exercise performance are well evidenced by several studies which induce mental fatigue mostly through the use of computer-based cognitively demanding tasks. Despite the growing body of evidence to support the impact, such literature has been critiqued regarding its lack of ecological validity.[46] Counterarguments propose that regardless of the inducement method, the same neurobiological changes occur, making the current literature largely translatable to the applied setting. Either way to apply the findings regarding the impact of mental fatigue on aspects of performance and invest time and resources into the management of mental fatigue and mental recovery, coaches, practitioners, and athletes themselves must identify and understand mental fatigue in their daily training and competition environments.[22] Accordingly, evidence which examines how athletes experience mental fatigue in sporting environments has emerged in recent years.

Qualitative research has informed some of the sports-specific causes and symptoms of mental fatigue and the perceived impact on performance. These findings justify that athletes perceive mental fatigue to be real with impact on their performance and recovery, both in competition and training periods. Russell, Jenkins, Rynne, Halson and Kelly[47] were the first to use qualitative approaches to research athlete perceptions of mental fatigue. Focus group discussions confirmed that athletes and practitioners perceive mental fatigue to negatively impact sporting performance. Signs and symptoms which may indicate athlete mental fatigue were also revealed (Figure 7.3) including disengagement, decreases in motivation and enthusiasm, increased displays of emotion, and withdrawal. Such indicators are also reinforced by Lam, Sproule, Turner, Murgatroyd, Gristwood, Richards and Phillips[48] who in a Delphi consensus project indicated mental fatigue to impact perceptual responses and emotional state in orienteering. Changes in concentration and feelings of a "full or active brain" were also reported by athletes as symptoms, in addition to an association with decreased discipline and attention to detail.[47] With regard to causes of mental fatigue (Figure 7.4), the presence and nature of

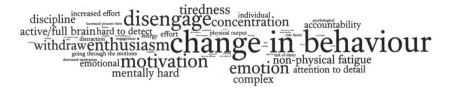

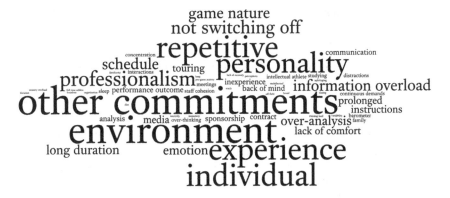

Figure 7.3 Worldcloud presenting the nature of perceived descriptors and symptoms of mental fatigue.

Source: Re-drawn from Russell S, Jenkins D, Rynne S, Halson S, Kelly V. *Eur J Sport Sci.* 2019;19(10):1367–1376.

Figure 7.4 Worldcloud presenting the nature of perceived causes or inducers of mental fatigue.

Source: Re-drawn from Russell S, Jenkins D, Rynne S, Halson S, Kelly V. *Eur J Sport Sci.* 2019;19(10):1367–1376.

other commitments, including activities such as external study, emotionally challenging work, media, sponsorship engagements, driving between commitments under time pressure, and challenges in managing relationship dynamics, have been raised as potential contributors.[47] Feelings of unfamiliarity or instability in the environment, such as travel to a new location or changing team members, are also indicated inducers. The professionalism of sport in addition to the repetitive nature and long duration of activities such as training drills, over analysis, and the need for constant problem solving were also cited. Further, constantly thinking about the sport in question and an inability to switch off were perceived to contribute to athlete mental fatigue. Many of these causes have been reinforced by the work of Thompson, Smith, Coutts, Skorski, Datson, Smith and Meyer,[49] where international female footballers indicated travel fatigue, an inability to switch off from football, team meetings, and pressure to succeed were causes of mental fatigue. Perceptions of the temporal nature of mental fatigue were also discussed in these qualitative studies. There is a strong perception from athletes and practitioners that mental fatigue exists in both an acute and cumulative manner.[47] Findings by Lam,

Sproule, Turner, Murgatroyd, Gristwood, Richards and Phillips[48] also further support the consensus that mental fatigue can be developed both acutely and chronically.

Athletes support the notion of perception of effort as a major mediator on performance, indicating activities to require increased effort when mentally fatigued.[47] The intent and intensity at which athletes engage with training may also be negatively influenced by mental fatigue, where they may be more likely to be "going through the motions" in addition to having slower response and reaction times. Impaired decision making, impulse control, emotional regulation, and diminished willpower have also been reported as perceived impacts by athletes and staff.

7.5.2 Athlete reports of mental fatigue in training, competition, and camp settings

Whilst early evidence has explored mental fatigue primarily via fundamental laboratory study designs, evidence which has explored athlete reports of mental fatigue has more recently emerged. As further discussed in the research approaches and limitations section of this chapter, feasibility barriers exist for the translation of neuro-physiological and behavioural assessment approaches to indicate mental fatigue in the applied setting. Accordingly, a large portion of the work exploring athlete experiences of mental fatigue in daily training and competition settings employs subjective indicators of mental fatigue. Nonetheless, this evidence base has begun to inform us about how athletes may experience mental fatigue during their daily pre-season, in-season, training or selection camps, and off-season settings. Overall, this evidence highlights to practitioners and researchers the importance of being cognisant of mental fatigue and mental recovery, and not just assessing but also managing these important factors across these phases.

Sport itself has been shown to demand various cognitive domains including information processing, working memory, response-inhibition, information recall, and sustained attention.[50] Evidence from Russell, Jenkins, Halson and Kelly[51] demonstrated mental fatigue in elite development athletes to increase significantly during a 60-minute netball match. This research obtained subjective ratings of mental fatigue within 30 minutes prior to, and following, 12 competitive matches during the season. The findings demonstrated that athletes report an increase in mental, as well as physical, fatigue during a 60-minute match. While further research should explore the extent of mental fatigue in differing sports, the duration of netball matches are comparative to other sports, and therefore indicate competitive fixtures in team sports are likely to cause elevations in athlete mental fatigue.

In addition to competition, athletes demonstrate fluctuations in self-reported mental fatigue across the pre-season phase. The pre-season phase is necessary to prepare athletes physically, technically, tactically, and psychologically for competition. Accordingly, fatigue and subsequent adaptation is a common and deliberate part of the pre-season phase. Work by Russell, Jenkins, Halson and Kelly[52] assessed athlete reports of mental fatigue across a 16-week pre-season. The findings demonstrated athletes to experience fluctuations in mental fatigue across the pre-season phase, with elevated levels reported during the later pre-season weeks.

As the evidence on how athletes experience mental fatigue has developed, a few studies have explored athlete reports of mental fatigue during the season. Russell, Jenkins, Halson, Juliff, Connick and Kelly[53] completed a league-wide study across two seasons and observed fluctuations in mental fatigue during both seasons. When accounting for individual heterogeneity and team, athletes reported higher ratings in round games towards the later part of each season. Abbott, Brownlee, Naughton, Clifford, Page and Harper[54] also assessed changes in perception of mental fatigue across a competitive season with academy soccer players. Athletes reported mental fatigue on match day and the days immediately following. Using this method, the ten players from the one team included in the study indicated higher mental fatigue reports during the early and mid-phase of the season, compared to the late season. While these findings differ from the prior league-wide outcomes, they support fluctuations and changes in athletes' experiences across phases. Further, a significant relationship with match outcome (win, draw, or loss) was found. Thus, contextual variables, such as outcome, hold potential to influence the phase-based observations.

Lastly, athlete reports of mental fatigue during differing international, competition, training, and preparation camps have been investigated.[55] Athlete reports of mental fatigue across eight training camps and six competition periods with international netballers revealed athletes to report elevated mental fatigue during training camps and preparation camps, compared to competition periods. The findings also revealed that, within specific individual camp and competition periods, differing levels of mental fatigue were reported by the group. Therefore, there is evidence to support that mental fatigue is not limited to competition, and elevations may be seen during intensified training and preparation periods, supporting the justification of regular monitoring and intentional proactive management.

> **Key point 7.7**
>
> *Athlete reports indicate fluctuations and instances of elevated mental fatigue in the daily training, competition, and camp settings.*

7.5.3 Differentiating mental fatigue and other common athlete self-report measures

As discussed throughout the chapter, mental fatigue is one of many aspects of fatigue worthy of consideration and management in sport and exercise. The multifaceted nature of fatigue makes identification and management of specific aspects challenging. This is especially true when individuals are exposed to both mental and physical demands concurrently, as is the case during sport and exercise. However, evidence from athletes indicates mental fatigue to be interactive with, yet a largely separate construct to, physical fatigue. Data obtained from athlete reports in daily training and competition environments indicated the shared variance between the aspects of fatigue to be 13.9%[51] and 14.3%.[52] The relationship of mental fatigue with other common athlete self-report measures has also been explored. Using ordinal regression models with two seasons of league-wide data, Russell, Jenkins, Halson, Juliff, Connick and Kelly[53] observed athlete reports of mental fatigue to significantly differ from physical fatigue, tiredness, stress, mood, and motivation. These are common self-report measures collected to indicate signs or symptoms of fatigue, with the findings demonstrating mental fatigue to be a unique aspect when reported by athletes. It is noted that in this study, there was no significant difference found between athlete reports of mental fatigue and sleep quality. However, single subjective assessment of sleep quality is not directly indicative of sleep efficiency, and the athletes completed these self-report measures within 30 minutes of waking. Accordingly, based on the proposed mechanisms behind mental fatigue, the potential increase in extracellular cerebral adenosine accumulation as a result of cognitive demand may have been countered by the effects of sleep in decreasing extracellular cerebral adenosine accumulation.[11] Athletes' experiences of mental fatigue largely differ from commonly collected athlete self-report measures, impressing the need for mental fatigue to be included as an independent measure indicative of athlete well-being and performance.

> **Key point 7.8**
>
> *Athlete reports indicate they perceive mental fatigue to differ to the majority of commonly obtained athlete self-report measures. This positions mental fatigue as a largely separate construct worthy of assessment and active management.*

7.6 Management of mental fatigue

Following the evidence demonstrating potentially negative consequences of mental fatigue on sport and exercise performance, attention has been directed towards strategies which may aid in the management of mental fatigue. Management of mental fatigue can take multiple approaches. Evidence supports a combination of employing acute mitigation countermeasures, strategies which enhance mental recovery, and the deliberate inducement to expose athletes to attempting to perform under mental fatigue. This brief section informs some of the available options for managing mental fatigue and mental recovery to help inform decisions around the practical application of these strategies.

7.6.1 *Acute countermeasures to mitigate mental fatigue and enhance mental recovery*

Proost, Habay, De Wachter, De Pauw, Rattray, Meeusen, Roelands and Van Cutsem[5] systematically reviewed acute countermeasures to mental fatigue, which had a physiological, behavioural, or psychological basis, and were employed prior to the performance task. The findings revealed that caffeine, odours, music, and extrinsic motivation appear most promising with regard to the acute mitigation (within seven days) of the effects of mental fatigue on subsequent performance. Several other strategies were identified, highlighting the broad range of techniques which have been investigated for this purpose. Such emerging evidence indicates promise for behavioural approaches such as listening to binaural beats, music, powernaps, or spending time in nature. Other physiological and nutritional aids with potential include creatine, cocoa flavanols, panax ginseng, and other substances mixed with caffeine. In addition to the provision of extrinsic motivation via feedback, other psychological strategies which may be of benefit include mindfulness and systematic breathing performed both with and without mental imagery.

7.6.2   Deliberate inducement of mental fatigue

In addition to acute mitigation of mental fatigue and enhancement of mental recovery, recent evidence suggests benefit of deliberately exposing individuals to mental fatigue to improve tolerance to performing under mental fatigue. Broadly, this concept has been coined 'brain endurance training' (BET), which involves engaging in cognitively fatiguing tasks. This can be delivered using differing modalities: in isolation following exercise, concurrently whilst continuously performing physical exercise, or intermittently rotating between cognitive and physical tasks. BET has been shown to be more effective at improving physical performance than physical training alone.[56,57] Specific protocols vary between studies with differing cognitive tasks and varying session durations employed. Current evidence indicates concurrent or post-exercise BET programmes lasting 20–30 minutes per session, three to four sessions per week, over four to six weeks, to be effective. Whilst specific mechanisms remain elusive, BET is proposed to support the development of resilience to mental fatigue and result in reduced mental effort experienced during physical activity.

> **Key point 7.9**
>
> *A range of strategies exist to manipulate mental fatigue and mental recovery to mitigate the potentially negative effects of mental fatigue on sport and exercise performance. Practitioners should be aware of available strategies and work to apply them on an individual basis where possible.*

7.7   Research approaches and limitations

There are several contextual factors to consider when interpreting the evidence around mental fatigue and applying them to practice and further research. The purpose of this section is not to provide an extensive overview of relevant considerations but to highlight a few key factors to consider when interpreting research on mental fatigue and sport and exercise performance.

Firstly, there has been considerable debate and discussion around the way in which mental fatigue is typically induced. Regardless of the choice of task, and whether it reflects the demands experienced by everyday exercisers and athletes, reporting of the targeted cognitive domains, and the duration and formation of the task are important for research translation. Secondly, inconsistencies in the way in which mental fatigue is identified or assessed can make interpretation and application challenging. Ideally, a combination of subjective, behavioural, and neuro-physiological markers should be used to indicate a state of mental fatigue. However, due to cost, access to equipment, and practical feasibility, it can be challenging to obtain markers from all three categories when assessing mental fatigue in a sport and exercise setting. Accordingly, large heterogeneity in use of markers is seen[5] which creates challenges in interpreting findings. Where possible, it is recommended that two or more indicators are used to assess mental fatigue.

Contextual differences may also need to be considered when interpreting responses to mental fatigue. Typically, large variability is seen with regard to responses to the deliberate inducement of mental fatigue, with varying severity of consequences and performance impact. For example, evidence from Martin, Thompson, Keegan and Rattray[58] demonstrated that individuals who reported higher levels of occupational cognitive demand better maintained physical endurance performance following mental exertion. This was one of the first projects to report influence of self-regulation as an individual moderating factor. The findings suggest that individuals who regularly engage in activities that require self-regulation may be protective towards the influence of mental fatigue. This work aligns with prior work which demonstrated professional cyclists to show greater resistance to the negative effects of mental fatigue than recreationally trained cyclists.[59] Another example of a contextual factor which may influence response to mental fatigue is sex. Jaydari Fard and Lavender[60] reported no significant differences in mental fatigue inducement between male and female groups; however, findings indicated task unfamiliarity had more of a negative influence on rection time for females than males. Lopes, Oliveira, Simurro, Akiba, Nakamura, Okano, Dias and Silva[61] found no sex differences in the impairment in aerobic running performance following inducement of mental fatigue. However, their findings indicated that perhaps being an athlete may make females more resistant to developing mental fatigue and experiencing the subsequent performance impacts in comparison to males, for which the athlete effect was not observed. Accordingly, whether performance level, sex differences, or the factors combined influence responses to mental fatigue remains largely elusive. Potential interindividual differences in susceptibility to mental fatigue have been systematically reviewed by Habay, Uylenbroeck, Van Droogenbroeck, De Wachter, Proost, Tassignon, De Pauw, Meeusen, Pattyn, Van Cutsem and Roelands.[62] They identified no effect of selected individual features (age, sex, body mass index, and performance level). However, these findings were likely attributed to methodological limitations. The authors suggested the under-reporting of participant characteristics, lack of standardisation across studies, and exclusion criteria of potentially influential variations may provide reasoning for the inconclusive effects. To enhance the capacity for practitioners to apply findings from research outputs on mental fatigue and mental recovery, future research should aim to clearly report these factors. Following guidelines such as the CONSORT,[63] STROBE,[64] CHERRIES,[65] and SAGER[66] for research undertaken within this field will allow practitioners to find relevant evidence to the individuals they are working with. At present, assessing response to mental fatigue and applying individual management strategies is recommended for practitioners.

Key point 7.10

To continue to progress the evidence base around mental fatigue and sport and exercise performance, researchers must intentionally report on relevant contextual factors to support practitioner interpretation and application of findings.

7.8   Practical applications and conclusions

- This chapter has introduced the concept of mental fatigue and mental recovery and provided background on the proposed physiological mechanisms behind mental fatigue.
- A summary of the impact on aspects of sport and exercise performance, athlete experiences of mental fatigue, management approaches, and future recommendations for research on the topic have been provided.

Key point 7.11

The relevance of mental fatigue and mental recovery to sport and exercise performance has gained scientific attention. Mental fatigue should be considered as an important aspect of fatigue in both research and practice, with critical thinking utilised when interpreting findings to inform evidence-based guidelines and practice.

- Mental fatigue and mental recovery have rapidly gained scientific attention in application to sport and exercise.
- In consideration of this, critical thinking should be applied when interpreting findings whilst research continues to develop practically applicable evidence-based guidelines.
- Nonetheless, mental fatigue should be an aspect of fatigue which practitioners are aware of and can consider in their practice.
- It is again noted that mental fatigue is one of many aspects of fatigue, and the perspective that multiple factors determine a state of fatigue should remain.

To think about case study

You are working with a soccer player contracted to a professional academy. Their regular pre-season training schedule consists of four on-field sessions, three strength-based sessions, two group tactical sessions, and one individual skill development session per week. Pre-season trial matches (which will inform final squad selection) commence in three weeks and the athlete has shared with you that they are feeling mentally fatigued, quoting perception of effort, decreased emotional regulation, and a reduction in discipline around many aspects of their training.

Based on the content of this chapter, how might you manage this athlete's mental fatigue and mental recovery? Consider how you may identify specific causes of their mental fatigue with regard to sports-specific lifestyle inducers, and the array of mitigation strategies available.

References

1 Di Giulio C, Daniele F, Tipton CM. Angelo Mosso and muscular fatigue: 116 years after the first congress of physiologists: IUPS commemoration. *Adv Physiol Educ*. Jun 2006;30(2):51–7. doi:10.1152/advan.00041.2005

2 Marcora SM, Staiano W, Manning V. Mental fatigue impairs physical performance in humans. *J Appl Physiol*. 2009;106(3):857–864.

3 Van Cutsem J, Marcora S, De Pauw K, Bailey S, Meeusen R, Roelands B. The effects of mental fatigue on physical performance: a systematic review. *Sports medicine (Auckland, NZ)*. 2017;47(8):1569–1588. doi:10.1007/s40279-016-0672-0

4 Lorist MM, Boksem MA, Ridderinkhof KR. Impaired cognitive control and reduced cingulate activity during mental fatigue. *Cogn Brain Res*. 2005;24(2):199–205.

5 Proost M, Habay J, De Wachter J, et al. How to tackle mental fatigue: a systematic review of potential countermeasures and their underlying mechanisms. *Sports Medicine*. 2022; 52(9):2129-2158. doi: 10.1007/s40279-022-01678-z

6 Chaudhuri A, Behan PO. Fatigue in neurological disorders. *The Lancet*. March 20, 2004;363(9413):978–988. doi: 10.1016/S0140-6736(04)15794-2

7 Boksem M, Tops M. Mental fatigue: costs and benefits. *Brain Res Rev*. 2008;59(1):125–139.

8 Qi P, Ru H, Gao L, et al. Neural mechanisms of mental fatigue revisited: new insights from the brain connectome. *Engineering*. April 1, 2019;5(2):276–286. doi: 10.1016/j.eng.2018.11.025

9 Kellmann M, Bertollo M, Bosquet L, et al. Recovery and performance in sport: consensus statement. *Int J Sports Physiol Perform*. February 1, 2018;13(2): 240–245. doi: 10.1123/ijspp.2017–0759

10 Roelands B, Kelly V, Russell S, Habay J. The physiological nature of mental fatigue: current knowledge and future avenues for sport science. *Int J Sports Physiol Perform*. 2021:1–2. doi: 10.1123/ijspp.2021–0524

11 Martin K, Meeusen R, Thompson KG, Keegan R, Rattray B. Mental fatigue impairs endurance performance: a physiological explanation. *Sports medicine (Auckland, NZ)*. September 2018;48(9):2041–2051. doi: 10.1007/s40279-018-0946-9

12 Van Cutsem J, Roelands B, Pluym B, et al. Can creatine combat the mental fatigue-associated decrease in visuomotor skills? *Med Sci Sports Exerc.* 2019;52(1): 120–130. doi: 10.1249/mss.0000000000002122

13 McMorris T. Cognitive fatigue effects on physical performance: the role of interoception. *Sports Med.* 2020;50(10):1703-1708. doi: 10.1007/s40279-020-01320-w. PMID: 32661840

14 McMorris T, Barwood M, Hale BJ, Dicks M, Corbett J. Cognitive fatigue effects on physical performance: a systematic review and meta-analysis. *Physiol Behav.* May 1, 2018;188:103–107. doi: 10.1016/j.physbeh.2018.01.029

15 Habay J, Van Cutsem J, Verschueren J, et al. Mental fatigue and sport-specific psychomotor performance: a systematic review. *Sports Med.* 2021;51(7):1527–1548. doi: 10.1007/s40279-021-01429-6

16 Sun H, Soh KG, Roslan S, Wazir MRWN, Soh KL. Does mental fatigue affect skilled performance in athletes? A systematic review. *PLoS One.* 2021;16(10):e0258307. doi: 10.1371/journal.pone.0258307

17 Yuan R, Sun H, Soh KG, Mohammadi A, Toumi Z, Zhang Z. The effects of mental fatigue on sport-specific motor performance among team sport athletes: a systematic scoping review. *Front Psychol.* 2023 Apr 11(14):1143618. doi: 10.3389/fpsyg.2023.1143618

18 Skala F, Zemková E. Effects of acute fatigue on cognitive performance in team sport players: does it change the way they perform? A scoping review. *Appl Sci.* 2022;12(3):1736.

19 Soylu Y, Arslan E, Kilit B. Psychophysiological responses and cognitive performance: a systematic review of mental fatigue on soccer performance. *Int J Sport Stud Health.* 2021;4(2).

20 Gonzalez-Villora S, Prieto-Ayuso A, Cardoso F, Teoldo I. The role of mental fatigue in soccer: a systematic review. *Int J Sports Sci Coaching.* 2022;17(4):903–916.

21 Cao S, Geok SK, Roslan S, Sun H, Lam SK, Qian S. Mental fatigue and basketball performance: a systematic review. *Front Psychol.* 2022;12:819081.

22 Russell S, Jenkins D, Smith M, Halson S, Kelly V. The application of mental fatigue research to elite team sport performance: new perspectives. *J Sci Med Sport.* June 2019;22(6):723–728. doi: 10.1016/j.jsams.2018.12.008

23 Smith M, Thompson C, Marcora S, Skorski S, Meyer T, Coutts A. Mental fatigue and soccer: current knowledge and future directions. *Sports medicine (Auckland, NZ).* April 5, 2018.doi: 10.1007/s40279-018-0908-2

24 Pires FO, Silva-Júnior FL, Brietzke C, et al. Mental fatigue alters cortical activation and psychological responses, impairing performance in a distance-based cycling trial. Original Research. *Front Physiol.* March 16, 2018;9(227).doi: 10.3389/fphys.2018.00227

25 MacMahon C, Schücker L, Hagemann N, Strauss B. Cognitive fatigue effects on physical performance during running. *J Sport Exerc Psychol.* 2014;36(4):375–381. doi: 10.1123/jsep.2013–0249

26 Pageaux B, Lepers R, Dietz KC, Marcora SM. Response inhibition impairs subsequent self-paced endurance performance. *Eur J Appl Physiol.* 2014;114(5):1095–1105.

27 Penna EM, Wanner SP, Campos BT, et al. Mental fatigue impairs physical performance in young swimmers. *Pediatr Exerc Sci.* 2017;20:1–8.

28 Brietzke C, Franco-Alvarenga P, Canestri R, et al. Carbohydrate mouth rinse mitigates mental fatigue effects on maximal incremental test performance, but not in cortical alterations. *Brain Sci.* 2020;10(8):493.

29 Smith M, Coutts A, Merlini M, Deprez D, Lenoir M, Marcora S. Mental fatigue impairs soccer-specific physical and technical performance. *Med Sci Sports Exerc.* February 2016;48(2):267–276. doi: 10.1249/MSS.0000000000000762

30 Veness D, Patterson SD, Jeffries O, Waldron M. The effects of mental fatigue on cricket-relevant performance among elite players. *J Sports Sci.* January 16, 2017;35(24):1–7. doi: 10.1080/02640414.2016.1273540

31 Dallaway N, Lucas SJE, Ring C. Cognitive tasks elicit mental fatigue and impair subsequent physical task endurance: effects of task duration and type. *Psychophysiology.* 2022;59(12):e14126. doi: 10.1111/psyp.14126

32 Gantois P, Lima-Júnior Dd, Fortes LdS, Batista GR, Nakamura FY, Fonseca FdS. Mental fatigue from smartphone use reduces volume-load in resistance training: a randomized, single-blinded cross-over study. *Percept Mot Skills.* 2021;128(4): 1640–1659.

33 Staiano W, Bonet LRS, Romagnoli M, Ring C. Mental fatigue: the cost of cognitive loading on weight lifting, resistance training, and cycling performance. *Int J Sports Physiol Perform.* May 1, 2023;18(5):465–473. doi: 10.1123/ijspp.2022–0356

34 Head JR, Tenan MS, Tweedell AJ, Price TF, LaFiandra ME, Helton WS. Cognitive fatigue influences time-on-task during bodyweight resistance training exercise. Original Research. *Front Physiol.* September 1, 2016;7. doi: 10.3389/fphys.2016.00373

35 Smith M, Marcora S, Coutts A. Mental fatigue impairs intermittent running performance. *Medicine and science in sports and exercise.* August 2015;47(8): 1682–1690. doi: 10.1249/mss.0000000000000592

36 Smith MR, Zeuwts L, Lenoir M, Hens N, De Jong LM, Coutts AJ. Mental fatigue impairs soccer-specific decision-making skill. *J Sports Sci.* 2016;34(14):1297–1304.

37 Filipas L, Rossi C, Codella R, Bonato M. Mental fatigue impairs second serve accuracy in tennis players. *Res Q Exerc Sport.* 2023:1–7. doi: 10.1080/02701367.2023.2174488

38 Le Mansec Y, Pageaux B, Nordez A, Dorel S, Jubeau M. Mental fatigue alters the speed and the accuracy of the ball in table tennis. *J Sports Sci.* 2018;36(23): 2751–2759. doi: 10.1080/02640414.2017.1418647

39 Englert C, Bertrams A. The effect of ego depletion on sprint start reaction time. *J Sport Exerc Psychol.* October 1, 2014;36(5):506–515. doi: 10.1123/jsep.2014-0029

40 Englert C, Persaud B, Oudejans R, Bertrams A. The influence of ego depletion on sprint start performance in athletes without track and field experience. Original Research. *Front Psychol.* August 17, 2015;6. doi: 10.3389/fpsyg.2015.01207

41 Van Cutsem J, De Pauw K, Vandervaeren C, Marcora S, Meeusen R, Roelands B. Mental fatigue impairs visuomotor response time in badminton players and controls. *Psychol Sport Exerc.* 2019;(45);101579

42 Coutinho D, Gonçalves B, Travassos B, Wong DP, Coutts AJ, Sampaio JE. Mental fatigue and spatial references impair soccer players' physical and tactical performances. *Front Psychol.* 2017;8:1645.

43 Kunrath CA, Nakamura FY, Roca A, Tessitore A, Teoldo Da Costa I. How does mental fatigue affect soccer performance during small-sided games? A cognitive, tactical and physical approach. *J Sports Sci.* August 2, 2020;38(15):1818–1828. doi: 10.1080/02640414.2020.1756681

44 Brown DM, Bray SR. Effects of mental fatigue on exercise intentions and behavior. *Ann Behav Med.* 2019;53(5):405–414.

45 Harris S, Bray SR. Effects of mental fatigue on exercise decision-making. *Psychology of Sport and Exercise*. September 1, 2019;44:1–8. doi: 10.1016/j.psychsport.2019.04.005

46 Thompson C, Fransen J, Skorski S, et al. Mental fatigue in football: Is it time to shift the goalposts? An evaluation of the current methodology. *Sports Med*. 2019;49(2):177–183.

47 Russell S, Jenkins D, Rynne S, Halson S, Kelly V. What is mental fatigue in elite sport? Perceptions from athletes and staff. *Eur J Sport Sci*. 2019;19(10):1367–1376.

48 Lam HKN, Sproule J, Turner AP, et al. International orienteering experts' consensus on the definition, development, cause, impact and methods to reduce mental fatigue in orienteering: a Delphi study. *J Sports Sci*. December 2, 2022;40(23): 2595–2607. doi: 10.1080/02640414.2023.2177027

49 Thompson C, Smith A, Coutts A, et al. Understanding the presence of mental fatigue in elite female football. *Res Q Exerc Sport*. 2021:1–12. doi: 10.1080/02701367.2021.1873224

50 Russell S, Kelly V, Halson S, Jenkins D. Cognitive Load in Sport. in Salmon, P.M., McLean, S., Dallat, C., Mansfield, N., Solomon, C., & Hulme, A. (Eds.). *Human Factors and Ergonomics in Sport: Applications and Future Directions* (1st ed.). CRC Press. 2020: 181-201 doi: 10.1201/9781351060073

51 Russell S, Jenkins D, Halson S, Kelly V. Changes in subjective mental and physical fatigue during netball games in elite development athletes. *J Sci Med Sport*. December 23, 2019;23(6):615–620. doi: 10.1016/j.jsams.2019.12.017

52 Russell S, Jenkins D, Halson S, Kelly V. Mental fatigue increases across a 16-week pre-season in elite female athletes. *J Sci Med Sport*. 2021;doi: 10.1016/j.jsams.2021.12.002

53 Russell S, Jenkins D, Halson S, Juliff L, Connick M, Kelly V. Mental fatigue over 2 elite netball seasons: a case for mental fatigue to be included in athlete self-report measures. *Int J Sports Physiol Perform*. January 1, 2021:1–10. doi: 10.1123/ijspp.2021–0028

54 Abbott W, Brownlee T, Naughton R, Clifford T, Page R, Harper L. Changes in perceptions of mental fatigue during a season in professional under-23 English Premier League soccer players. *Res Sports Med*. 2020;28(4):529–539.

55 Russell S, Jenkins D, Halson S, Juliff L, Kelly V. How do elite female team sport athletes experience mental fatigue? Comparison between international competition, training and preparation camps. *Eur J Sport Sci*. 2021:1–11. doi: 10.1080/17461391.2021.1897165

56 Dallaway N, Lucas SJE, Ring C. Concurrent brain endurance training improves endurance exercise performance. *J Sci Med Sport*. 2021;24(4):405–411. doi: 10.1016/j.jsams.2020.10.008

57 Staiano W, Merlini M, Romagnoli M, Kirk U, Ring C, Marcora S. Brain endurance training improves physical, cognitive, and multitasking performance in professional football players. *Int J Sports Physiol Perform*. December 1, 2022;17(12): 1732–1740. doi: 10.1123/ijspp.2022-0144

58 Martin K, Thompson KG, Keegan R, Rattray B. Are individuals who engage in more frequent self-regulation less susceptible to mental fatigue? *J Sport Exerc Psychol*. 2019:1–9. doi: 10.1123/jsep.2018-0222

59 Martin K, Staiano W, Menaspà P, et al. Superior inhibitory control and resistance to mental fatigue in professional road cyclists. *PLoS One*. 2016;11(7):e0159907.

60 Jaydari Fard S, Lavender AP. A comparison of task-based mental fatigue between healthy males and females. *Fatigue: Biomedicine, Health & Behavior.* January 2, 2019;7(1):1–11. doi: 10.1080/21641846.2019.1562582

61 Lopes TR, Oliveira DM, Simurro PB, et al. No sex difference in mental fatigue effect on high-level runners' aerobic performance. *Med Sci Sports Exerc.* April 1, 2020;52(10):2207–2216. doi: 10.1249/mss.0000000000002346

62 Habay J, Uylenbroeck R, Van Droogenbroeck R, et al. Interindividual variability in mental fatigue-related impairments in endurance performance: a systematic review and multiple meta-regression. *Sports Med Open.* February 20, 2023;9(1):14. doi: 10.1186/s40798-023-00559-7

63 Moher D, Hopewell S, Schulz KF, et al. CONSORT 2010 explanation and elaboration: updated guidelines for reporting parallel group randomised trials. *Int J Surgery.* 2012;10(1):28–55.

64 Von Elm E, Altman DG, Egger M, et al. The strengthening the reporting of observational studies in epidemiology (STROBE) statement: guidelines for reporting observational studies. *Int J Surgery.* 2014;12(12):1495–1499.

65 Eysenbach G. Improving the quality of web surveys: the checklist for reporting results of internet e-surveys (CHERRIES). *J Med Internet Res.* September 29, 2004;6(3):e34. doi:10.2196/jmir.6.3.e34

66 Heidari S, Babor TF, De Castro P, Tort S, Curno M. Sex and gender equity in research: rationale for the SAGER guidelines and recommended use. *Research Integrity and Peer Review.* May 3, 2016;1(1):2. doi: 10.1186/s41073-016-0007-6

Section 3

Fatigue

Is it the same for everyone?

8 Influence of sport and exercise demand on fatigue mechanisms

8.1 Introduction

Section 2 of this book discussed some primary candidates behind the development of fatigue during sport and exercise. For clarity, the influence of factors that could modulate these candidates was not discussed. It is beyond the scope of this book to provide information on all potential modulating factors. For example, the influence of health, illness, and disease on fatigue would warrant multiple books to itself. Similarly, while we know that many aspects of human performance decline with advancing age, this is not necessarily due to the onset of novel fatigue mechanisms.

Three primary factors that modulate fatigue processes even when things like health and age are accounted for are the specific demands of the sport and exercise, biological sex, and training status. Therefore, Section 3 will focus on these factors, beginning with sport and exercise demand. The chapter will be structured differently to those in Section 2. The information in Section 2 will be heavily referenced, but not reiterated. Therefore, some parts of this chapter will be more concise than others, and the reader should read this chapter with reference to Section 2 to maximise their understanding. The chapter will highlight types of sport and exercise that have different physical requirements and potential fatigue mechanisms from Section 2 will be linked to each type. Of course, there will be significant crossover of some fatigue mechanisms across different types of sport and exercise. Furthermore, human physiology does not neatly compartmentalise to external sport and exercise categorisations. However, aligning the physiology as closely as possible to these categorisations should help your understanding.

A few important points before reading this chapter: firstly, for ease of communication potential fatigue mechanisms will be presented almost in a 'standalone' fashion. Remember that physiological and biochemical function is extremely complex and highly integrated, and it is unlikely that just one of the mechanisms highlighted will be solely responsible for fatigue in any sport and exercise situation. Secondly, as has been touched upon in previous chapters, the relative influence of a particular fatigue mechanism may depend in part on the environmental conditions. For example, a hot and humid environment is going to place greater emphasis on fatigue mechanisms associated with dehydration

DOI: 10.4324/9781003326137-11

and hyperthermia compared to a cool environment. For clarity, this chapter will discuss sport and exercise taking place in a thermoneutral environment, in a situation that is not excessively humid or subject to any other external factors that could influence fatigue processes (unless specifically stated). Thirdly, only those mechanisms that are likely to contribute significantly to fatigue will be discussed. If a fatigue mechanism is not discussed it is because existing research does not support it as a major source of fatigue during that form of sport/exercise; however, it does not mean that the mechanism should be completely or permanently discounted (remember, knowledge on fatigue processes is ever changing).

8.2   The influence of sport and exercise demand on fatigue mechanisms

8.2.1   *Prolonged submaximal exercise*

At first glance, it appears easy to define prolonged submaximal exercise. However, there are still considerations that need to be made regarding the duration and intensity of the activity. Prolonged sport/exercise can be completed below, at, or above key physiological thresholds that significantly impact physiological responses and hence fatigue processes. Two key thresholds are the lactate threshold, which represents the boundary between moderate and heavy-intensity activity, and the critical power (cycling) or speed (running) which represents the boundary between heavy- and severe-intensity activity.

> **Key point 8.1**
>
> *Prolonged submaximal activity can be categorised as moderate, heavy, or severe-intensity, and the intensity domain has a significant impact on the prevalent fatigue mechanisms.*

It is beyond the scope of this book to provide detailed insights into these thresholds, and interested readers are recommended to consult Faude *et al.*[1] and Poole *et al.*[2] However, what is important is that transitioning between moderate, heavy, and severe-intensity domains drives distinct physiological changes that have direct and significant impacts on performance and influence fatigue. Therefore, this section will discuss prolonged submaximal sport and exercise in the moderate, heavy, and severe-intensity domains (despite its name, the severe-intensity domain can be considered submaximal as you 'enter' this domain at an intensity below $\dot{V}O_2max$).

8.2.1.1   *What are the likely causes of fatigue during prolonged submaximal sport and exercise in the moderate-intensity domain?*

The key performance requirements and associated fatigue mechanisms during moderate-intensity prolonged sport and exercise are summarised in Figure 8.1.

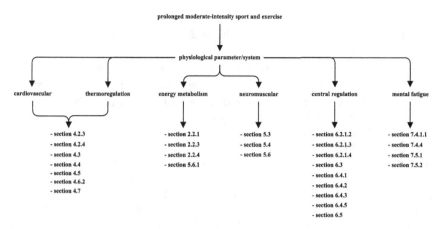

Figure 8.1 Potential causes of fatigue during prolonged moderate-intensity submaximal sport and exercise. Only those performance requirements that may play a direct, significant role in the fatigue process are highlighted. The section numbers refer to sections of this book that discuss the potential causes of fatigue associated with each of the identified performance requirements.

Moderate-intensity prolonged sport/exercise is characterised by the attainment of a physiological steady state. After the first few minutes, $\dot{V}O_2$, heart rate, substrate-level phosphorylation, and blood lactate concentration stabilise and there is no breakdown of phosphocreatine (PCr). Of course, changes in intensity within the moderate-intensity domain will cause changes in heart rate, $\dot{V}O_2$, and metabolism as appropriate to match the energy demand, but these parameters will quickly stabilise again. The attainment of a physiological steady state has important implications for fatigue processes and sport/exercise tolerance. In fact, it can be challenging to study fatigue processes during moderate-intensity sport/exercise in detail because the intensity allows activity to continue for many hours, meaning that the activity is almost always stopped before significant performance impairment takes place.[3]

During prolonged moderate-intensity submaximal sport and exercise, fluid loss via sweating (among other avenues) may decrease blood plasma volume. Reduced plasma volume may reduce the volume of blood entering the heart in each cardiac cycle which could reduce stroke volume and cardiac output, meaning that heart rate must increase (termed cardiovascular drift) to maintain the necessary O_2 delivery to working tissue (Section 4.2.3 and Figure 4.2). These alterations represent a reduction in cardiac efficiency which could lead to impaired performance.[4] Cardiovascular drift is a common explanation for the loss of cardiac steady state that may occur during prolonged moderate-intensity sport and exercise.

If body water loss continues, reduced plasma volume may generate competition for blood flow among core organs, working tissues, and the skin. It is biologically imperative that core organs receive sufficient blood flow to maintain function, therefore skin blood flow may be reduced to the extent that evaporative heat loss is impaired and core temperature subsequently increases. However, it is questionable whether the attainment of a

> **Key point 8.2**
>
> *Increases in skin temperature may be a more important component of fatigue during prolonged submaximal activity than increases in core temperature.*

'critical' high core temperature is a direct cause of fatigue during sport and exercise (Section 4.7.3). Instead, increases in skin temperature (which can occur due to reduced sweat rate and evaporative heat loss) may be more important than high core temperature in contributing to hyperthermia-induced fatigue. High skin temperatures require a higher skin blood flow, which may impair cardiac efficiency, reduce $\dot{V}O_2$max, and increase the relative intensity, causing the athlete to fatigue earlier (Section 4.7.3).

Prolonged activity in the moderate-intensity domain is by definition completed at a lower intensity than the heavy or severe-intensity domains. Therefore, under equal environmental conditions, the rate of fluid loss will be lower, meaning that potential performance limitations due to fluid loss may take longer to manifest. However, these issues should not be discounted.

Prolonged submaximal sport and exercise in the moderate-intensity domain is fuelled solely by aerobic metabolism of carbohydrate (via glycogen and blood glucose) and fat, if any temporary and short-lived deviations in intensity are discounted. The relative contribution of carbohydrate and fat to metabolism is dependent on factors such as gender, dietary intake, training status, and environmental conditions, but the most important determinants are duration and intensity (changing intensity even within the moderate-intensity domain will change the contribution of carbohydrate and fat oxidation). Maximal fat oxidation rates occur at around 40%–65% $\dot{V}O_2$max, indicating significant individual variability.[5,6] At these intensities, fat can be the dominant contributor to energy requirements.[6] However, the intensity range for maximal fat oxidation is lower than the intensity at which the majority of endurance activities would be undertaken, certainly in competitive athletes (for example, estimated intensity for a mountain ultramarathon run lasting between 8 and 14 hours is 63% $\dot{V}O_2$max, near the likely upper limit of maximal fat oxidation rate; this intensity will naturally increase with decreasing activity duration).[7] Therefore, carbohydrate oxidation (and by extension carbohydrate availability) is a consideration during prolonged submaximal sport and exercise in the moderate-intensity domain (Section 2.2.3).

Muscle glycogen depletion can occur after approximately 2 hours of sport/exercise, although this is a very general timeframe that is influenced by intensity, environmental conditions, baseline muscle glycogen concentration, and athlete training status. Well-trained endurance athletes show an enhanced ability to metabolise fat at a given intensity which may allow them to 'spare' muscle glycogen and maintain a higher intensity for longer. While muscle glycogen depletion will impair the intensity at which prolonged moderate-intensity sport and exercise can be com-

> **Key point 8.3**
>
> *Well-trained endurance athletes oxidise more fat and less carbohydrate at a given relative intensity. This may enable endurance athletes to spare glycogen stores and delay the onset of fatigue associated with glycogen depletion. However, it is becoming more likely that the role of glycogen depletion in muscle fatigue is dependent on the specific site of depletion.*

pleted, or even cause cessation of the activity, the specific mechanisms behind this impairment are still debated (Section 2.2.3).

Hypoglycaemia can occur during prolonged submaximal sport and exercise, secondary to liver glycogen depletion. The extent of hypoglycaemia will depend on activity duration and intensity (liver glucose release increases linearly with intensity and is also higher later in long duration sport and exercise when muscle glycogen stores become depleted), the pre-activity energy status of the athlete, and whether or not the athlete consumes carbohydrate during the activity (which may spare liver glycogen and/ or independently maintain blood glucose levels). The development of hypoglycaemia can contribute to fatigue during prolonged submaximal sport and exercise by limiting fuel

> **Key point 8.4**
>
> *Hypoglycaemia may contribute to the development of central fatigue during prolonged sport and exercise. However, the role of hypoglycaemia in fatigue is inconsistent, and dependent on factors pre- and during activity.*

supply to working muscles and/or contributing to central fatigue (Section 2.2.3.2.2). However, it should be remembered that the influence of hypoglycaemia on muscle carbohydrate oxidation, endurance capacity, and fatigue development is debated (Section 2.2.3.2.2). Specific to prolonged moderate-intensity sport and exercise, hypoglycaemia may need to be a consideration due to the duration of the activities that would likely be undertaken in this intensity domain. However, hypoglycaemia remains an unlikely issue in the majority of athletes,[8] although appropriate athlete preparation and event management is likely a factor in the relative risk of hypoglycaemia.

Significant impairments in sarcoplasmic reticulum (SR) calcium (Ca^{2+}) release and reuptake have been found following prolonged submaximal exercise,[9] and these impairments have been linked to fatigue.[10] Section 5.6.1 discussed the potential importance of muscle glycogen on SR function due to mechanisms related or unrelated to the traditional role of glycogen as a fuel

> **Key point 8.5**
>
> *Prolonged submaximal sport and exercise is probably impaired by sarcoplasmic reticulum dysregulation and altered Ca^{2+} kinetics, but the mechanisms behind this have not been conclusively determined.*

source (the specific mechanisms are still debated).[10] Muscle glycogen depletion can occur during prolonged moderate-intensity sport and exercise, meaning impairments in SR function may occur.

The potential for a central/anticipatory regulation of sport and exercise performance was introduced in Section 6.3. The observations highlighted in support of such performance regulation can also be related to prolonged moderate-intensity sport and exercise[11] (general absence of catastrophic homeostatic failure at exhaustion, significant increases in intensity in the final stages of the activity, and the employment of varied pacing strategies depending on intensity, environmental conditions, and the expected difficulty of the activity). The psychobiological model of sport and exercise regulation may apply to the type of activities that would likely be completed in the moderate-intensity domain, particularly by trained athletes (namely ultra-endurance type activities). It is perhaps easy to see how an individual competing in such activities could reach the point where the effort required to continue is equal to the maximum effort they are willing to give or how an individual could reach their perceived true maximal effort and feel unable to continue (Section 6.5). The potential ability of the psychobiological model to explain the impact of psychological influences on performance also aligns it to long duration activities, which undoubtably require certain psychological skills/traits for success that are outside of the scope of this book. It would be interesting to see the psychobiological model explored in this context in more detail.

Research has demonstrated that the loss of maximal voluntary contraction force in skeletal muscle following prolonged moderate-intensity activity is central rather than peripheral in origin.[12-14] Therefore, it appears that fatigue during this type of activity may be more central than peripheral in nature. However, as Burnley and Jones[3] point out, we should be careful when interpreting this data as in these studies the activities were conducted for a fixed distance/duration, rather than to exhaustion.

8.2.1.2   What are the likely causes of fatigue during prolonged submaximal sport and exercise in the heavy-intensity domain?

The key physiological differences between moderate (below lactate threshold) and heavy (above lactate threshold) intensity activity are the $\dot{V}O_2$ slow

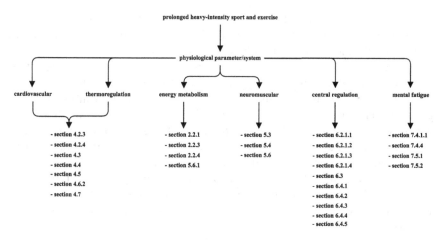

prolonged heavy-intensity sport and exercise

physiological parameter/system

cardiovascular	thermoregulation	energy metabolism	neuromuscular	central regulation	mental fatigue
- section 4.2.3		- section 2.2.1	- section 5.3	- section 6.2.1.1	- section 7.4.1.1
- section 4.2.4		- section 2.2.3	- section 5.4	- section 6.2.1.2	- section 7.4.4
- section 4.3		- section 2.2.4	- section 5.6	- section 6.2.1.3	- section 7.5.1
- section 4.4		- section 5.6.1		- section 6.2.1.4	- section 7.5.2
- section 4.5				- section 6.3	
- section 4.6.2				- section 6.4.1	
- section 4.7				- section 6.4.2	
				- section 6.4.3	
				- section 6.4.4	
				- section 6.4.5	

Figure 8.2 Potential causes of fatigue during prolonged heavy-intensity submaximal sport and exercise. Only those performance requirements that may play a direct, significant role in the fatigue process are highlighted. The section numbers refer to sections of this book that discuss the potential causes of fatigue associated with each of the identified performance requirements.

component and increase in blood lactate concentration. These variables stabilise but take approximately 10–20 minutes to do so. As a result, the O_2 cost of heavy-intensity activity is increased. Heavy-intensity activity commonly ranges from 60% to 85% $\dot{V}O_2$max and can be sustained for around 40 minutes to 3 hours,[3] although this range is influenced by a number of factors. The key performance requirements and associated fatigue mechanisms during heavy-intensity prolonged sport and exercise are summarised in Figure 8.2.

As with moderate-intensity sport and exercise, prolonged activity in the heavy-intensity domain can leave individuals susceptible to negative impairment in cardiovascular function and thermoregulation due to body heat gain and/or fluid loss. As intensity is greater in the heavy-intensity domain, it is logical to assume that the potential risk of these issues would be greater than in the moderate-intensity domain. However, the duration of moderate-intensity activity can be considerably longer than in the heavy domain. Of course, factors including the prevailing environmental conditions and fluid intake strategies will play a significant role.

Muscle glycogen depletion may be a primary source of fatigue during heavy-intensity sport and exercise. The higher intensity, greater $\dot{V}O_2$ due to the slow component, and use of glycogen by type I and II muscle fibres will tax muscle glycogen stores and it could be for these reasons that exhaustion in the heavy-intensity domain is often linked with low muscle glycogen.[3,15] The greater intensity and associated demand placed on skeletal muscles in the heavy-intensity domain also causes fatigue in individual muscle fibres which in turn requires the recruitment of more (mainly type II) fibres to take up the shortfall (it is this additional recruitment that at least partly drives the $\dot{V}O_2$ slow component).[16] This implies that localised muscle glycogen depletion (as discussed in Section 2.2.3) may meaningfully contribute to fatigue during heavy-intensity prolonged sport and exercise, without significant reductions in whole-muscle adenosine triphosphate (ATP) supply.[3]

Extracellular potassium (K^+) concentration increases with increasing intensity and with the recruitment of type II fibres (Section 5.3). Heavy-intensity activity is more intense than moderate-intensity activity and can involve progressive recruitment of type II fibres, indicating that fatigue in the heavy-intensity domain may be related to extracellular K^+ accumulation. This appears to be the case as significant increases in extracellular K^+ concentration have been found during heavy-intensity activity lasting around 44 minutes, and the increased extracellular K^+ was related to reduced muscle fibre excitability.[17] It is also possible that the reduced excitability reduced SR Ca^{2+} release, which would impair excitation-contraction coupling and muscle force production (Section 5.6).[17]

If localised muscle glycogen depletion occurs during heavy-intensity prolonged activity, as is likely, then glycogen-related impairments in Ca^{2+} dynamics are also a probable cause of fatigue (Section 5.6.1). It is probable that only glycogen-dependent Ca^{2+} movement from the SR is impaired, as while reductions in PCr are seen in approximately the first 6 minutes of heavy-intensity activity PCr concentration then stabilises, meaning inorganic phosphate (Pi) does not accumulate and will not impair Ca^{2+} dynamics (Section 5.6.2).[18] Similarly, hydrogen (H^+) does not accumulate in the muscle during heavy-intensity activity,[18] making any H^+-related impairments in Ca^{2+} dynamics or function unlikely (Section 5.6.1). The interactive effect of changes in K^+, muscle excitability, muscle glycogen concentration, and Ca^{2+} dynamics suggests that as heavy-intensity activity progresses the negative impact of muscle glycogen depletion and changes in Ca^{2+} dynamics may become more important determinants of fatigue.

The maximal voluntary contraction of a muscle can decline by around 25% following heavy-intensity activity,[19] suggesting the presence of central fatigue. Potential central fatigue mechanisms were discussed in Section 6.2, but it is not clear to what extent any of these apply to heavy-intensity prolonged activity, particularly as most of these mechanisms have significant limitations/conflicting data. Extracellular K^+ accumulation during heavy-intensity activity could contribute to central fatigue via stimulation of group IV afferents (Section 6.2.1.1), however this needs further investigation. The multifaceted fatigue mechanisms at play during heavy-intensity activity will also make it difficult to establish cause and effect relationships between isolated variables.

Key point 8.6

Prolonged submaximal sport and exercise in the heavy-intensity domain is complex and incorporates peripheral and central mechanisms via combined ionic and metabolic pertubations.

8.2.1.3 What are the likely causes of fatigue during prolonged submaximal sport and exercise in the severe-intensity domain?

The defining characteristic of activity in the severe-intensity domain is the inability to achieve a steady-state $\dot{V}O_2$, metabolic response, or acid-base balance. Oxygen (O_2) consumption will progressively increase to $\dot{V}O_2$max, blood lactate, H^+, and Pi will continue to rise, and PCr will continue to fall until termination of the activity. Severe-intensity activity is commonly at an intensity >85% $\dot{V}O_2$max and can be sustained for no more than around 40 minutes depending on how far above critical power the activity is taking place, and other factors. The key performance requirements and associated fatigue mechanisms during severe-intensity prolonged sport and exercise are summarised in Figure 8.3.

Activity in the severe domain impairs the contractile function of muscle fibres, likely via the mechanisms discussed later in this section. This inexorable loss of contractile function necessitates the progressive recruitment of additional motor units in order to continue at the target intensity.[3,20] Additional recruitment of motor units is thought to contribute to the $\dot{V}O_2$max component and explain why the slow component develops more rapidly and continually in the severe-intensity domain.[3]

Upon reaching $\dot{V}O_2$max and the ceiling of O_2 utilisation continued motor unit recruitment would involve the recruitment of muscle fibres predisposed to non-oxidative metabolism. Recruitment of these fibres would exacerbate

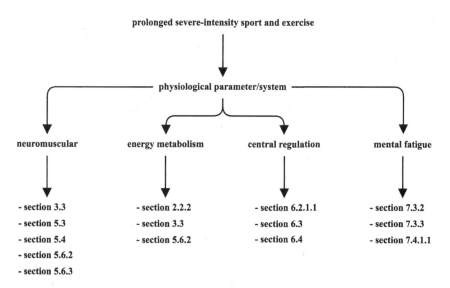

Figure 8.3 Potential causes of fatigue during prolonged severe-intensity submaximal sport and exercise. Only those performance requirements that may play a direct, significant role in the fatigue process are highlighted. The section numbers refer to sections of this book that discuss the potential causes of fatigue associated with each of the identified performance requirements.

many of the fatigue processes discussed later in this section. Therefore, the slow component of $\dot{V}O_2$ present in severe-domain activity has broad implications for fatigue processes. Tolerance of severe-domain activity once $\dot{V}O_2$max is reached is limited to at most a few minutes.[3]

Above critical power, muscle and blood lactate concentration progressively increase even if intensity remains stable. While lactate per se is likely not a significant contributor to fatigue (Section 3.3), its progressive accumulation is concurrent with that of H^+ and, by definition, reductions in pH. The reduction in pH throughout activity in the severe domain can be three times greater than in the heavy domain[18] and reaches its lowest point at task failure.[3] Therefore, potential fatigue mechanisms associated with metabolic acidosis may be prevalent during severe-intensity activity (Section 3.3.3).

Depletion of muscle glycogen is not a significant contributor to fatigue in severe-intensity activity, mainly because the activity does not last long enough. However, the rate of reduction in PCr concentration is around twice as fast in the severe-intensity domain vs. the heavy-intensity domain,[18] with PCr concentration at exhaustion around 23%–26% of resting values.[17,18] There is also a PCr slow component in the severe-intensity domain, indicative of a progressively increasing phosphate cost of muscle force production possibly due to increased ATP cost of contraction and/or greater type II muscle fibre contribution.[18,21] The rapid reduction in PCr concentration in the severe-intensity domain could contribute to fatigue by reducing substrate available to fill the shortfall in energy metabolism between that required to maintain intensity and that which can be provided oxidatively (Section 2.2.2). It is also entirely plausible that some muscle fibres would experience even greater reductions in PCr concentration, which could have a significant negative impact on the function of the whole muscle.

Depletion of PCr also leads to accumulation of Pi, which has been shown to increase more rapidly during severe vs. heavy-intensity activity and reach values more than 500% greater than at rest.[18] Inorganic phosphate accumulation may contribute to fatigue via direct action on cross-bridges and by inhibition of Ca^{2+} release from the SR (Section 5.6.2). The synergistic nature of the role of Pi and acidosis on myofilament Ca^{2+} sensitivity (Section 3.3.3.1) suggests that this fatigue process could be particularly pertinent to severe-intensity activity, as high Pi and low pH is exactly the metabolic profile observed during sport and exercise in this intensity domain.[3]

The intense nature of severe-domain muscle contractions, along with significant recruitment of type II muscle fibres, strongly implicates extracellular K^+ accumulation in the fatigue process (Section 5.3). Plasma K^+ concentration has been shown to progressively increase during severe-intensity activity, which may be indicative of increases in interstitial K^+ concentration.[17] Muscle excitability also reduced in parallel with increased metabolic stress, and this was attributed at least in part to increased extracellular K^+ concentration.[17] Of course, extracellular K^+ accumulation can directly impair action potential propagation along the sarcolemma, but this will also subsequently impair SR Ca^{2+} release and ultimately muscle cross-bridge formation and force production (Section 5.3).

Severe-intensity activity is associated with significant reductions in ATP (at least locally) and pH and increases in adenosine diphosphate (ADP), H^+, and extracellular K^+. All of these changes stimulate group III and IV afferent fibres, which provide sensory feedback about the mechanical and metabolic status of the working muscle tissue (Section 6.2.1.1). This stimulation is a crucial part of the exercise pressor reflex, but elevated firing of these afferents due to significant accumulation of metabolites reduces corticospinal excitability and hence muscle activation. As a result, severe-intensity activity may be limited by central fatigue mediated by group III/IV afferent stimulation. There is research evidence for increased central neural engagement during severe-intensity activity in an attempt to compensate for peripheral fatigue development.[17] As severe-intensity activity continues, the central nervous system (CNS) will continue to receive inhibitory feedback from group III/IV afferents while simultaneously attempting to drive the fatiguing muscles harder in order to maintain intensity.[3] In this situation, fatigue and/or exhaustion will occur if the CNS is unable to compensate for the loss of muscle force production/excitability.[3,22]

The highly interactive nature of peripheral and central regulation of performance in the severe-intensity domain, mediated by group III/IV afferents, brings about a 'chicken and egg' scenario. It is very difficult to elucidate whether fatigue is due directly to peripheral limitations associated with metabolic perturbation, central fatigue via afferent feedback, or a combination of the two.[17] Most current thinking points towards peripheral events as more important in the fatigue process during severe-intensity activity.[23]

It is also worth mentioning that blood H^+ accumulation and associated reductions in arterial pH significantly increase ventilation via increased breathing frequency.[24] This increased respiratory muscle work can impair limb blood flow as more blood is required by the respiratory muscles[3,25] and potentially by respiratory muscle fatigue.[26] However, more work is required here.

> **Key point 8.7**
>
> *Prolonged submaximal sport and exercise in the severe-intensity domain is limited by predominantly peripheral mechanisms linked to the inability to achieve a physiological steady-state.*

8.2.1.4 Summary

Potential fatigue mechanisms are influenced by the intensity domain in which sport and exercise take place. Fatigue in the moderate domain is predominantly centrally mediated, perhaps with contributions from muscle glycogen depletion and hyperthermia (in some situations). Fatigue in the heavy-intensity domain is the most complex, with both peripheral and central fatigue evident via the combined influences of multiple ionic and metabolic perturbations and depletion of muscle glycogen (certainly at the micro level) that have an direct impact on muscle contractile function and impair the ability of the CNS to drive muscle fibres.[17] In the severe domain, physiological and metabolic steady state is impossible, leading to a progressive reduction in PCr concentration and tissue pH and increases in Pi, H^+, blood lactate concentration, extracellular K^+, and $\dot{V}O_2$. The need for continued recruitment of primarily type II fibres to compensate for fatiguing fibres exacerbates all of these negative metabolic and ionic changes, which impair both peripheral and central processes required for muscle contraction. Essentially, the power/torque required by the muscles exceeds that which can be supplied by the neuromuscular system due to anaerobic substrate depletion, accumulation of metabolic by-products, attainment of $\dot{V}O_2$max, or a combination of these.[3,17] Peripheral factors appear to play a more important role in severe-intensity activity, although the specific mechanisms at play may depend on how far above critical power/speed/torque the activity takes place.[23]

8.2.2 Field-based team games

This section focusses on field-based team games such as soccer, rugby, and field hockey. Low-intensity work (standing, walking, jogging) is predominant in most field-based team games. However, the requirement to perform several hundred brief intense actions along with rapid, continuous changes of activity suggests a notable stress on aerobic and anaerobic energy pathways. The requirement to rapidly and forcefully activate skeletal muscle for short periods of time is a crucial difference between team games and prolonged submaximal sport and exercise and may influence the fatigue processes at work in team games.

Average heart rate during field-based team games is approximately 75%–95% of maximum heart rate,[27,28] and the estimated mean $\dot{V}O_2$ during a soccer match is 70%–80% $\dot{V}O_2$max.[29] Mean blood lactate concentration ranges from approximately 2.8–10 mmol.L. Carbohydrate is the primary fuel source during team games, despite the predominance of low-intensity work. The extent of muscle glycogen depletion is variable and likely affected by playing position, game intensity, environmental conditions, muscle fibre type recruitment, and pre-game glycogen concentrations.[30,31]

Team games appear to impose a similar average physiological stress to that observed in prolonged submaximal sport and exercise. Aerobic metabolism is dominant, but anaerobic contribution is crucial to successful performance. However, the moment-to-moment demand of team games requires a notable high- and maximal-intensity component, making it significantly different to steady-state sport and exercise.

8.2.2.1 What are the likely causes of fatigue during field-based team games?

Research investigating the physical demand and determinants of fatigue during team games has discovered two 'forms' of fatigue during this type of activity. It appears that team games players experience temporary fatigue following periods of high-intensity activity; this is referred to as transient fatigue.[32] A progressive fatigue also develops that results in less high-intensity activity, sprinting, and overall distance covered towards the end of a match.[33–35]

> **Key point 8.8**
>
> *There are two distinct "forms" of fatigue during team games exercise. One is a temporary fatigue that occurs following high-intensity periods of a game (transient fatigue); the other is a progressive fatigue that impairs high-intensity exercise and distance covered towards the end of a match.*

8.2.2.1.1 TRANSIENT FATIGUE

The performance requirements of field-based team games and the fatigue mechanisms associated with transient fatigue are in Figure 8.4. Notable blood lactate concentrations have been reported during team games, suggesting significant use of anaerobic glycolysis. Therefore, fatigue during team games may be associated with intramuscular acidosis.[31] This suggestion has some support from studies demonstrating significant increases in muscle lactate and acidosis, and weak but statistically significant correlations between muscle lactate concentration and decreased sprint performance, following intense periods of play.[36]

While H^+ accumulation has been put forward as a candidate for transient fatigue, decreases in muscle pH during soccer are only moderate[29] and these changes have not been related to impaired per-

> **Key point 8.9**
>
> *Neither high muscle lactate concentration nor reduced muscle pH appear to be a cause of transient fatigue during team games.*

formance.[29,37] Also, there is evidence to show that muscle pH levels 1.5 minutes before exhaustion during intense intermittent exercise were not different to those values seen at exhaustion.[38] It therefore appears that reduced tissue pH is not a likely cause of transient fatigue during team games.[29]

Section 2.2.2.2 discussed the significant positive relationship between the ability to resynthesise PCr and the recovery of power output during repeated sprinting. However, correlation studies between PCr recovery and repeated sprint performance also show that PCr recovery is associated with about 45%–71% of the recovery of power output, suggesting that there are other factors that also contribute to intermittent exercise performance.

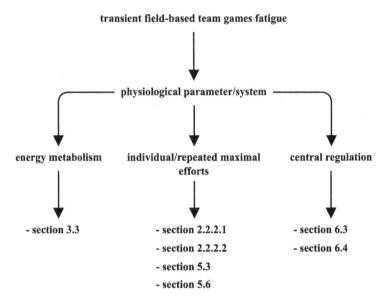

Figure 8.4 Potential causes of transient fatigue during field-based team games. Only those performance requirements that may play a direct significant role in the fatigue process are highlighted. The section numbers refer to sections of this book that discuss the potential causes of fatigue associated with each of the identified performance requirements.

Following intense periods of activity during team games the decrease in muscle PCr concentration is correlated with impaired sprinting ability.[31,37] However, muscle PCr depletion following high-intensity periods of team games appears to be moderate,[39,40] and other research has shown no changes in muscle PCr concentration towards the end of intermittent exercise tests designed to replicate the repeated

> **Key point 8.10**
>
> *Despite correlations between reduced muscle PCr and impaired sprinting performance, available evidence suggests that PCr depletion is not responsible for transient fatigue during team games.*

sprint nature of team games.[38] The bulk of the available evidence appears to suggest that depletion of muscle PCr is not the cause of transient fatigue during team games.[29,31,39]

Dysregulation of the SR can occur during prolonged exercise (Section 5.6), and this may be linked to accumulation of Pi (Section 5.6.2) and muscle glycogen depletion (Section 5.6.1). Therefore, it is plausible that SR dysregulation could contribute to fatigue during field-based team games. However, specific data confirming this is currently lacking.

Extracellular K^+ accumulation may be implicated in transient fatigue during team games. While we know that intense short-term sport and exercise causes sufficient extracellular K^+ accumulation to depolarise the muscle membrane potential and reduce force production, very little work has been done investigating K^+ turnover during team games.[31] For example, we know that blood K^+ levels are elevated during a soccer match,[36] but this study did not provide information on the accumulation of K^+ in the muscle interstitium. Caffeine ingestion improved the performance of intense intermittent exercise similar to that undertaken during team games and caused a reduction in interstitial K^+ concentration.[41] These authors suggested that improved performance with caffeine ingestion indicates a role of interstitial K^+ accumulation in impairing performance during team games type activity. However, the authors also note that other influences of caffeine ingestion, such as elevated catecholamine concentrations and/or reduced central fatigue, may have contributed to improved performance with reduced interstitial K^+ concentration a coincidental finding. This possibility is further supported by the finding that interstitial K^+ concentrations in the control trial were not high enough to contribute to fatigue.[41] As a result, it cannot be conclusively determined whether extracellular K^+ accumulation plays a role in transient fatigue during team games, and in elite female soccer it has not been implicated in transient fatigue.[40]

> **Key point 8.11**
>
> *Blood K^+ levels are elevated during a soccer match, which may indicate a net loss of K^+ from the muscle and possible K^+ accumulation in the interstitium. However, this has not been measured in team games exercise. There is some indirect evidence that extracellular K^+ accumulation may play a role in transient during team games, but not enough to come to a conclusive decision.*

The specific cause(s) of transient fatigue during team games is currently unknown. While there are candidates, none of these has been consistently or clearly shown to cause transient fatigue. An interesting consideration is that transient fatigue may represent a form of pacing to enable the player to complete a full game without excessive performance loss or the requirement for a long recovery period, which is rarely available in field-based team games. The discussions in Chapter 6 focussed on the concept of regulation of performance via real-time interpretation of exercise demands (Sections 6.3 and 6.4). Given that transient fatigue is often observed following high-intensity periods of activity the concept of a continual regulation of intensity based on existing exercise demands would appear to fit the nature of transient fatigue during team games. However, to date, insufficient research has investigated the potential role of perceptual regulation in transient fatigue during team games.

8.2.2.1.2 PROGRESSIVE FATIGUE

The performance requirements of field-based team games and the fatigue mechanisms associated with progressive fatigue are in Figure 8.5. The extent of muscle glycogen depletion during team games is variable and likely affected by playing position, game intensity, environmental conditions, muscle fibre type recruitment, and pre-game muscle glycogen concentration.[30,31,42] However, it is generally accepted that muscle glycogen concentration during team games can fall to a level where performance, particularly in the latter stages of the game, might be impaired.[37,43] This suggestion is supported by the wealth of research documenting performance improvements and a delay in the onset of fatigue when carbohydrate supplements are used during team games (Section 2.2.3.2.3). However, the critique of the carbohydrate supplementation literature (summarised in Table 2.1) should be considered.

Progressive increases in blood-free fatty acid concentrations during the second half of team games[36,42] suggests an increased reliance on fat as a fuel source, perhaps due to reduced glycogen availability.[29] When players start a soccer match with partial glycogen depletion significant reductions occur by half-time and stores are almost fully depleted at the end of the game, in contrast to players who start with full glycogen stores.

While muscle glycogen concentrations can be significantly reduced during team games, this does not necessarily imply a causative relationship between muscle glycogen depletion and progressive fatigue. Some studies have shown reductions in muscle glycogen during team games to levels that are insufficient to maintain maximal glycolytic rate (approximately 200 mmol.kg dry weight),[29] whereas other studies demonstrate much less muscle glycogen depletion. For example, Krustrup *et al.*[36] found that muscle glycogen concentrations

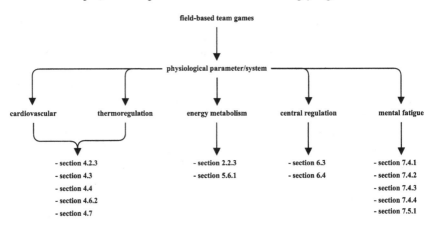

Figure 8.5 Potential causes of fatigue that develops towards the end of field-based team games. Only those performance requirements that may play a direct significant role in the fatigue process are highlighted. The section numbers refer to sections of this book that discuss the potential causes of fatigue associated with each of the identified performance requirements.

at the end of a football game ranged from 150 to 350 mmol.kg dry weight. However, the authors looked more closely and found that about half of type I and type II quadriceps muscle fibres were almost or completely depleted of muscle glycogen following the match. Findings such as this have led to the sug-

Key point 8.12

It is likely that muscle glycogen depletion plays some role(s) in progressive fatigue during team games. The exact nature of this role is still under investigation, but may relate to depletion of glycogen in specific locations within individual muscle fibres. Under normal circumstances, hypoglycaemia is not a cause of fatigue during team games.

gestion that fatigue towards the end of a game could be related to muscle glycogen depletion in individual muscle fibres. This relates back to the discussions in Sections 2.2.3 and 5.6.1 that there is certainly a link between muscle glycogen depletion and fatigue, but that the nature of this link is not fully known. Section 5.6.1 discussed the potential for localised muscle glycogen depletion to contribute to impaired Ca^{2+} kinetics via reduced ATP concentrations in areas of the cell responsible for Ca^{2+} release and uptake, or by means unrelated to glycogen's role as an energy source. Therefore, localised muscle glycogen depletion in individual fibres could contribute to fatigue development during team games via these mechanisms. However, no research studies have specifically investigated this possibility. As a result, we are currently left with the conclusion that muscle glycogen depletion does likely play a role in progressive fatigue during team games, but the extent of this role and the exact mechanisms behind it are not yet known.

During competitive field-based team games in thermoneutral conditions, fluid losses of up to 3 litres have been reported, increasing to 4–5 litres in hot and humid environments.[44-46] Fluid losses during 90-minute soccer training equate to about 1.4%–1.6% of pre-exercise body mass (BM),[44,46] with fluid deficits of 1%–2% BM typical during competition across the majority of environmental conditions.[47]

As discussed in Section 4.3, a belief has existed for a long time that fluid losses of ≥ 2% BM can impair physiological and psychological function during sport and exercise. However, Section 4.3 discussed issues with the early research that was used to 'promote' this 2% threshold and introduced more recent studies that appear to refute the notion of the

Key point 8.13

Typical fluid losses during team games training and competition amount to 1-2% body mass. This is unlikely to contribute to a significant reduction in performance.

2% threshold. Of course, it is likely that large volumes of fluid loss could impact negatively on team games performance. However, as mentioned above, typical fluid losses during team games training and competition, particularly soccer, are only 1%–2% BM.

There is some supporting evidence regarding dehydration and performance decrements in field-based team games, with reductions in sprint-dribbling performance and decision making in soccer seen when players were dehydrated by ~2% of their BM.[48,49] However, there is also research that has not found team games performance decrements with dehydration. Given the huge range of factors (related to the individual, sport/activity, outcome measure, environmental conditions, etc.) that can influence the findings of sport and exercise hydration research it would be useful for a comprehensive meta-analysis to be carried out, controlling for as many of these confounding variables as possible.

Section 4.3 discussed how drinking according to the dictate of individual thirst may be an effective approach to hydration. If this is the case, it poses a problem for team games players that may impact their performance. For the majority of field-based team games such as soccer, rugby, and hockey, there are no scheduled breaks in play to consume fluid. Therefore, players are limited to consuming fluid at half-time and during any unforeseen breaks in play. As a result, team games players may not be able to respond to their own thirst drive. This suggestion was put forward by Edwards and Noakes[47] who proposed that rather than a direct cause of fatigue, dehydration is one in a number of dynamic markers within the central governor/ anticipatory feedback model of performance (Section 6.3 and 6.4). This self-pacing hypothesis is supported by observations of similar sweat rates across team games played in widely different environmental conditions, minimal to moderate fluid losses during games, no difference in core temperature between the first and second halves of games,[50] lack of attainment of a 'critical' core temperature during soccer matches (Section 4.7.3),[51] the ability of individuals of wide fitness levels to complete a full match, and that *ad libitum* drinking maximises performance despite varying levels of dehydration.[52] To date, the influence of the thirst drive on team games performance, independent of changes in hydration status or thermoregulation, has not been closely investigated.

It appears that team games players (at least well-conditioned players) rarely reach a core temperature that could be considered 'critical' for performance impairment.[47] However, Section 4.7.3 mentioned that high skin temperatures can impair performance independently from changes in core temperature. Therefore, skin temperature response may play a role in the development of fatigue during team games. While there are studies that have shown improved performance when increases in skin temperature are reduced or prevented,[53,54] there is currently not much data reporting the skin temperature responses to team games, independent from changes in core temperature. Therefore, it is not possible to determine whether or not skin temperature is a potential cause of fatigue during team games or whether strategies to reduce skin temperature would improve team games performance.

Research has reported reductions in electromyography (EMG, Section 1.4.2) activity of the quadriceps muscles during and after actual and simulated soccer, and reductions in maximal voluntary contraction force (MVC, Section 1.3.1) immediately following soccer.[55-57] These findings imply a central aspect to fatigue. However, implying a central component as the cause of reduced muscle EMG activity is speculative as changes to EMG activity of a muscle do not necessarily signify altered central neural drive, and muscle EMG activity can change during and after exercise but these changes do not necessarily alter muscle force production.[58] Despite this, evidence for reduced MVC during and after team games exercise does suggest a central component to the fatigue process in team games. The exact causes of this central fatigue component require further study.

> **Key point 8.14**
>
> *There may be a central component to progressive fatigue during team games. However, this requires more robust study, particularly regarding the nature of the possible central fatigue in the absence of hyperthermia.*

Over the last 5–10 years, a large body of work has investigated the potential impact of mental fatigue on aspects of team games performance, particularly soccer (Section 7.4). This work demonstrates that mental fatigue can impair technical, tactical, and physical performance in soccer.[59-63] The potential impact of mental fatigue on team games may be due to the high physical and cognitive demand required by these sports (Section 7.4.2). However, the outcomes of mental fatigue research should be interpreted in the context of known issues such as the ecological validity of methods used to induce mental fatigue and the methods used to measure mental fatigue (Section 7.7).[64]

8.2.3 Sport and exercise lasting approximately 90 seconds to 5 minutes

This section deals with sport and exercise where the aim is to achieve the best performance over a duration of 90 seconds to 5 minutes. The best example of this type of activity would be middle-distance running (800 to 1500 metres). For this reason, the rest of this section will refer to activities lasting around 90 seconds to 5 minutes as middle-distance activities, although the information in this section applies beyond running. Attempting to achieve a best performance in this timeframe would place the individual in the severe-intensity or even the extreme-intensity domain, which as the name implies is an intensity greater than severe-intensity activity and is characterised by task failure (exhaustion) before attainment of $\dot{V}O_2$max (maximum tolerable duration approximately 3 minutes or less).[65] Therefore, many of the fatigue mechanisms

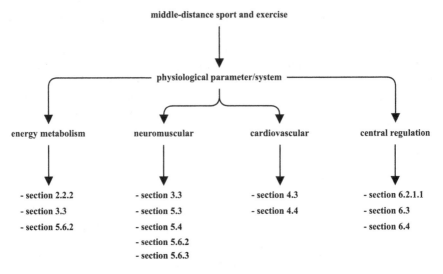

Figure 8.6 Potential causes of fatigue during sport and exercise lasting approximately 90 seconds to 5 minutes. Only those performance requirements that may play a direct significant role in the fatigue process are highlighted. The section numbers refer to sections of this book that discuss the potential causes of fatigue associated with each of the identified performance requirements.

highlighted in Section 8.2.1.3 would be relevant here. The key performance requirements and associated fatigue mechanisms during middle-distance activities are in Figure 8.6.

Peak muscle lactate concentrations occur following activity that causes exhaustion in approximately 3–7 minutes. Therefore, it is not surprising that both an 800- metre and 1,500-metre run require notable contributions from the aerobic and anaerobic energy pathways. For an 800-metre run, the approximate percentage contribution of aerobic/anaerobic energy systems to total ATP resynthesis is 60%–70%/30%–40%.[66,67] For the 1,500-metre run, the approximate aerobic/anaerobic contribution is 84/16%.[67] For both the 800- and 1,500-metre distance, the 'crossover' from a predominantly anaerobic to a predominantly aerobic ATP resynthesis occurs between 15 and 30 seconds into the run.[67] The importance of the anaerobic energy system diminishes as activity duration increases.[68]

Research has identified the relationship between $\dot{V}O_2$max and running economy, $\dot{V}O_2$ at the second ventilatory threshold, and running speed at the second ventilatory threshold as important indicators of middle-distance performance.[69,70] Measurement and interpretation of these variables appear to enable discrimination between an athlete's predisposition as either a middle- or long-distance runner.[70] The known importance of these physiological markers to performance during middle-distance activities may also help identify relevant fatigue mechanisms.

8.2.3.1 What are the likely causes of fatigue during middle-distance activities?

Aerobic metabolism is crucial for performance in middle-distance events. Therefore, factors that impair cardiovascular responses, and hence the ability to deliver O_2 to working muscles, could be a source of fatigue during middle-distance activities.

The primary factors addressed in this book that could impair cardiovascular function during sport and exercise are dehydration and hyperthermia. Both dehydration and hyperthermia are usually associated with longer duration activity as it takes time for both of these conditions to develop. It is highly unlikely that either dehydration or hyperthermia would negatively impact the cardiovascular response of athletes during an event lasting 90 seconds to 5 minutes.

> **Key point 8.15**
>
> *Under normal circumstances, it is unlikely that impairments to cardiovascular function are a cause of fatigue during middle-distance activity.*

There may be some situations where either dehydration or hyperthermia could impact middle-distance performance, for example, if an athlete began without appropriate preparation (i.e. significant pre-existing hypohydration) and/or if the event took part in extreme conditions (particularly regarding temperature and humidity). However, in the majority of situations, it is unlikely that impaired function of the cardiovascular system would play a role in fatigue development during middle-distance activity.

Due to the intensity of middle-distance activities, many of the metabolic and ionic perturbations discussed in Section 8.2.1.3 are possible fatigue mechanisms. Middle-distance activity requires significant contributions from the anaerobic energy pathways, which will lead to production of muscle lactate and H^+. The reader is referred to Sections 3.2 and 3.3 for a more focussed discussion of lactate and fatigue. Potentially of more relevance to middle-distance activity is H^+ production. During severe-intensity activity, muscle pH can drop to below 6.5, which would indicate increased acidosis via H^+ production. As discussed in Section 3.3.3, at physiological temperatures and pH levels metabolic acidosis has a smaller impact on SR Ca^{2+} release, muscle membrane excitability, and glycolytic rate than was originally thought. However, this impact could still be enough to impair severe-intensity performance. Also, reductions in tissue pH can stimulate group III and IV muscle afferents, potentially increasing sensations of muscular pain/discomfort, inhibiting central drive, and thereby contributing to the development of central fatigue (Section 3.3.3.4).

Many studies have shown an improvement in severe-intensity performance following ingestion of sodium bicarbonate.[71-74] Sodium bicarbonate is a compound that makes the blood more alkaline. This increased alkalinity creates a greater pH gradient between the muscle and blood, allowing the blood to more readily 'accept' greater amounts of H^+ from the muscle which would allow greater H^+ production before any potentially fatiguing issues arise. The performance benefit seen with sodium bicarbonate ingestion is very similar to the performance decrement seen when ammonium chloride (a compound that increases the acidity of the blood) is ingested.[73] However, it is interesting that some studies which found performance improvements with sodium bicarbonate ingestion also reported no difference in muscle pH at the end of exercise with or without sodium bicarbonate.[75] The lack of influence of sodium bicarbonate on muscle pH in the face of a performance improvement suggests that there may be other mechanisms by which sodium bicarbonate improves performance (Section 3.3.3.4).[76–78]

> **Key point 8.16**
>
> *The significant H^+ production and associated muscle pH reduction during middle-distance activity may contribute to fatigue by alterations in Ca^{2+} kinetics, muscle membrane excitability, and glycolysis. However, the influence of pH on these factors in vivo is less than previously thought. Hydrogen production may induce central fatigue either via stimulation of type III and IV muscle afferents and/or causing arterial oxygen desaturation and cerebral hypoxia.*

Extracellular K^+ accumulation can occur after 1 minute of severe-intensity activity.[17] This rate of accumulation suggests that any role of extracellular K^+ accumulation on fatigue may exert an effect within the timeframe of middle-distance activity. Such effects could be peripheral (reduced sarcolemmal membrane excitability and subsequent reductions in SR Ca^{2+} release) (Section 5.3) or central via stimulation of group III/IV afferents (Sections 5.3 and 6.2.1.1).

> **Key point 8.17**
>
> *Notable extracellular K^+ accumulation may occur during middle-distance activity, which may impair muscle membrane excitability and muscle function. However, many mechanisms exist to reduce the effect of extracellular K^+ accumulation on muscle membrane excitability. Potassium accumulation may influence the CNS and contribute to central fatigue, however more research is needed before this can be confirmed.*

As well as extracellular K^+-induced alterations in Ca^{2+} kinetics, the known effects of intramuscular Pi on SR Ca^{2+} release and myofilament Ca^{2+} sensitivity, as well as the interactive impact of Pi and acidosis on myofilament Ca^{2+}

dynamics, could play a significant role in peripheral fatigue in middle-distance activities. During severe-intensity activity, PCr concentration can fall by ~50% in 3 minutes and ~66% in 5 minutes.[18] Not only

> **Key point 8.18**
>
> *Impaired Ca^{2+} kinetics, possibly via Pi and mg^{2+} accumulation and/or localised ATP depletion, may play a role in muscle fatigue during middle-distance activity.*

does this indicate a reduced availability of anaerobic substrate for ATP resynthesis (itself a potential avenue for fatigue), but it also indicates a significant increase in Pi (Section 8.2.1.3) and associated fatigue mechanisms.

8.2.4 Sport and exercise lasting 30–60 seconds

This section deals with sport and exercise where the aim is to achieve the best performance over a duration of 30–60 seconds (referred to in this section as long distance sprinting). A good example of this type of activity would be 400-metre running. Attempting to achieve a best performance in this timeframe would place the individual in the extreme-intensity domain. The key performance requirements of this type of activity are in Figure 8.7.

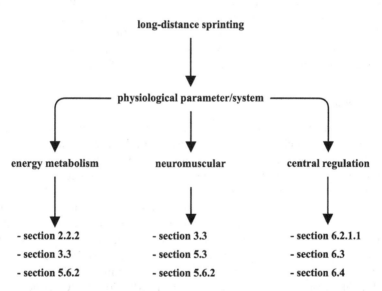

Figure 8.7 Potential causes of fatigue during sport and exercise lasting 30–60 seconds. Only those performance requirements that may play a direct significant role in the fatigue process are highlighted. The section numbers refer to sections of this book that discuss the potential causes of fatigue associated with each of the identified performance requirements.

Long distance sprinting is dependent on high rates of anaerobic metabolism, a high $\dot{V}O_2$max, and neuromuscular function to generate large muscle power.[68] It may be surprising to read that a high $\dot{V}O_2$max has been associated with performance during activity of this nature; however, the aerobic/anaerobic energy contribution to a 400-metre run is approximately 35%–45%/55%–65%.[66,67] Indeed, it is worth remembering that Spencer and Gastin[67] show the crossover from predominantly anaerobic to predominantly aerobic energy supply occurs between 15 and 30 seconds in middle-distance running. During a 400-metre run, PCr degradation is the predominant source of ATP resynthesis during the first 100 metres, followed by glycolysis from 100 to 300 metres, with almost no contribution from PCr in the final quarter of the run.[68,79,80] The notable contribution of glycolysis to ATP resynthesis may explain why there is a strong correlation between 400-metre performance and both anaerobic energy contribution[41] and peak blood lactate concentration.[80] Peak running velocity occurs 50–100 metres into the run, followed by a progressive decrease in velocity until 300 metres, and a notable reduction in velocity in the final 100 metres.[81] This velocity pattern appears to be similar regardless of ability level, and in fact the greatest decrement in velocity during the final 100 metres is seen in world-class 400-metre runners.[81] The difference is that peak running velocity is greater in higher quality runners, and velocity remains significantly higher for at least the first half of the race.[81]

A high anaerobic capacity may relate to performance in long distance sprinting by increasing power output and running velocity, as the rate at which ATP can be supplied anaerobically influences both of these factors.[66] This suggestion is supported by research showing that greater explosive strength, strength endurance, and power leads to better 400-metre performance.[68,82]

8.2.4.1   *What are the likely causes of fatigue during long distance sprinting?*

The role of lactate production and pH changes on fatigue during long distance sprinting is likely similar to that during middle-distance activity (Section 8.2.3.1), so will only be discussed briefly. The importance of anaerobic metabolism to sprinting performance increases as sprint distance decreases. During a 400-metre run, which resides near the upper limit of the 30–60-second range discussed in this section (at least for sub-elite individuals), blood pH significantly declines.[83] It could therefore be implied that there is a significant intramuscular acidosis during events of this duration, which may contribute to myofilament contractile impairment and hence muscle force production. This could be exacerbated in the face of increased intramuscular Pi concentration which is likely present due to the significant reduction in PCr concentration seen during 400-metre running, with the greatest reduction observed over the first 100 metres.[79] This suggestion is supported by research showing that running velocity during a 400-metre run in world-class athletes does not begin to decline until 11–13 seconds into the run,[81] which is longer than the time taken for velocity to drop during a short-distance sprint (Section 8.2.5). Therefore, the combined impact of acidosis and Pi could directly impair muscle cross-bridge function and Pi could also impair SR Ca^{2+} concentration and release. Of course, depletion of PCr would also reduce the rate at which ATP could be re-synthesised and would necessitate a slowing of running velocity (i.e. fatigue).

The rapid accumulation of extracellular K^+ during intense activity (Section 8.2.3.1) means that K^+ accumulation in the interstitium or the t-tubules should be considered as a potential cause of fatigue during long distance sprinting. Studies have found that muscle membrane excitability appears to be preserved following a long duration sprint.[84] Also, the time course of recovery of muscle torque (more than 30 minutes) is far longer than would be expected if reduced muscle membrane excitability due to extracellular K^+ accumulation was a significant cause of fatigue.[84,85] Long distance sprinting may be too short to experience negative effects of extracellular K^+ accumulation, but it would be useful to have specific data on this issue.

Section 8.2.3.1 also discussed how increased acidosis, extracellular K^+ concentration, and ADP concentration might stimulate group III and IV muscle afferents and potentially cause central fatigue. Research has shown notable reductions in MVC force immediately following a 400-metre run (Section 1.3.1)[84]; however, notable reductions in muscle torque production via electrical stimulation of the muscle were also found (Section 1.3.1). It therefore appears that reductions in muscle force production following a 400-metre run are mainly due to peripheral causes, with central causes having less of an influence.[84]

> **Key point 8.19**
>
> *Reductions in muscle force production following sport and exercise lasting 30-60 seconds are probably due to peripheral causes rather than central fatigue.*

Pacing strategies are arguably present in the majority of sporting events, whether as a conscious attempt to maximise performance or as a subconscious effort to prevent significant homeostatic disruption to body systems (Section 6.4.3). Pacing strategies are observed during all-out cycling lasting approximately 45 seconds.[86] This pacing strategy consists of

> **Key point 8.20**
>
> *Extracellular K^+ accumulation probably does not play a notable role in fatigue during long distance sprinting. However, Ca^{2+} kinetics may be impaired during this form of activity.*

> **Key point 8.21**
>
> *Phosphocreatine depletion probably does contribute to fatigue during long distance sprinting.*

a lower peak power output and initial mean power output (0–10 seconds of the test) and reduced fatigue in the first 15 seconds of the test compared with 15- and 30-second all-out cycling bouts. Interestingly, there appears to be a relationship between rating of perceived exertion (RPE) and blood lactate concentration during long all-out sprints, suggesting the possibility of lactate acting as an afferent signal that influences RPE and the pacing strategy employed.[86] If this were the case, it would indicate that anticipatory regulation might play a role in modulating long distance sprint performance (Sections 6.3.2 and 6.4).

8.2.5   Sport and exercise lasting 10–30 seconds

The key performance requirements and associated fatigue mechanisms during sport and exercise lasting 10–30 seconds (referred to in this section as short-distance sprinting) are in Figure 8.8. Short-distance sprinting is defined as the equivalent of a 100–200-metre sprint (approximately 10–30 seconds of maximal effort). For optimal performance in short-distance sprinting, it is crucial for athletes to obtain and maintain their maximum- or near-maximum velocity throughout the race.[68] However, decrements in velocity of about 8% and 20% occur during 100 and 200-metre races, respectively.[84] In 100-metre running peak, velocity is attained about 40–60 metres into the race, after which it begins to decline.[87] A similar pattern is seen in the 200-metre race, except peak velocity tends to be lower and the drop-off in velocity

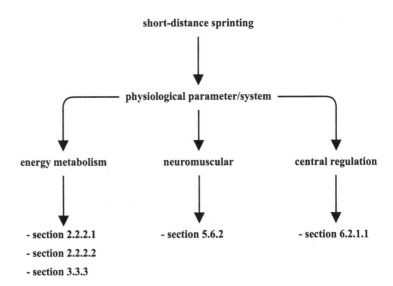

Figure 8.8 Potential causes of fatigue during sport and exercise lasting 10–30 seconds. Only those performance requirements that may play a direct significant role in the fatigue process are highlighted. The section numbers refer to sections of this book that discuss the potential causes of fatigue associated with each of the identified performance requirements.

smaller but of course going on for longer.[88] This velocity trend helps to explain how Usain Bolt set the 100 metre world record of 9.58 seconds in 2009, as during that race Bolt was able to maintain his peak velocity from 50 to 80 metres before beginning to slow. This indicates that the person most likely to win a short-duration sprint is the person who slows down the least during the race.

> **Key point 8.22**
>
> *Phosphocreatine contributes a significant amount of the ATP required during short distance sprinting, and strong associations are present between PCr availability and short-duration sprint performance. Therefore, PCr depletion has a performance limiting role during short distance sprinting.*

The aerobic/anaerobic energy contribution to a 100-metre run is approximately 10%–20%/80%–90%[89] and for a 200-metre run approximately 30%/70%.[67] Unsurprisingly, anaerobic metabolism is dominant, but the aerobic contribution of 10%–30% suggests that the aerobic system should not be completely ignored when training for short-distance sprinting.[67] Despite this suggestion, aerobic capacity does not appear to be related to performance in either the 100- or 200-metre run.[68] In contrast, performance in both distances is significantly related to anaerobic capacity.[68,89,90] Neuromuscular function and muscle power are also primary factors in performance during short-distance sprinting.[68]

8.2.5.1 What are the likely causes of fatigue during short-distance sprinting?

The short time to complete short-distance sprints may give the perspective that there are fewer and less complex causes of fatigue in this type of activity compared to endurance-based exercise. However, it is almost certain that the causes of fatigue during short-distance sprints are still multi-factorial.[91]

Phosphocreatine contributes approximately 50% of the ATP resynthesised during a 6-second sprint and 25% of the ATP during a 20-second sprint, with the remainder supplied by glycolysis and aerobic metabolism (Section 2.2.2.1 and Figure 2.2). The rapid reduction in PCr during sprinting may reduce the rate at which ATP can be resynthesised, thereby necessitating a reduction in running velocity. This suggestion is partly

> **Key point 8.23**
>
> *The concentrations of muscle and blood lactate, and reduction in blood pH, following a 100 m sprint are not sufficient to be a cause of fatigue. Significant reductions in muscle pH following a 20 second cycle sprint suggest that reduced pH may contribute to fatigue during sprints of this duration.*

supported by research showing a significant increase in running velocity during a 100-metre sprint following a period of creatine supplementation, which can increase muscle PCr concentrations.[92] Greater PCr availability could improve sprint performance by maintaining ATP resynthesis via high-energy phosphates for longer into the sprint.[92] The association between PCr resynthesis and subsequent sprint performance (Section 2.2.2.2) indicates that PCr depletion does play a limiting role in short-distance sprint performance.

While acidosis does not appear to play a significant role in fatigue during the 100-metre sprint, in the 200-metre sprint athletes are required to continue running maximally for a further 10 seconds or so. Following 20 seconds of cycle sprinting, muscle pH falls significantly.[93] This reduction in pH may be sufficient to impair performance via the mechanisms discussed elsewhere (Section 3.3.3).

Significant increases in muscle Pi concentrations have been reported following 10- and 20-second sprints.[93] However, it is very difficult to establish the time course of Pi accumulation *in vivo* during short-duration maximal sprinting. Therefore, it is difficult to know whether a sufficient intramuscular accumulation of Pi would occur quickly enough to cause any disturbances in Ca^{2+} kinetics or cross-bridge force production during, for example, a 100-metre sprint (Section 5.6.2).

Impaired membrane excitability does not appear to be a cause of fatigue for short-distance sprints.[84] In fact, no significant correlations have been found between speed decrement and peripheral metabolic or neuromuscular changes during short-distance sprinting.[84] Nevertheless, significant decreases in EMG activity of the leg muscles have been found following 100- and 200-metre sprints.[94] These changes may relate to suboptimal output from the motor cortex (perhaps due to reduced motor neuron/muscle responsiveness, Section 6.2.1.1), peripheral fatigue (see the above sections), or decreased sensitivity of the stretch reflex following short-distance sprints, perhaps via stimulation of type III and IV muscle afferents.[84,95] Reduced stretch reflex activity would impair the propulsive force of the athletes muscles, reducing muscle power, and, hence, speed.

8.2.6   Resistance exercise

Discussing fatigue mechanisms associated with resistance exercise requires a different approach to the previous sections. Resistance exercise is more of a training exercise as opposed to a competitive activity. Therefore, it is difficult to describe the performance requirements associated with success at resistance exercise, in contrast to highlighting the specific performance requirements of, say, prolonged submaximal activity vs. long distance sprinting. However, anyone who has tried resistance exercise will know that fatigue does occur, usually manifesting in muscle pain/discomfort, a reduction in the speed at which the resistance can be moved, and perhaps even a complete inability to continue moving the resistance. Specific causes of fatigue may differ depending on the type of resistance exercise that is being done, but the current body of literature investigating fatigue processes during different forms of whole-body resistance exercise is smaller than that for other activities. Therefore, this section will focus on resistance exercise that would elicit maximal- or near-maximal muscle contraction forces. The key performance requirements and associated fatigue mechanisms during resistance exercise are in Figure 8.9.

Recovery following maximal- or near-maximal lifting (i.e. strength exercise) appears to occur more quickly than recovery following submaximal lifting to failure.[96] This may appear paradoxical due to the possible perception that maximal lifting is 'tougher' than submaximal lifting. Importantly, though, it may indicate that fatigue processes in maximal strength exercise are different to those in submaximal endurance resistance exercise.

Key point 8.24

Recovery from maximal or near-maximal lifting is faster than recovery from submaximal lifting to failure. This suggests that fatigue processes in maximal lifting may be different to those during submaximal lifting.

Maximal strength exercise is generally carried out at a low repetition range (usually 1–5), interspersed with long recovery durations (2–5 minutes).[96] Due to this work/rest pattern, a set of maximal strength exercise will generally take no longer than approximately 10 seconds, followed by substantial recovery. Despite a short work bout, a maximal effort is required, therefore it is likely that substantial PCr depletion is seen following a set of maximal strength lifts.[96,97] This PCr depletion would reduce the rate of ATP resynthesis and could account at least partly for the decreased lifting velocity and reduced muscle torque seen following maximal- or near-maximal muscle activation.[98,99] This could also explain the more rapid recovery of muscle strength; by the time, the next set of lifting is required a notable resynthesis of PCr will have occurred, which would enable the athlete to achieve maximal lifting loads.[97] Therefore, PCr kinetics could play a role in performance during maximal strength training.

Significant correlations have also been found between reductions in muscle force and blood lactate concentration.[100] This correlation has led to the suggestion that fatigue during hypertrophy resistance exercise may be related to significant

Key point 8.25

Phosphocreatine depletion may contribute to reductions in lifting velocity and muscle torque during following maximal and near-maximal lifting. Inorganic phosphate accumulation and associated dysregulation of Ca^{2+} kinetics may also play a role, but this requires further study.

anaerobic glycolysis, H^+ production, and reduced muscle pH.[97] However, the issues with this hypothesis have been covered elsewhere (Section 3.3.3). A higher level of voluntary muscle activation (such as during maximal strength exercise) will lead to more rapid energy depletion and metabolite accumulation.[98] In the case of maximal strength exercise, one of the key metabolites to accumulate could be Pi via PCr breakdown. Accumulation of Pi may impair SR Ca^{2+} release, reducing muscle contractile force (Section 5.6.2).[98,101] However, direct measurements of such effects during maximal strength exercise are lacking. Furthermore, many studies have used electrical stimulation techniques on individual muscle groups as a model for the study of fatigue during maximal muscle contractions, and findings from such studies should be interpreted with this in mind.

Central and peripheral fatigue have been documented during maximal voluntary muscle contractions.[102] During a maximal isometric voluntary contraction muscle force production begins to fall almost immediately and the force increase induced by electrical stimulation increases, indicating the presence of central fatigue (Section 1.2.2).[103,104] A slowing of motor unit firing rates has been shown during sustained and repeated maximal muscle contractions,[105] and the mechanisms behind this are crucial for the understanding of central fatigue development during maximal muscle activation.[104] The potential mechanisms are quite complex; however, slowing of motor unit firing rate likely relates to one or more of the following: (1) A decrease in excitatory input through the motor neurons; (2) An increase in inhibitory input to the motor neurons; and (3) A decrease in the responsiveness of the motor neurons themselves to stimulation.[104] Evidence suggests that the slowing of motor unit firing rates is most likely due to a combination of decreased responsiveness of the motor neurons and inhibition of motor neuron firing (perhaps via group III and IV afferent stimulation and reduced muscle spindle activity, Section 6.2.1.1).[106,107] Excitatory input may not decrease but may become suboptimal by failing to compensate for changes to motor neuron function caused by reduced responsiveness and increased inhibition.[104]

Some studies have reported a lack of central fatigue during resistance exercise, implying an importance of peripheral fatigue.[100] However, the extent of peripheral fatigue may depend on muscle fibre

> **Key point 8.26**
>
> *Central fatigue may develop during maximal and near-maximal lifting via a number of potential changes in excitatory or inhibitory inputs to the motor neurons and/or decreased motor neuron responsiveness.*

> **Key point 8.27**
>
> *The relative influence of central and peripheral fatigue processes during resistance exercise may depend on factors such as muscle fibre type, resistance load, and training status.*

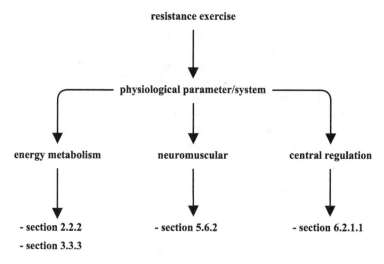

Figure 8.9 Potential causes of fatigue during resistance exercise. Only those performance requirements previously discussed in the book that may play a direct
significant role in the fatigue process are highlighted. The section numbers
refer to sections of this book that discuss the potential causes of fatigue associated with each of the identified performance requirements.

type, with type II fibres potentially more affected by peripheral fatigue,[108]
and the degree of central fatigue may depend on training status, with more
highly resistance-trained individuals capable of 'generating' more central fatigue.[100] Yet more evidence for the complexity of studying fatigue and drawing
conclusions.

8.3 Summary

- Prolonged submaximal sport and exercise should be considered relative to
  its intensity domain, particularly moderate-, heavy-, and severe-intensity
  domains, as fatigue mechanisms are likely to differ across these domains.
- During prolonged submaximal sport and exercise in the moderate-intensity
  domain, central fatigue is prominent, although there may be a contribution
  from muscle glycogen depletion and hyperthermia/hypohydration.
- Fatigue is most complex in the heavy-intensity domain. A range of peripheral and central mechanisms are at play that have direct impact on
  muscle contractile function and the ability of the CNS to drive muscle
  fibres.
- In the severe domain, physiological and metabolic steady state is impossible, leading to a progressive reduction in PCr concentration and tissue
  pH and increases in Pi, H^+, blood lactate concentration, extracellular K^+,
  and $\dot{V}O_2$. Anaerobic substrate depletion, accumulation of metabolic by-
  products, attainment of $\dot{V}O_2max$, or a combination of these contributes to
  fatigue, with peripheral mechanisms more important than central factors.

- During field-based team games, a transient fatigue occurs following high-intensity periods of activity and a more progressive fatigue develops towards the end of a game.
- The cause of transient fatigue during team games is not known, and it appears that decreased muscle and blood pH, PCr depletion, and altered muscle membrane excitability are not strong causative factors. It is interesting to consider the possibility of transient fatigue as a form of pacing during team games, perhaps as part of a central/anticipatory regulation of performance. However, this suggestion needs to be investigated.
- Progressive fatigue during team games may be influenced by muscle glycogen depletion, limitations to fluid intake (but not necessarily actual fluid loss), and central fatigue.
- Middle-distance activities may be impaired by H^+ production and reduced pH stimulating group III and IV afferents and/or desaturating arterial haemoglobin and inducing cerebral hypoxia, both of which would contribute to central fatigue. Significant extracellular K^+ accumulation can occur within the timeframe of middle-distance activity, which may impair muscle function. Inorganic phosphate and Mg^{2+} accumulation in muscle may also impair Ca^{2+} kinetics.
- Long distance sprinting may be impaired by altered excitation-contraction coupling, possibly via impaired SR function and Ca^{2+} kinetics, and PCr depletion. There may also be an aspect of anticipatory regulation of performance during long-distance sprinting and altered muscle contractile ability within 10 seconds of the onset of long-distance sprints.

Short-distance sprinting is impaired by PCr depletion. Performance in 200-metre sprinting may be impaired by reductions in muscle pH, but this is not a cause of fatigue in the 100-metre sprint. More research is required to determine the potential influence of Pi accumulation and altered Ca^{2+} kinetics on short sprint performance. Short sprint performance can also be impaired by alterations in neuromuscular function, possibly mediated by changes to motor neuron responsiveness, peripheral fatigue, or decreased stretch reflex sensitivity.

High-load resistance exercise may be impaired by PCr depletion and intramuscular metabolite accumulation. High-load resistance exercise may also be influenced by the development of central fatigue, although the relative influence of peripheral and central fatigue may depend on muscle fibre type and training status.

Test yourself

Answer the following questions to the best of your ability. Try to understand the information gained from answering these questions before you progress with the book.

1 What are the key physiological characteristics of prolonged sport and exercise performed in the moderate-, heavy-, and severe-intensity domains?
2 Outline and contrast the potential fatigue mechanisms during prolonged moderate-, heavy-, and severe-intensity activity.
3 Summarise the potential causes of fatigue during each of these activity types: field-based team games, middle-distance exercise, long distance sprinting, short-distance sprinting, and resistance exercise.

References

1 Faude O, Kindermann W, Meyer T. Lactate threshold concepts: how valid are they? *Sports Med.* 2009;39(6):469–490.
2 Poole DC, Burnley M, Vanhatalo A, Rossiter HB, Jones AM. Critical Power: an important fatigue threshold in exercise physiology. *Med Sci Sports Exerc.* 2016;48(11):2320–2334.
3 Burnley M, Jones AM. Power-duration relationship: physiology, fatigue, and the limits of human performance. *Eur J Sport Sci.* 2018;18(1):1–12.
4 Casa DJ, Armstrong LE, Hillman SK, et al. National athletic trainers' association position statement: fluid replacement for athletes. *J Athl Train.* 2000;35(2):212–224.
5 Hargreaves M, Spriet LL. Skeletal muscle energy metabolism during exercise. *Nat Metab.* 2020;2(9):817–828.
6 Purdom T, Kravitz L, Dokladny K, Mermier C. Understanding the factors that effect maximal fat oxidation. *J Int Soc Sports Nutr.* 2018;15:3.
7 Fornasiero A, Savoldelli A, Fruet D, Boccia G, Pellegrini B, Schena F. Physiological intensity profile, exercise load and performance predictors of a 65-km mountain ultra-marathon. *J Sports Sci.* 2018;36(11):1287–1295.
8 Hoffman MD, Rogers IR, Joslin J, Asplund CA, Roberts WO, Levine BD. Managing collapsed or seriously ill participants of ultra-endurance events in remote environments. *Sports Med.* 2015;45(2):201–212.
9 Leppik JA, Aughey RJ, Medved I, Fairweather I, Carey MF, McKenna MJ. Prolonged exercise to fatigue in humans impairs skeletal muscle Na+-K+-ATPase activity, sarcoplasmic reticulum Ca2+ release, and Ca2+ uptake. *J Appl Physiol (1985).* 2004;97(4):1414–1423.
10 Wada M, Kuratani M, Kanzaki K. Calcium kinetics of sarcoplasmic reticulum and muscle fatigue. *J Phys Fitness Sports Med.* 2013;2:169–178.
11 Noakes TD. The central governor model of exercise regulation applied to the marathon. *Sports Med.* 2007;37(4–5):374–377.
12 Davies CT, Thompson MW. Physiological responses to prolonged exercise in ultra-marathon athletes. *J Appl Physiol (1985).* 1986;61(2):611–617.
13 Martin V, Kerherve H, Messonnier LA, et al. Central and peripheral contributions to neuromuscular fatigue induced by a 24-h treadmill run. *J Appl Physiol (1985).* 2010;108(5):1224–1233.
14 Lepers R, Maffiuletti NA, Rochette L, Brugniaux J, Millet GY. Neuromuscular fatigue during a long-duration cycling exercise. *J Appl Physiol (1985).* 2002;92(4):1487–1493.
15 Coyle EF, Coggan AR, Hemmert MK, Ivy JL. Muscle glycogen utilization during prolonged strenuous exercise when fed carbohydrate. *J Appl Physiol (1985).* 1986;61(1):165–172.

16 Krustrup P, Soderlund K, Mohr M, Bangsbo J. The slow component of oxygen uptake during intense, sub-maximal exercise in man is associated with additional fibre recruitment. *Pflugers Arch.* 2004;447(6):855–866.

17 Black MI, Jones AM, Blackwell JR, et al. Muscle metabolic and neuromuscular determinants of fatigue during cycling in different exercise intensity domains. *J Appl Physiol (1985).* 2017;122(3):446–459.

18 Jones AM, Wilkerson DP, DiMenna F, Fulford J, Poole DC. Muscle metabolic responses to exercise above and below the "critical power" assessed using 31P-MRS. *Am J Physiol Regul Integr Comp Physiol.* 2008;294(2):R585–R593.

19 Sahlin K, Seger JY. Effects of prolonged exercise on the contractile properties of human quadriceps muscle. *Eur J Appl Physiol Occup Physiol.* 1995;71(2–3):180–186.

20 Burnley M, Vanhatalo A, Jones AM. Distinct profiles of neuromuscular fatigue during muscle contractions below and above the critical torque in humans. *J Appl Physiol (1985).* 2012;113(2):215–223.

21 Rossiter HB, Ward SA, Howe FA, Kowalchuk JM, Griffiths JR, Whipp BJ. Dynamics of intramuscular 31P-MRS P(i) peak splitting and the slow components of PCr and O2 uptake during exercise. *J Appl Physiol (1985).* 2002;93(6):2059–2069.

22 Dideriksen JL, Enoka RM, Farina D. Neuromuscular adjustments that constrain submaximal EMG amplitude at task failure of sustained isometric contractions. *J Appl Physiol (1985).* 2011;111(2):485–494.

23 Schafer LU, Hayes M, Dekerle J. The magnitude of neuromuscular fatigue is not intensity dependent when cycling above critical power but relates to aerobic and anaerobic capacities. *Exp Physiol.* 2019;104(2):209–219.

24 Guyenet PG, Bayliss DA. Neural control of breathing and CO2 homeostasis. *Neuron.* 2015;87(5):946–961.

25 Romer LM, Polkey MI. Exercise-induced respiratory muscle fatigue: implications for performance. *J Appl Physiol (1985).* 2008;104(3):879–888.

26 Aliverti A. The respiratory muscles during exercise. *Breathe.* 2016;12:165–168.

27 Duthie G, Pyne D, Hooper S. Applied physiology and game analysis of rugby union. *Sports Med.* 2003;33(13):973–991.

28 Gabbett T, King T, Jenkins D. Applied physiology of rugby league. *Sports Med.* 2008;38(2):119–138.

29 Bangsbo J, Mohr M, Krustrup P. Physical and metabolic demands of training and match-play in the elite football player. *J Sports Sci.* 2006;24(7):665–674.

30 Abt G, Zhou S, Weatherby R. The effect of a high-carbohydrate diet on the skill performance of midfield soccer players after intermittent treadmill exercise. *J Sci Med Sport.* 1998;1(4):203–212.

31 Mohr M, Krustrup P, Bangsbo J. Fatigue in soccer: a brief review. *J Sports Sci.* 2005;23(6):593–599.

32 Schimpchen J, Gopaladesikan S, Meyer T. The intermittent nature of player physical output in professional football matches: an analysis of sequences of peak intensity and associated fatigue responses. *Eur J Sport Sci.* 2021;21(6):793–802.

33 Bangsbo J, Norregaard L, Thorso F. Activity profile of competition soccer. *Can J Sport Sci.* 1991;16(2):110–116.

34 Bangsbo J, Mohr M. Variations in running speed and recovery time after a sprint during top-class soccer matches. *Med Sci Sports Exerc.* 2005;37:S87.

35 Mohr M, Krustrup P, Bangsbo J. Match performance of high-standard soccer players with special reference to development of fatigue. *J Sports Sci.* 2003;21(7):519–528.

36 Krustrup P, Mohr M, Steensberg A, Bencke J, Kjaer M, Bangsbo J. Muscle metabolites during a football match in relation to a decreased sprinting ability. Fifth World Congress of Soccer and Science; 2003; Lisbon, Portugal.

37 Krustrup P, Mohr M, Steensberg A, Bencke J, Kjaer M, Bangsbo J. Muscle and blood metabolites during a soccer game: implications for sprint performance. *Med Sci Sports Exerc.* 2006;38(6):1165–1174.

38 Krustrup P, Mohr M, Amstrup T, et al. The yo-yo intermittent recovery test: physiological response, reliability, and validity. *Med Sci Sports Exerc.* 2003;35(4):697–705.

39 Bangsbo J, Iaia FM, Krustrup P. Metabolic response and fatigue in soccer. *Int J Sports Physiol Perform.* 2007;2(2):111–127.

40 Krustrup P, Mohr M, Nybo L, et al. Muscle metabolism and impaired sprint performance in an elite women's football game. *Scand J Med Sci Sports.* 2022;32(Suppl 1):27–38.

41 Mohr M, Nielsen JJ, Bangsbo J. Caffeine intake improves intense intermittent exercise performance and reduces muscle interstitial potassium accumulation. *J Appl Physiol (1985).* 2011;111(5):1372–1379.

42 Balsom PD, Gaitanos GC, Soderlund K, Ekblom B. High-intensity exercise and muscle glycogen availability in humans. *Acta Physiol Scand.* 1999;165(4):337–345.

43 Mohr M, Vigh-Larsen JF, Krustrup P. Muscle glycogen in elite soccer – a perspective on the implication for performance, fatigue, and recovery. *Front Sports Act Living.* 2022;4:876534.

44 Maughan RJ, Shirreffs SM, Merson SJ, Horswill CA. Fluid and electrolyte balance in elite male football (soccer) players training in a cool environment. *J Sports Sci.* 2005;23(1):73–79.

45 Reilly T. Energetics of high-intensity exercise (soccer) with particular reference to fatigue. *J Sports Sci.* 1997;15(3):257–263.

46 Shirreffs SM, Aragon-Vargas LF, Chamorro M, Maughan RJ, Serratosa L, Zachwieja JJ. The sweating response of elite professional soccer players to training in the heat. *Int J Sports Med.* 2005;26(2):90–95.

47 Edwards AM, Noakes TD. Dehydration: cause of fatigue or sign of pacing in elite soccer? *Sports Med.* 2009;39(1):1–13.

48 McGregor SJ, Nicholas CW, Lakomy HK, Williams C. The influence of intermittent high-intensity shuttle running and fluid ingestion on the performance of a soccer skill. *J Sports Sci.* 1999;17(11):895–903.

49 Fortes LS, Nascimento-Junior JRA, Mortatti AL, Lima-Junior D, Ferreira MEC. Effect of dehydration on passing decision making in soccer athletes. *Res Q Exerc Sport.* 2018;89(3):332–339.

50 Edwards AM, Clark NA. Thermoregulatory observations in soccer match play: professional and recreational level applications using an intestinal pill system to measure core temperature. *Br J Sports Med.* 2006;40(2):133–138.

51 Aughey RJ, Goodman CA, McKenna MJ. Greater chance of high core temperatures with modified pacing strategy during team sport in the heat. *J Sci Med Sport.* 2014;17(1):113–118.

52 Robinson TA, Hawley JA, Palmer GS, et al. Water ingestion does not improve 1-h cycling performance in moderate ambient temperatures. *Eur J Appl Physiol Occup Physiol.* 1995;71(2–3):153–160.

53 Schlader ZJ, Simmons SE, Stannard SR, Mundel T. Skin temperature as a thermal controller of exercise intensity. *Eur J Appl Physiol.* 2011;111(8):1631–1639.

54 Temfemo A, Carling C, Ahmaidi S. Relationship between power output, lactate, skin temperature, and muscle activity during brief repeated exercises with increasing intensity. *J Strength Cond Res.* 2011;25(4):915–921.

55 Rahnama N, Lees A, Reilly T. Electromyography of selected lower-limb muscles fatigued by exercise at the intensity of soccer match-play. *J Electromyogr Kinesiol.* 2006;16(3):257–263.

56 Rampinini E, Bosio A, Ferraresi I, Petruolo A, Morelli A, Sassi A. Match-related fatigue in soccer players. *Med Sci Sports Exerc.* 2011;43(11):2161–2170.

57 Robineau J, Jouaux T, Lacroix M, Babault N. Neuromuscular fatigue induced by a 90-minute soccer game modeling. *J Strength Cond Res.* 2012;26(2):555–562.

58 Gandevia SC. Spinal and supraspinal factors in human muscle fatigue. *Physiol Rev.* 2001;81(4):1725–1789.

59 Badin OO, Smith MR, Conte D, Coutts AJ. Mental fatigue: impairment of technical performance in small-sided soccer games. *Int J Sports Physiol Perform.* 2016;11(8):1100–1105.

60 Kunrath CA, Nakamura FY, Roca A. How does mental fatigue affect soccer performance during small-sided games? A cognitive, tactical and physical approach. *J Sports Sci.* 2020;38(15):1818–1828.

61 Coutinho D, Goncalves B, Travassos B, Wong DP, Coutts AJ, Sampaio JE. Mental fatigue and spatial references impair soccer players' physical and tactical performances. *Front Psychol.* 2017;8:1–12.

62 Trecrori A, Boccolini G, Duca M, Formenti D, Alberti G. Mental fatigue impairs physical activity, technical and decision-making performance during small-sided games. *PLoS ONE.* 2020;15(9):1–12.

63 Gonzalez-Villora S, Prieto-Ayuso A, Cardoso F, Teoldo I. The role of mental fatigue in soccer: a systematic review. *Int J Sports Sci Coaching.* 2022;17(4):903–916.

64 Thompson C, Fransen J, Skorski S, et al. Mental fatigue in football: is it time to shift the goalposts? An evaluation of the current methodology. *Sports Med.* 2019;49:177–183.

65 Mezzani A, Hamm LF, Jones AM, et al. Aerobic exercise intensity assessment and prescription in cardiac rehabilitation: a joint position statement of the European association for cardiovascular prevention and rehabilitation, the American association of cardiovascular and pulmonary rehabilitation and the Canadian association of cardiac rehabilitation. *Eur J Prev Cardiol.* 2013;20(3):442–467.

66 Duffield R, Dawson B, Goodman C. Energy system contribution to 400-metre and 800-metre track running. *J Sports Sci.* 2005;23:299–307.

67 Spencer MR, Gastin PB. Energy system contribution during 200- to 1500-m running in highly trained athletes. *Med Sci Sports Exerc.* 2001;33:157–162.

68 Dal Pupo J, Arins FB, Guglielmo LGA, Da Silva R, Moro ARP, Santos SG. Physiological and neuromuscular indices associated with sprint running performance. *Res Sports Med.* 2013;21:124–135.

69 Ingham SA, Whyte GP, Pedlar C, Bailey DM, Dunman N, Nevill AM. Determinants of 800-m and 1500-m running performance using allometric models. *Med Sci Sports Exerc.* 2008;40:345–350.

70 Rabadan M, Diaz V, Calderon FJ, Benito PJ, Peinado AB, Maffulli N. Physiological determinants of speciality of elite middle- and long-distance runners. *J Sports Sci.* 2011;29:975–982.

71 Bird SR, Wiles J, Robbins J. The effect of sodium bicarbonate ingestion on 1500-m racing time. *J Sports Sci.* 1995;13:399–403.

72 Carr AJ, Gore CJ, Hopkins WG. Effects of acute alkalosis and acidosis on performance: a meta-analysis. *Sports Med.* 2011;41:801–814.

73 McNaughton LR, Siegler J, Midgley A. Ergogenic effects of sodium bicarbonate. *Curr Sports Med Rep.* 2008;7:230–236.

74 Wilkes D, Gledhill N, Smyth R. Effect of acute induced metabolic alkalosis on 800-m racing time. *Med Sci Sports Exerc.* 1983;15:277–280.

75 Bishop D, Edge J, Davis C, Goodman C. Induced metabolic alkalosis affects muscle metabolism and repeated-sprint ability. *Med Sci Sports Exerc.* 2004;36:807–813.

76 Knicker AJ, Renshaw I, Oldham ARH, Cairns SP. Interactive processes link the multiple symptoms of fatigue in sport competition. *Sports Med.* 2011;41:307–328.

77 Nybo L, Secher NH. Cerebral perturbations provoked by prolonged exercise. *Prog Neurobiol.* 2004;72:223–261.

78 Nielsen HB, Bredmose PR, Stromstad M, Volianitis S, Quistorff B, Secher NH. Bicarbonate attenuates arterial desaturation during maximal exercise in humans. *J Appl Physiol* 2002;93:724–731.

79 Hirvonen J, Nummela A, Rusko H, Rehunen S, Harkonen M. Fatigue and changes of ATP, creatine phosphate, and lactate during the 400-m sprint. *Can J Sport Sci.* 1992;17(2):141–144.

80 Nummela A, Vuorimaa T, Rusko H. Changes in force production, blood lactate and EMG activity in the 400-m sprint. *J Sports Sci.* 1992;10(3):217–228.

81 Hanon C, Gajer B. Velocity and stride parameters of world-class 400-meter athletes compared with less experienced runners. *J Strength Cond Res.* 2009;23(2):524–531.

82 Miguel PJ, Reis VM. Speed strength endurance and 400m performance. *New Stud Athlet.* 2004;19:39–45.

83 Hanon C, Lepretre PM, Bishop D, Thomas C. Oxygen uptake and blood metabolic responses to a 400-m run. *Eur J Appl Physiol.* 2010;109(2):233–240.

84 Tomazin K, Morin JB, Strojnik V, Podpecan A, Millet GY. Fatigue after short (100-m), medium (200-m) and long (400-m) treadmill sprints. *Eur J Appl Physiol.* 2012;112(3):1027–1036.

85 Lattier G, Millet GY, Martin A, Martin V. Fatigue and recovery after high-intensity exercise part I: neuromuscular fatigue. *Int J Sports Med.* 2004;25(6):450–456.

86 Wittekind AL, Micklewright D, Beneke R. Teleoanticipation in all-out short-duration cycling. *Br J Sports Med.* 2011;45(2):114–119.

87 Mackala K. Optimisation of performance through kinematic analysis of the different phases of the 100 metres. *New Stud Athlet.* 2007;22:7–16.

88 Mureika JR. Modelling wind and altitude effects in the 200 m sprint. *Can J Physiol.* 2003;81:895–910.

89 Duffield R, Dawson B, Goodman C. Energy system contribution to 100-m and 200-m track running events. *J Sci Med Sport.* 2004;7(3):302–313.

90 Nevill AM, Ramsbottom R, Nevill ME, Newport S, Williams C. The relative contributions of anaerobic and aerobic energy supply during track 100-, 400- and 800-m performance. *J Sports Med Phys Fitness.* 2008;48(2):138–142.

91 Maughan R, Gleeson M. *The Biochemical Basis of Sports Performance.* Oxford: Oxford University Press; 2004.

92 Skare OC, Skadberg, Wisnes AR. Creatine supplementation improves sprint performance in male sprinters. *Scand J Med Sci Sports.* 2001;11(2):96–102.

93 Bogdanis GC, Nevill ME, Lakomy HK, Boobis LH. Power output and muscle metabolism during and following recovery from 10 and 20 s of maximal sprint exercise in humans. *Acta Physiol Scand.* 1998;163(3):261–272.

94 Mero A, Peltola E. Neural activation in fatigued and non-fatigued conditions of short and long sprint running. *Biol Sport.* 1989;6:43–58.

95 Ross A, Leveritt M, Riek S. Neural influences on sprint running: training adaptations and acute responses. *Sports Med.* 2001;31(6):409–425.

96 Willardson JM. A brief review: factors affecting the length of the rest interval between resistance exercise sets. *J Strength Cond Res.* 2006;20:978–984.

97 Sahlin K, Ren JM. Relationship of contraction capacity to metabolic changes during recovery from a fatiguing contraction. *J Appl Physiol (1985).* 1989;67(2): 648–654.

98 Nordlund MM, Thorstensson A, Cresswell AG. Central and peripheral contributions to fatigue in relation to level of activation during repeated maximal voluntary isometric plantar flexions. *J Appl Physiol (1985).* 2004;96(1):218–225.

99 van den Tillaar R, Saeterbakken A. Effect of fatigue upon performance and electromyographic activity in 6-RM bench press. *J Hum Kinet.* 2014;40:57–65.

100 Ahtiainen JP, Hakkinen K. Effect of fatigue upon performance and electromyographic activity in 6-RM bench press. *J Strength Cond Res.* 2009;23:1129–1134.

101 Westerblad H, Allen DG. Recent advances in the understanding of skeletal muscle fatigue. *Curr Opin Rheumatol.* 2002;14(6):648–652.

102 Taylor JL, Allen GM, Butler JE, Gandevia SC. Supraspinal fatigue during intermittent maximal voluntary contractions of the human elbow flexors. *J Appl Physiol (1985).* 2000;89(1):305–313.

103 Gandevia SC, Allen GM, Butler JE, Taylor JL. Supraspinal factors in human muscle fatigue: evidence for suboptimal output from the motor cortex. *J Physiol.* 1996;490 (Pt 2)(Pt 2):529–536.

104 Taylor JL, Gandevia SC. A comparison of central aspects of fatigue in submaximal and maximal voluntary contractions. *J Appl Physiol (1985).* 2008;104(2):542–550.

105 Rubinstein S, Kamen G. Decreases in motor unit firing rate during sustained maximal-effort contractions in young and older adults. *J Electromyogr Kinesiol.* 2005;15(6):536–543.

106 Andersen B, Westlund B, Krarup C. Failure of activation of spinal motoneurones after muscle fatigue in healthy subjects studied by transcranial magnetic stimulation. *J Physiol.* 2003;551(Pt 1):345–356.

107 Butler JE, Taylor JL, Gandevia SC. Responses of human motoneurons to corticospinal stimulation during maximal voluntary contractions and ischemia. *J Neurosci.* 2003;23(32):10224–10230.

108 Boerio D, Jubeau M, Zory R, Maffiuletti NA. Central and peripheral fatigue after electrostimulation-induced resistance exercise. *Med Sci Sports Exerc.* 2005;37(6):973–978.

9 Influence of biological sex and training status on fatigue

9.1 Introduction

Chapter 8 discussed the crucial role that sport and exercise demand plays in the fatigue process. There are other factors that can also influence the how and why of fatigue, even within the same sport/exercise. This chapter will provide an overview of two of these factors: biological sex and training status. As with everything to do with sport and exercise physiology, biological sex and training status will also have interactive influences on fatigue.

9.2 Biological sex

As discussed throughout this book, the causes of fatigue during sport and exercise are specific to the demands of the task. This task specificity can vary between males and females because of biological sex differences in physiological responses to sport and exercise.[1,2] Much is yet to be discovered about the sex differences in fatigue during dynamic, whole-body sport and exercise.[1]

9.2.1 How does fatigue differ between males and females?

During sustained or intermittent isometric contractions at the same relative intensity, females appear to be less fatigable than males.[1,3] Fatigability between sexes seems to be influenced by muscle group, with less fatigability seen in females for the elbow flexors, back extensors, knee extensors, and respiratory muscles,[2-5] less of a sex difference for the dorsi flexors and plantar flexors,[6,7] and no sex difference for the elbow extensors.[8] The effect of sex on fatigability in specific muscle groups may depend on the neural, metabolic, and contractile make-up of each muscle group (discussed below). Sex differences in fatigability during isometric contractions also greatly diminish as the intensity of the contraction increases,[1-3,6,8,9] or when males and females are matched for muscle strength.

A similar pattern is seen during concentric muscle contractions, with females showing less fatigability than males, although the extent of the sex difference is smaller than for isometric contractions.[2] For concentric contractions,

DOI: 10.4324/9781003326137-12

sex differences in fatigability can be lessened by independently increasing the intensity and speed of contraction.[10,11] For eccentric contractions, a slightly different picture is seen. Muscle force reduction after repeated eccentric contractions is either similar between sexes[12] or is actually greater in females compared to males.[13]

Recent data compared for the first time the fatigue profile of males and females relative to the critical intensity (analogous to the critical power) during intermittent isometric knee extension exercise.[14] While absolute critical intensity was greater in males, relative critical intensity was actually greater in females. Interestingly, females lasted approximately twice as long during open-ended intermittent isometric contractions at 110% of critical intensity and showed less fatigability during a fixed-intensity task. The greater endurance in females was associated with less contractile impairment and faster recovery, which the authors attributed to less deoxygenation of the knee extensor muscles.[14]

Investigating the fatigue response to specific contraction types in isolated muscle groups is interesting but perhaps not the most relevant to sport and exercise contexts. A more externally valid model of research has investigated the fatigue response of males and females to repeated cycle sprints. This work has found that females are generally less fatigable (they show smaller reductions in power output) than males.[15] However, this is not a universal finding as some work shows no significant difference between sexes,[16] particularly when males and females are matched for initial power output. Females also seem to recover from repeated cycle sprints more quickly than males.[17]

> **Key point 9.1**
>
> *During sustained and intermittent isometric contractions, concentric contractions, and repeated sprints, females are less fatigable than males. However, less fatigability in females is dependent on the muscle group tested and is greatly reduced as the intensity of the contraction increases, or when sexes are matched for muscle strength.*

9.2.2   *What might explain sex differences in sport and exercise fatigue?*

From a physiological standpoint, numerous potential explanations exist for sex differences in fatigability. These are summarised in the following text, and in Figure 9.1.

In Section 9.2.1, it was mentioned that when males and females are matched for strength or power output, sex differences in fatigability are greatly reduced or even negated. There are minimal sex differences in strength per unit of muscle.[1] Therefore, it seems that a potential cause of sex differences in fatigability relates to absolute strength differences between males and females. The

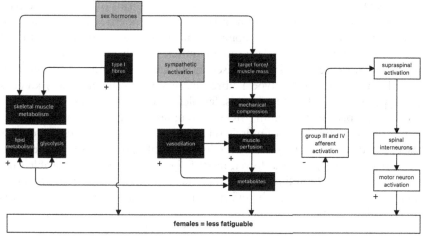

Figure 9.1 Potential physiological mechanisms behind the sex differences in muscle fatigability during sport and exercise. The relative impact of specific mechanisms will depend on the task (particularly type and intensity/strength of contraction, and muscle group(s) used). Black boxes = intramuscular processes; white boxes = nervous system processes; grey boxes = hormonal and sympathetic processes.

Source: Re-drawn from Hunter SK. *Acta Physiol (Oxf)*. 2014;210(4):768–789.

larger muscle mass and greater force exerted by males can generate mechanical and metabolic consequences that could exacerbate fatigue compared with females.[1]

Reduced blood flow to working muscle could exacerbate fatigue via changes in intramuscular metabolic and contractile conditions. Females have better muscle perfusion than males during low- to moderate-intensity isometric contractions (at least for some muscle groups).[5] Better perfusion in females may be due to less contraction-induced compression of the arteries supplying muscle with blood. The difference in arterial compression between sexes occurs because males generally exert greater absolute muscle force than females, thereby exerting more pressure on intramuscular arterial blood routes during contractions.[18] Alterations in muscle perfusion between sexes may also help to explain why sex differences in fatigability are reduced when the intensity of muscle contraction increases and when sexes are matched for strength. During high-intensity contractions, blood flow will be occluded to a similar level for both sexes,[9] as it would be if contraction strength was similar. However, females also have a greater ability to dilate the arteries that supply muscles with blood[19] and have greater capillarisation of certain muscle groups (particularly those with more type I fibres), which may also help them to perfuse their muscles better than males. Greater vasodilation in females is independent of strength.[1]

It is well known that males and females differ in terms of muscle fibre type and size, and therefore metabolism and contractile properties. Any one of these differences could influence fatigability. Females have a greater proportion of type I muscle fibres than males in many muscles involved in locomotion and functional movements.[20] Type I muscle fibres are more fatigue resistant than type II fibres. Specifically, type I fibres show slower calcium (Ca^{2+}) kinetics than type II fibres.[21] In line with this, females have been shown to have slower rates of sarcoplasmic reticulum (SR) Ca^{2+} reuptake than males,[22] which would contribute to a slower rate of muscle relaxation. Less muscle fatigue in females has been correlated with slower muscle contractile properties.[23] It therefore seems that females possess a slower, more fatigue-resistant muscle profile than males.[1] However, the influence of muscle fibre type on Ca^{2+} kinetics and rate of contraction indicate that the effect of these mechanisms on sex differences in fatigability will be muscle specific.[1]

Sex differences in muscle fibre type and contractile properties are also suggestive of differences in muscle metabolism during sport and exercise. Indeed, it has been shown that females use glycolysis to a lesser extent than males during high-intensity isometric contractions[24] and produce less blood lactate and a smaller reduction in adenosine triphosphate (ATP) during sprinting, probably due to greater type I fibre content.[25] Conversely, no sex difference is seen for phosphocreatine (PCr) or oxidative metabolism.[24] Females oxidise more fat and less carbohydrate than males during sport and exercise at the same relative intensity.[20] Again, this may relate in part to the greater type I fibre content of females as type I fibres are more suited to aerobically oxidising lipid. Taken together, the metabolic response of females to sport and exercise may be indicative of a more fatigue-resistant state, due to less production of potentially fatigue-inducing metabolites from anaerobic glycolysis and a lesser reliance on finite glycogen and blood glucose as an energy source (Sections 2.2.3 and 3.2).

Investigation of sex differences in voluntary muscle activation suggests that sex differences in fatigability may reside more in the periphery. There seem to be minimal sex differences in voluntary activation during brief maximal contractions of upper body muscles,[26] and no sex difference in the extent of central fatigue following low- and high-intensity isometric contractions of upper body muscles.[1] However, it does seem that males show a greater reduction than females in the ability to voluntarily activate lower limb muscles during maximal contractions.[27] A speculative suggestion for this upper-lower body sex difference is that males may generate

Key point 9.2

Females may be less fatigable than males due to differences in muscle perfusion, type I muscle fibre content, muscle energy metabolism and metabolite production, and, potentially, differences in voluntary muscle activation (at least of lower limb muscles).

greater peripheral afferent feedback from group III and IV muscle afferents in the lower limbs than females, perhaps due to the differences in muscle perfusion and metabolism discussed earlier.[1,28]

Finally, it is appropriate to address the potential influence of the female menstrual cycle on fatigability during sport and exercise. Currently, there is no clear evidence that fatigability is influenced by stages of the menstrual cycle,[29] at least during sport and exercise in normal environmental conditions. However, menstrual cycle stage may influence physiological and perceptual responses to prolonged submaximal sport and exercise in hot and humid conditions.[30]

9.3   Training status

In this section, training status refers to the predominant requirements/ qualities that an athlete wishes to develop/maximise through training in order to succeed in their sport. Once again, this is not as simple as it initially appears! Clearly, some sports overtly require great focus on endurance-based characteristics (often termed aerobic sports), for example, marathon running. Other sports have a clear focus on explosive power (often [and often erroneously] termed anaerobic sports), for example, the 100-metre sprint or field sports such as the shot-put. However, a huge range of sports require a combination of these "aerobic" and "anaerobic" qualities, for example, team games such as soccer and rugby. As with many aspects of physiology and fatigue, it would be incredibly complicated and perhaps counter-productive to try to align fatigue processes across the full spectrum of training statuses required in different sport and exercise situations. Instead, this section will highlight key aspects of physiology and psychophysiology and provide an overview of how differences in training status may affect these aspects and by extension fatigue processes.

9.3.1   *The influence of training status on fatigue mechanisms*

Different types of training can generate different and often quite specific physiological adaptations. Of course, training also increases the physical capacity of the body to perform sport and exercise. If different types of training yield different physiological adaptations, then it stands to reason that training *per se*, and specific types of training, may influence the fatigue mechanisms that can impair sport and exercise performance. For ease of reference, this section will specifically address the potential fatigue mechanisms discussed in Section 2 of this book and does not provide an all-encompassing overview of the myriad potential influences of training status on sport and exercise performance.

9.3.1.1   *Energy metabolism*

Classic adaptations to endurance training include increased muscle mitochondrial density, aerobic enzyme concentration and activity, and muscle capillarisation and perfusion that together improve the ability of the muscles to aerobically resynthesise ATP. Endurance training also increases the expression and activity of intramuscular fatty acid transport proteins and metabolic enzymes. Collectively, these adaptations enable an endurance-trained individual to oxidise more fat and less carbohydrate at a given relative intensity.[31,32]

Increased fat and reduced carbohydrate oxidation suggest that endurance-trained individuals may be able to reduce the rate at which they deplete endogenous glycogen stores during sport and exercise, and thereby be less affected by potential fatigue mechanisms associated with glycogen depletion (Section 2.2.3). For instance, one of the ways in which muscle glycogen depletion is thought to impair performance is by reducing SR Ca^{2+} release due to depletion of intramyofibrillar glycogen and an associated impairment of ATP resynthesis near the muscle triads (Section 2.2.3.2.1). Type I muscle fibres contain more subsarcolemmal and intramyofibrillar glycogen than type II fibres.[33] As endurance-trained athletes will likely have a greater proportion of type I muscle fibres, this may confer an advantage by increasing the amount of time before intramyofibrillar glycogen is depleted. The subcellular localisation of glycogen is influenced by training status,[34] with subsarcolemmal glycogen accumulating most rapidly through training.[33] However, while subsarcolemmal and intermyofibrillar glycogen can be increased after several weeks of endurance training, intramyofibrillar glycogen concentration may only increase after long-term training or in highly trained athletes.[33] Highly endurance-trained athletes do still show impairment in SR Ca^{2+} release that is associated with low intramyofibrillar glycogen content[35]; however, the association between low muscle glycogen and fatigue is less pronounced in more highly trained people.[35] While endurance training may not increase intramyofibrillar glycogen concentrations, it could be speculated that it may attenuate the rate of intramyofibrillar glycogen depletion, thereby delaying the onset of potential dysregulation of SR Ca^{2+} kinetics. While some authors have implicated differences in training status as a reason for different study findings,[35] more specific research is required that compares subcellular glycogen use and associated SR dysfunction in people of differing training states.

Performance during repeated-sprint sport and exercise is related to the ability to break down PCr during the sprint and replenish it during the subsequent recovery period (Section 2.2.2.2). Sprint-trained athletes have the highest PCr degradation rates,[36] probably due in part to greater activity of creatine kinase in type II muscle fibres,[37] of which sprint-trained athletes will likely have a greater proportion. Conversely, endurance-trained athletes have the greatest PCr resynthesis rates.[38] Replenishment of PCr stores is reliant on the aerobic resynthesis of ATP, and strong positive correlations have been found between submaximal measures of endurance performance, $\dot{V}O_2max$, and PCr resynthesis rates.[39,40] The relationship between aerobic fitness and PCr resynthesis rate suggests that during repeated-sprint sport and exercise more aerobically fit individuals would begin each sprint with higher PCr concentrations, which may attenuate reductions in sprint performance attributed to PCr depletion. Indeed, it has been shown that endurance-trained people maintain power output significant better than team games players during ten 6 second sprints interspersed with 30 seconds recovery.[41] The greater rate of PCr depletion in sprint/power-trained people and greater rate of resynthesis of PCr in endurance-trained people suggest that sprint/power athletes may be more susceptible to any fatiguing effects of

> **Key point 9.3**
>
> *Endurance-trained people oxidise more fat and less carbohydrate at a given relative intensity which may reduce, or delay, the influence of fatigue mechanisms associated with glycogen depletion. Endurance training may also increase the rate of PCr resynthesis, enabling better maintenance of performance during repeated-sprint activity.*

PCr depletion, particularly during repeated-sprint exercise (Sections 2.2.2.1 and 2.2.2.2). These findings also suggest that from a training perspective, it is important for team games players to develop aerobic fitness as well as sprint speed/power, as this may improve PCr resynthesis rate and enable better high-intensity performance throughout a match. This suggestion is supported by research showing improvements in sprint number and overall match intensity following 8 weeks of aerobic interval training in soccer players.[42] However, it is not possible to conclusively attribute this improved performance to mechanisms associated with PCr kinetics (Section 8.2.2.1.1).[43]

9.3.1.2 Metabolic acidosis

Team games athletes have a greater muscle hydrogen (H^+) buffering capacity than endurance-trained or untrained people.[44] Greater muscle buffer capacity may enable greater performance during high-intensity sport and exercise, particularly involving repeated sprints. This suggestion is supported by work showing a correlation between muscle buffer capacity and work completed during repeated sprints, meaning that the greater the muscle buffer capacity the more work could be completed.[45] Greater muscle buffer capacity of team games players may be an adaptation to the type of training they carry out, which would involve repeated bouts of high-intensity sport and exercise that may stimulate adaptations to buffering processes.[44]

Sprint-trained athletes tend to have a higher prevalence of type II muscle fibres. These muscle fibres contain high concentrations of glycogen and anaerobic enzymes and are therefore able to generate energy via anaerobic glycolysis more effectively than type I fibres. Anaerobic glycolysis produces lactate and H^+ (Section 3.3) and it appears to be important for optimal function to remove particularly H^+ from the muscle. Type II muscle fibres contain a much larger concentration of monocarboxylate transporter 4 (MCT4) protein than type I fibres.[46] These transporters function to remove lactate and H^+ from the muscle cells and move it either into the blood or into adjacent muscle cells for use in aerobic ATP resynthesis (Sections 3.3 and 3.3.1).[47] Therefore, individuals with a greater type II fibre profile may be more effective at removing lactate and H^+ from working muscle.

While sprint-trained athletes may have specific mechanisms for buffering and transporting lactate and H^+, it appears that endurance training also causes adaptations that may influence lactate and H^+ production and removal. Firstly, endurance athletes tend to have greater proportions of type I muscle fibres which are more suited to oxidative metabolism. As a result, endurance-trained athletes produce less muscle lactate at a given intensity than non-endurance-trained athletes.[48,49] Secondly, endurance training is designed to potentiate the aerobic capacity of these muscle fibres. The ability to remove blood lactate has been strongly correlated with muscle oxidative capacity.[50] This may relate to the finding that the expression of MCT1 is greater in type I muscle fibres and that aerobic training increases the expression of MCT1 protein in the sarcolemma and mitochondria of skeletal muscle.[47,51] Sarcolemmal MCT1 may contribute to lactate and H^+ uptake into type I fibres from the blood and removal to other muscle fibres in the cell-cell lactate shuttle, and mitochondrial MCT1 could facilitate intracellular transport of lactate and H^+ into the mitochondria to take part in oxidative ATP resynthesis.[47,52,53]

The nature of lactate and H^+ movement into and out of the blood and skeletal muscle is complex, influenced by muscle morphology and the sport and exercise demand, and is still being investigated. However, the fundamental role of training status is that sprint-trained and team games athletes have more effective muscle lactate/H^+ buffering and removal processes than endurance-trained athletes, and in turn, endurance-trained athletes are more effective at transporting lactate and H^+ into adjacent muscle fibres for use in aerobic ATP resynthesis, and have muscle fibre profiles that produce less lactate and H^+ at a given relative intensity.

> **Key point 9.4**
>
> *Team games athletes have a greater muscle H^+ buffering capacity than endurance or sprint-trained athletes. Sprint-trained athletes are able to move lactate and H^+ out of the muscle very effectively. Endurance-trained athletes produce less lactate and H^+ at a given relative intensity and have an enhanced ability to move lactate and H^+ into muscle mitochondria for use in the aerobic resynthesis of ATP.*

9.3.1.3 *Thermoregulation*

There is some suggestion that people with greater aerobic fitness are better able to tolerate sport and exercise in high ambient temperatures than less aerobically fit people.[54] More aerobically fit people begin exercise in hot conditions with a lower core temperature, are able to continue exercising for significantly longer, and end exercise with a significantly higher core temperate than less fit people.[55] If aerobic fitness is able to offset some of the negative influences of hyperthermia (Section 4.6), it may be of benefit to performance, particularly prolonged sport and exercise as recent work indicates that aerobic fitness has a positive impact on evaporative heat loss only up to moderate-intensity activity.[56] Neuroendocrine markers of central fatigue appear to follow a temperature-dependent increase and be similarly present in trained and untrained people at exhaustion during exercise in the heat.[57]

Unsurprisingly, the ability of more aerobically fit people to better tolerate sport and exercise in the heat has been attributed to the regular exercise that is likely undertaken by fitter people. More specifically, aerobically fitter people are able to tolerate a higher core temperature during sport and exercise, suggesting that a given core temperature increase generates a greater relative thermal strain in less-fit individuals.[57] Aerobically fitter people encounter a lower circulatory strain at a given core temperature during sport and exercise in the heat due to their greater blood volume and stroke volume,[58] which also enables increased skin blood flow for a given core temperature.[54] However, cardiovascular responses of trained and untrained people during sport and exercise in the heat do not support the suggestion that less cardiovascular strain enables fitter people to better tolerate sport and exercise in the heat.[59] Endurance training facilitates cutaneous vasodilation at a lower core temperature, reduces the internal temperature threshold for sweating, increases sweat rate at a given core temperature, and increases maximal sweat rate.[54] All of these adaptations would facilitate greater heat loss earlier on in a sport and exercise bout.

The perception of physiological strain during sport and exercise in the heat is also lower for more aerobically trained individuals.[57] This finding again suggests that trained people are able to tolerate higher core temperatures during sport and exercise due to the familiarity of regular increases in core temperature during training.[59] Intriguingly, this suggestion links greater exercise tolerance of aerobically fit people to the anticipatory model of sport and exercise regulation, particularly the use of prior exercise experience in developing a perception of the bout to come (Section 6.3.2, Figure 6.4, and Table 6.1). It is also possible that lower body fat enables a greater tolerance to sport and exercise in the heat, as fat has a greater capacity for heat storage than

> **Key point 9.5**
>
> *Aerobically trained people have a greater ability to tolerate sport and exercise in high temperatures which is linked to the ability to tolerate higher core temperatures. This ability may be related to lower cardiovascular strain, reduced perception of physical strain, and lower body fat levels.*

lean tissue.[59] The influence of body fat on tolerance to sport and exercise in the heat may be independent of aerobic fitness.[59]

As is generally the case with the intricate and interrelated human physiological responses to sport and exercise, it is likely that the mechanisms behind aerobically fitter people's ability to better tolerate sport and exercise in the heat are multifaceted. It must also be considered that not all research supports the influence of aerobic fitness on greater tolerance to sport and exercise in the heat.[60]

9.3.1.4   Calcium and potassium kinetics

Type II muscle fibres have a faster Ca^{2+} release from and uptake into the SR, a greater rate of Ca^{2+} release per muscle action potential, and more Ca^{2+} binding sites on troponin C than type I fibres.[61,62] These differences contribute to the greater force production and faster contraction velocity of type II fibres and demonstrate how the mechanics of a muscle fibre are suited to its function. However, type I muscle fibres have greater SR Ca^{2+} concentrations which would better facilitate Ca^{2+} release by increasing the open probability of SR release channels.[63] The greater open probability of Ca^{2+} release channels may also make the SR of type I fibres less susceptible to potentially inhibiting effects of Mg^{2+} (Sections 5.6.2 and 5.6.3)[64] and less susceptible to fatigue.[62] Furthermore, type II muscle fibres show greater increases in Pi concentration than type I muscle fibres due to their ability to break down ATP and PCr at faster rates.[65] Greater intramuscular Pi concentration in type II fibres may make them more susceptible to Ca^{2+}-Pi precipitation in the SR (Section 5.6.2).

Despite the potentially beneficial properties of type I muscle fibres with regard to Ca^{2+} kinetics, fatigue significantly impairs SR Ca^{2+} release and uptake in endurance-trained, resistance-trained, and untrained individuals.[21] However, the decline in SR function is greater in untrained compared with endurance-trained people. Furthermore, the extent of impairment in SR function is correlated with the percentage of type II fibres, suggesting a greater functional impairment in this fibre type.[21] Interestingly, short-term endurance training causes a reduction in the rate of SR Ca^{2+} release and uptake.[66] While at first glance this may be counter-intuitive and suggestive of a negative training adaptation, reduced Ca^{2+} kinetics may actually represent the beginning of functional changes geared towards improving the oxidative capacity of the muscle.[66] Indeed, longer duration endurance training

---

Key point 9.6

The function of the sarcoplasmic reticulum of type I muscle fibres may be less impaired by Mg^{2+} and Pi accumulation than that of type II fibres. Indeed, the decline in sarcoplasmic reticulum function during sport and exercise is related to type II fibre content. Endurance, resistance, and sprint training all increase Na^+, N^+ pump content, suggesting all forms of training may improve the ability to attenuate extracellular K^+ accumulation

increases levels of proteins involved in skeletal muscle Ca^{2+} handling,[67] and similar findings have also been reported in type II muscle fibres.[68]

High-intensity intermittent training reduces extracellular potassium (K^+) accumulation during incremental single-leg exercise to exhaustion.[69] It appears that reduced extracellular K^+ accumulation following training is due to greater reuptake of K^+ into the muscle via increased activity of sodium (Na^+), K^+ pumps.[51,69] Density of skeletal muscle Na^+, K^+ pumps is increased by about 14%–20% by endurance training, 16% by sprint training, and 10%–18% by high-intensity intermittent and resistance training.[51,70–72] It therefore appears that individuals involved in most forms of training may be able to improve their ability to attenuate extracellular K^+ accumulation. However, this may be of most importance to sprint/power-based athletes, as type II muscle fibres may be more susceptible to extracellular K^+ accumulation.[62]

9.3.1.5 Central governor/anticipatory regulation of performance

As mentioned in Section 6.5, central/anticipatory regulation of performance as proposed by existing models (Section 6.3.2 and Figure 6.4) is controversial, complex, and very difficult to experimentally study. Therefore, perhaps unsurprisingly, the influence of training status on central/anticipatory regulation has not been sufficiently well isolated in a research setting.

The employment of a pacing strategy during sport and exercise (Section 6.4.3) may provide support for central/anticipatory regulation of performance, as it is proposed that continual adjustment of intensity occurs in line with a pre-developed template rating of perceived exertion (RPE) which is developed by peripheral afferent feedback, knowledge of expected sport and exercise demands, and prior exercise experience (Figure 6.4). It has been shown that the ability to refine a pacing strategy in order to complete a given task more quickly or efficiently is improved with training and experience (Section 6.4.3). If pacing strategies are indeed part of a central/anticipatory regulation of performance designed to enable sport and exercise completion without significant physical damage, then training experience may be crucial to the success of this regulatory system.

Afferent peripheral feedback is also proposed to contribute to the generation of conscious RPE that is used as a regulator of sport and exercise performance (Section 6.3.2,

Key point 9.7

Training status and prior sport and exercise experience improve the ability to pace during sport and exercise. If pacing strategies are indicative of central/anticipatory regulation, then training experience may be beneficial in this process. People with greater training status may also generate less peripheral afferent feedback, potentially improving the comparison between conscious RPE and template RPE, and hence performance.

Figure 6.4). Training, particularly high-intensity aerobic and more traditional endurance training, may attenuate the potential influence of sport and exercise-induced peripheral metabolic, ionic, and thermoregulatory alterations on fatigue at a given intensity. Therefore, it could be suggested that individuals of a higher training status may generate less peripheral afferent feedback at a given intensity which could translate to a more favourable comparison between conscious and template RPE during sport and exercise, and hence, better performance. This suggestion is supported by research showing lower RPE at a given relative intensity in aerobically fitter individuals compared to those of lower fitness levels.[73]

9.3.1.6   *Mental fatigue*

Research investigating the impact of mental fatigue on sport and exercise performance is in its relative infancy (Chapter 7). However, there is some evidence which suggests that training status may influence the impact of mental fatigue on performance. Martin *et al.*[74] demonstrated that professional road cyclists were more resistant to the negative performance impact of mental fatigue than recreational road cyclists. Whether or not this difference is underpinned by physiological, psychological, or psychophysiological differences, and whether any of these differences are genetic and/or developed through training and lifestyle is yet to be determined. More work needs to be done which sheds light on the mechanisms underpinning the impact of mental fatigue on sport and exercise performance; then, armed with this knowledge, future investigations can better study the potential impact of training status on mental fatigue.

> **Key point 9.8**
>
> *Greater endurance training status may reduce the impact of mental fatigue on sport and exercise performance. However, more research in this area is required.*

9.4   Summary

* Females appear less fatigable than males during sustained and intermittent isometric contractions, concentric contractions, and repeated sprinting. The better fatigability of females is greatly reduced or negated with increasing contraction intensity, or when sexes are matched for strength.
* Reasons for the greater fatigability of females include better muscle perfusion, greater type I muscle fibre content, differences in metabolic responses to sport and exercise, and better voluntary activation of the lower limb muscles.

- Endurance-trained individuals oxidise more fat and less carbohydrate at a given relative intensity and are able to replenish PCr at a faster rate. This may negate, or at least delay, fatigue processes associated with glycogen depletion and enable better maintenance of performance during repeated-sprint activity.
- Team games athletes have a greater ability to buffer muscle H^+ production than endurance-trained or untrained people, which may enable greater repeated-sprint performance. Type II muscle fibres contain greater MCT4 content, which may allow sprint-trained athletes to move lactate and H^+ out of the muscle more effectively. Endurance-trained athletes not only tend to have a muscle fibre profile that favours reduced lactate and H^+ production but also have greater muscle MCT1 content, which may allow better transport of lactate and H^+ from cell to cell, and also transport into the mitochondria for use in aerobic ATP resynthesis.
- Individuals with a higher aerobic fitness can better tolerate sport and exercise in high temperatures, seemingly due to a greater tolerance for high core temperatures and a host of adaptations that facilitate heat loss at lower intensities and greater heat loss for a given intensity.
- Type I muscle fibres have greater SR Ca^{2+} concentrations, which will facilitate Ca^{2+} release and make the SR less susceptible to inhibitory influences during sport and exercise. Type II fibres show greater increases in Pi concentration, which may increase susceptibility to Ca^{2+}-Pi precipitation in the SR.
- Endurance-trained individuals report a lower RPE at a given relative intensity and demonstrate training adaptations that may attenuate potential afferent feedback from peripheral changes in metabolic, ionic, and thermoregulatory status. If central/anticipatory performance regulation is governed by afferent peripheral feedback and conscious RPE, then it may mean that endurance-trained people are less "held-back" by this performance-regulating system. However, this suggestion requires experimental study.
- Initial work suggests that endurance training status may reduce the impact of mental fatigue on performance. However, more work is required in the field of mental fatigue and sport and exercise performance in order to confirm and expand on these initial findings.

Test yourself

Answer the following questions to the best of your ability. Try to understand the information gained from answering these questions before you progress with the book.

1 List the potential reasons why females show less fatigability than males during some forms of sport and exercise.
2 Why might the sex difference in fatigability be reduced, or even negated, with greater muscle contraction intensities or when sexes are matched for strength?

3 How might endurance training reduce the impact of fatigue processes associated with glycogen depletion? How may it enable better maintenance of repeated-sprint performance?
4 How might different types of training influence potential fatigue mechanisms associated with metabolic acidosis?
5 Summarise the influence of endurance training on the tolerance to sport and exercise in the heat.
6 How are Ca^{2+} kinetics influenced by muscle fibre type? How does this relate to specific training statuses?
7 How might training status be speculated to influence the potential role of central/anticipatory regulation and mental fatigue on sport and exercise performance?

References

1 Hunter SK. Sex differences in human fatigability: mechanisms and insight to physiological responses. *Acta Physiol (Oxf)*. 2014;210(4):768–789.
2 Hunter SK. Sex differences and mechanisms of task-specific muscle fatigue. *Exerc Sport Sci Rev.* 2009;37(3):113–122.
3 Guenette JA, Romer LM, Querido JS, et al. Sex differences in exercise-induced diaphragmatic fatigue in endurance-trained athletes. *J Appl Physiol (1985)*. 2010;109(1):35–46.
4 Fulco CS, Rock PB, Muza SR, et al. Slower fatigue and faster recovery of the adductor pollicis muscle in women matched for strength with men. *Acta Physiol Scand.* 1999;167(3):233–239.
5 Hunter SK, Enoka RM. Sex differences in the fatigability of arm muscles depends on absolute force during isometric contractions. *J Appl Physiol (1985)*. 2001;91(6):2686–2694.
6 Avin KG, Naughton MR, Ford BW, et al. Sex differences in fatigue resistance are muscle group dependent. *Med Sci Sports Exerc.* 2010;42(10):1943–1950.
7 Donguk J, M. G, Bioldeau M. Sex differences in central and peripheral fatigue induced by sustained isometric ankle plantar flexion. *J Electromyogr Kinesiol.* 2022;65:1–10.
8 Dearth DJ, Umbel J, Hoffman RL, Russ DW, Wilson TE, Clark BC. Men and women exhibit a similar time to task failure for a sustained, submaximal elbow extensor contraction. *Eur J Appl Physiol.* 2010;108(6):1089–1098.
9 Yoon T, Schlinder Delap B, Griffith EE, Hunter SK. Mechanisms of fatigue differ after low- and high-force fatiguing contractions in men and women. *Muscle Nerve.* 2007;36(4):515–524.
10 Maughan RJ, Harmon M, Leiper JB, Sale D, Delman A. Endurance capacity of untrained males and females in isometric and dynamic muscular contractions. *Eur J Appl Physiol Occup Physiol.* 1986;55(4):395–400.
11 Senefeld J, Yoon T, Bement MH, Hunter SK. Fatigue and recovery from dynamic contractions in men and women differ for arm and leg muscles. *Muscle Nerve.* 2013;48(3):436–439.
12 Power GA, Dalton BH, Rice CL, Vandervoort AA. Delayed recovery of velocity-dependent power loss following eccentric actions of the ankle dorsiflexors. *J Appl Physiol (1985)*. 2010;109(3):669–676.

13 Sewright KA, Hubal MJ, Kearns A, Holbrook MT, Clarkson PM. Sex differences in response to maximal eccentric exercise. *Med Sci Sports Exerc.* 2008;40(2):242–251.

14 Ansdell P, Brownstein CG, Skarabot J, et al. Sex differences in fatigability and recovery relative to the intensity-duration relationship. *J Physiol.* 2019;597(23):5577–5595.

15 Billaut F, Bishop DJ. Mechanical work accounts for sex differences in fatigue during repeated sprints. *Eur J Appl Physiol.* 2012;112(4):1429–1436.

16 Smith KJ, Billaut F. Tissue oxygenation in men and women during repeated-sprint exercise. *Int J Sports Physiol Perform.* 2012;7(1):59–67.

17 Laurent CM, Green JM, Bishop PA, et al. Effect of gender on fatigue and recovery following maximal intensity repeated sprint performance. *J Sports Med Phys Fitness.* 2010;50(3):243–253.

18 Hunter SK, Griffith EE, Schlachter KM, Kufahl TD. Sex differences in time to task failure and blood flow for an intermittent isometric fatiguing contraction. *Muscle Nerve.* 2009;39(1):42–53.

19 Parker BA, Smithmyer SL, Pelberg JA, Mishkin AD, Herr MD, Proctor DN. Sex differences in leg vasodilation during graded knee extensor exercise in young adults. *J Appl Physiol (1985).* 2007;103(5):1583–1591.

20 Roepstorff C, Thiele M, Hillig T, et al. Higher skeletal muscle alpha2AMPK activation and lower energy charge and fat oxidation in men than in women during submaximal exercise. *J Physiol.* 2006;574(Pt 1):125–138.

21 Li JL, Wang XN, Fraser SF, Carey MF, Wrigley TV, McKenna MJ. Effects of fatigue and training on sarcoplasmic reticulum Ca(2+) regulation in human skeletal muscle. *J Appl Physiol (1985).* 2002;92(3):912–922.

22 Harmer AR, Ruell PA, Hunter SK, et al. Effects of type 1 diabetes, sprint training and sex on skeletal muscle sarcoplasmic reticulum Ca2+ uptake and Ca2+-ATPase activity. *J Physiol.* 2014;592(3):523–535.

23 Wust RC, Morse CI, de Haan A, Jones DA, Degens H. Sex differences in contractile properties and fatigue resistance of human skeletal muscle. *Exp Physiol.* 2008;93(7):843–850.

24 Russ DW, Lanza IR, Rothman D, Kent-Braun JA. Sex differences in glycolysis during brief, intense isometric contractions. *Muscle Nerve.* 2005;32(5):647–655.

25 Esbjornsson M, Sylven C, Holm I, Jansson E. Fast twitch fibres may predict anaerobic performance in both females and males. *Int J Sports Med.* 1993;14(5):257–263.

26 Keller ML, Pruse J, Yoon T, Schlinder-Delap B, Harkins A, Hunter SK. Supraspinal fatigue is similar in men and women for a low-force fatiguing contraction. *Med Sci Sports Exerc.* 2011;43(10):1873–1883.

27 Martin PG, Rattey J. Central fatigue explains sex differences in muscle fatigue and contralateral cross-over effects of maximal contractions. *Pflugers Arch.* 2007;454(6):957–969.

28 Tiller NB, Elliott-Sale KJ, Knechtle B, Wilson PB, Roberts JD, Millet GY. Do sex differences in physiology confer a female advantage in ultra-endurance sport? *Sports Med.* 2021;51:895–915.

29 Janse de Jonge XA. Effects of the menstrual cycle on exercise performance. *Sports Med.* 2003;33(11):833–851.

30 Janse DEJXA, Thompson MW, Chuter VH, Silk LN, Thom JM. Exercise performance over the menstrual cycle in temperate and hot, humid conditions. *Med Sci Sports Exerc.* 2012;44(11):2190–2198.

31 Phillips SM, Green HJ, Tarnopolsky MA, Heigenhauser GF, Hill RE, Grant SM. Effects of training duration on substrate turnover and oxidation during exercise. *J Appl Physiol (1985).* 1996;81(5):2182–2191.

32 Venables MC, Achten J, Jeukendrup AE. Determinants of fat oxidation during exercise in healthy men and women: a cross-sectional study. *J Appl Physiol (1985)*. 2005;98(1):160–167.

33 Nielsen J, Holmberg HC, Schroder HD, Saltin B, Ortenblad N. Human skeletal muscle glycogen utilization in exhaustive exercise: role of subcellular localization and fibre type. *J Physiol*. 2011;589(Pt 11):2871–2885.

34 Nielsen J, Ortenblad N. Physiological aspects of the subcellular localization of glycogen in skeletal muscle. *Appl Physiol Nutr Metab*. 2013;38(2):91–99.

35 Ortenblad N, Nielsen J, Saltin B, Holmberg HC. Role of glycogen availability in sarcoplasmic reticulum Ca2+ kinetics in human skeletal muscle. *J Physiol*. 2011;589(Pt 3):711–725.

36 Hirvonen J, Rehunen S, Rusko H, Harkonen M. Breakdown of high-energy phosphate compounds and lactate accumulation during short supramaximal exercise. *Eur J Appl Physiol Occup Physiol*. 1987;56(3):253–259.

37 Yamashita K, Yoshioka T. Profiles of creatine kinase isoenzyme compositions in single muscle fibres of different types. *J Muscle Res Cell Motil*. 1991;12(1):37–44.

38 Takahashi H, Inaki M, Fujimoto K, et al. Control of the rate of phosphocreatine resynthesis after exercise in trained and untrained human quadriceps muscles. *Eur J Appl Physiol Occup Physiol*. 1995;71(5):396–404.

39 Bogdanis GC, Nevill ME, Boobis LH, Lakomy HK, Nevill AM. Recovery of power output and muscle metabolites following 30 s of maximal sprint cycling in man. *J Physiol*. 1995;482 (Pt 2)(Pt 2):467–480.

40 Yoshida T, Watari H. Metabolic consequences of repeated exercise in long distance runners. *Eur J Appl Physiol Occup Physiol*. 1993;67(3):261–265.

41 Hamilton AL, Nevill ME, Brooks S, Williams C. Physiological responses to maximal intermittent exercise: differences between endurance-trained runners and games players. *J Sports Sci*. 1991;9(4):371–382.

42 Helgerud J, Engen LC, Wisloff U, Hoff J. Aerobic endurance training improves soccer performance. *Med Sci Sports Exerc*. 2001;33(11):1925–1931.

43 Glaister M. Multiple sprint work: physiological responses, mechanisms of fatigue and the influence of aerobic fitness. *Sports Med*. 2005;35(9):757–777.

44 Edge EJ, Bishop D, Hill-Haas S, Dawson B, Goodman C. Comparison of muscle buffer capacity and repeated-sprint ability of untrained, endurance-trained and team-sport athletes. *Eur J Appl Physiol*. 2006;96(3):225–234.

45 Bishop D, Edge J, Davis C, Goodman C. Induced metabolic alkalosis affects muscle metabolism and repeated-sprint ability. *Med Sci Sports Exerc*. 2004;36(5):807–813.

46 Juel C, Halestrap AP. Lactate transport in skeletal muscle – role and regulation of the monocarboxylate transporter. *J Physiol*. 1999;517(Pt 3):633–642.

47 Dubouchaud H, Butterfield GE, Wolfel EE, Bergman BC, Brooks GA. Endurance training, expression, and physiology of LDH, MCT1, and MCT4 in human skeletal muscle. *Am J Physiol Endocrinol Metab*. 2000;278(4):E571–E579.

48 Berg K. Endurance training and performance in runners: research limitations and unanswered questions. *Sports Med*. 2003;33(1):59–73.

49 Holloszy JO, Coyle EF. Adaptations of skeletal muscle to endurance exercise and their metabolic consequences. *J Appl Physiol Respir Environ Exerc Physiol*. 1984;56(4):831–838.

50 Thomas C, Sirvent P, Perrey S, Reynaud E, Mercier J. Relationships between maximal muscle oxidative capacity and blood lactate removal after supramaximal exercise and fatigue indexes in humans. *J Appl Physiol* 2004;97:2132–2138.

51 Juel C. Training-induced changes in membrane transport proteins of human skeletal muscle. *Eur J Appl Physiol.* 2006;96(6):627–635.

52 Gladden LB. Lactate metabolism: a new paradigm for the third millennium. *J Physiol.* 2004;558(Pt 1):5–30.

53 Thomas C, Perrey S, Lambert K, Hugon G, Mornet D, Mercier J. Monocarboxylate transporters, blood lactate removal after supramaximal exercise, and fatigue indexes in humans. *J Appl Physiol (1985).* 2005;98(3):804–809.

54 Periard JD, Eijsvogels TMH, Daanen HAM. Exercise under heat stress: thermoregulation, hydration, performance implications, and mitigation strategies. *Physiol Rev.* 2021;101(4):1873–1979.

55 Cheung SS, McLellan TM. Heat acclimation, aerobic fitness, and hydration effects on tolerance during uncompensable heat stress. *J Appl Physiol (1985).* 1998;84(5):1731–1739.

56 Notley SR, Lamarche DT, Meade RD, Flouris AD, Kenny GP. Revisitng the influence of individual factors in heat exchange during exercise in dry heat using direct calorimetry. *Exp Physiol.* 2019;104(7):1038–1050.

57 Wright HE, Selkirk GA, Rhind SG, McLellan TM. Peripheral markers of central fatigue in trained and untrained during uncompensable heat stress. *Eur J Appl Physiol.* 2012;112(3):1047–1057.

58 Hopper MK, Coggan AR, Coyle EF. Exercise stroke volume relative to plasma-volume expansion. *J Appl Physiol (1985).* 1988;64(1):404–408.

59 Selkirk GA, McLellan TM. Influence of aerobic fitness and body fatness on tolerance to uncompensable heat stress. *J Appl Physiol (1985).* 2001;91(5):2055–2063.

60 Mora-Rodriguez R. Influence of aerobic fitness on thermoregulation during exercise in the heat. *Exerc Sport Sci Rev.* 2012;40(2):79–87.

61 Allen DG, Lamb GD, Westerblad H. Skeletal muscle fatigue: cellular mechanisms. *Physiol Rev.* 2008;88(1):287–332.

62 Stephenson DG, Lamb GD, Stephenson GM. Events of the excitation-contraction-relaxation (E-C-R) cycle in fast- and slow-twitch mammalian muscle fibres relevant to muscle fatigue. *Acta Physiol Scand.* 1998;162(3):229–245.

63 Sitsapesan R, Williams AJ. The gating of the sheep skeletal sarcoplasmic reticulum Ca(2+)-release channel is regulated by luminal Ca2+. *J Membr Biol.* 1995;146(2):133–144.

64 Fryer MW, Stephenson DG. Total and sarcoplasmic reticulum calcium contents of skinned fibres from rat skeletal muscle. *J Physiol.* 1996;493(Pt 2):357–370.

65 Fitts RH. The cross-bridge cycle and skeletal muscle fatigue. *J Appl Physiol (1985).* 2008;104(2):551–558.

66 Green HJ, Burnett M, Kollias H, Ouyang J, Smith I, Tupling S. Malleability of human skeletal muscle sarcoplasmic reticulum to short-term training. *Appl Physiol Nutr Metab.* 2011;36(6):904–912.

67 Ferreira JC, Bacurau AV, Bueno CR, Jr., et al. Aerobic exercise training improves Ca2+ handling and redox status of skeletal muscle in mice. *Exp Biol Med (Maywood).* 2010;235(4):497–505.

68 Morissette MP, Susser SE, Stammers AN, et al. Differential regulation of the fiber type-specific gene expression of the sarcoplasmic reticulum calcium-ATPase isoforms induced by exercise training. *J Appl Physiol (1985).* 2014;117(5):544–555.

69 Nielsen JJ, Mohr M, Klarskov C, et al. Effects of high-intensity intermittent training on potassium kinetics and performance in human skeletal muscle. *J Physiol.* 2004;554(Pt 3):857–870.

70 Fraser SF, Li JL, Carey MF, et al. Fatigue depresses maximal in vitro skeletal muscle Na(+)-K(+)-ATPase activity in untrained and trained individuals. *J Appl Physiol (1985)*. 2002;93(5):1650–1659.

71 McKenna MJ, Schmidt TA, Hargreaves M, Cameron L, Skinner SL, Kjeldsen K. Sprint training increases human skeletal muscle Na(+)-K(+)-ATPase concentration and improves K+ regulation. *J Appl Physiol (1985)*. 1993;75(1):173–180.

72 Green H, Dahly A, Shoemaker K, Goreham C, Bombardier E, Ball-Burnett M. Serial effects of high-resistance and prolonged endurance training on Na+-K+ pump concentration and enzymatic activities in human vastus lateralis. *Acta Physiol Scand*. 1999;165(2):177–184.

73 Travlos AK, Marisi DQ. Perceived exertion during physical exercise among individuals high and low in fitness. *Percept Mot Skills*. 1996;82(2):419–424.

74 Martin K, Staiano W, Menaspa P, et al. Superior inhibitory control and resistance to mental fatigue in professional road cyclists. *PLoS One*. 2016;11(7):1–15.

Section 4

Summary

Where next?

10 Conclusion

10.1 Where next?

Chapter 1 introduced some of the main ways in which fatigue can be measured and quantified. The importance of ensuring that measured variables reflect potentially fatigue-causing mechanisms, and the difficulty in measuring some potential modulators of fatigue, was discussed. New and emerging technology that is being implemented in the study of fatigue in sport and exercise was also introduced. Technological advances and the development of new measurement procedures enable access to new avenues of study and a greater understanding and appreciation of a research area, and such advances have driven many of the recent developments in the study of the physiological regulation of sport and exercise.

Technological developments usually move at quite a rapid pace. Therefore, future research into fatigue in sport and exercise should, and almost certainly will, make use of these developments. It would be futile to suggest which specific mechanisms, organs, or variables should be focussed on, as often the technological advance leads us to the next fatigue candidate, as opposed to the candidate necessitating the technological development. Therefore, the targets of fatigue research in the coming years may not have even been identified yet. However, there is certainly scope for further investigation into potential mechanisms of fatigue that have already been identified. For example, how we perceive the sensation of effort during sport and exercise, the sensing of various peripheral biochemical and metabolic changes, how these signals may be integrated and contribute to the development of fatigue, and the role of the brain in fatigue (dependent and independent of peripheral signalling and effort perception) all require better understanding and a clearer application to the fatigue process. This is just one example of ongoing study that needs to be developed and explored further, as it may lead us in new directions of investigation.

Throughout this book, it has been stated that fatigue in almost all situations is likely to be an integrated, complex, and multifaceted occurrence. Traditional experimental research involves manipulating a single variable and measuring

DOI: 10.4324/9781003326137-14

the effect of that change on a specific outcome measure, while carefully controlling for any other factors that could also influence the outcome measure. While this level of control is beneficial for producing valid results regarding the effect of the manipulated variable, it is not reflective of the way the body functions during sport and exercise. The human response to sport and exercise is complex and highly integrated (particularly as sport and exercise influences almost all body organs and systems). Therefore, it is important that research attempts to reflect this complexity as much as possible, as changing or focussing on only one variable at a time will not give the full picture of the influence of that change, such as the "knock on" influence of the change on other variables/organs/body systems. An example of this is the association between lactate/lactic acid production and the development of fatigue (both lactate and lactic acid are referred to on purpose; see Section 3.3). Isolated measurement of high rates of lactate/lactic acid production at the point of fatigue led to the conclusion that lactate/lactic acid production causes fatigue. However, wider investigation into the dynamics of anaerobic glycolysis and the fate of intramuscular lactate has completely reshaped our understanding of the role of lactate/lactic acid in the fatigue process (Chapter 3). This change in thinking may have also encouraged the development of other lines of enquiry into fatigue development, as we could no longer fall back on the traditional explanation of lactate/lactic acid as the fatigue-inducing culprit.

There are examples in the literature of studies that attempt to "re-create" the integrated human sport and exercise response, and the authors of such studies should be commended. The reason why this is not routinely done is that it is extremely difficult to retain the experimental control necessary for the results to have meaning. However, if fatigue research is to truly understand its subject and provide answers as well as more questions, then new technologies and measurement tools must maximise our ability to study the development of a multifaceted phenomenon in the most appropriate way possible. Progress in this direction since publication of the first edition of this book is visible, and hopefully will continue.

While specific research designs should try to use an integrative approach, so should fatigue researchers themselves. One of the hindrances when trying to assimilate fatigue research on a particular topic is the different procedures and measurements used by different research groups, even when those groups are studying a very similar topic. If someone reads two articles on a particular aspect of fatigue that appear to contradict one another, can that person be assured that the contrasting results represent genuine conflict about the topic or could it simply be due to the different protocols used in the two studies? It is of course inappropriate to state that every research study on a particular topic should use the same methodology. However, it would be useful for research into fatigue in sport and exercise to be more collaborative so that different research groups could confer on the best ways in which to study a particular topic, and then conduct those studies in a way that generates larger and more cohesive data sets which can be compared and contrasted with greater meaning, as opposed to study findings being compared on the basis of differences in the research approach. This may further knowledge in a more economical and time-efficient manner. It must be said that research groups in most areas of research would be happy to collaborate more with colleagues, but logistical issues (finance/funding, time, institutional restrictions etc.) often get in the way. Therefore, this suggestion is made from an "ideal world" perspective. Nevertheless, if it could happen, then it may significantly benefit the study of fatigue in sport and exercise.

Aside from the use of emerging technologies, many of the discussion points above could to some extent be negated by using the paradigm of fatigue as a global symptom of the disease caused by sport and exercise (Section 1.2.4). One of the main tenets of this paradigm is that fatigue should not be compartmentalised or fragmented, meaning that it may become easier to establish common methodologies on which to study fatigue. Similarly, the use of more well-defined outcome measures, alongside the self-reporting of fatigue, could overcome issues related to the selection of study outcome measures. At the time of writing, this alternative perspective of fatigue has gained some traction in the literature but has not become the dominant paradigm on which fatigue research is based. Therefore, it is difficult to judge the impact that the paradigm has had/will have on fatigue. Hopefully, in the coming years, more work will use this paradigm as a basis for studying fatigue. It will be interesting to observe how the findings of this research build on, and perhaps require us to re-evaluate, the knowledge gained from the wealth of more "traditional" fatigue research.

10.2 A word of caution

The preface of this book mentioned that it was not possible to encompass the full scope of sport and exercise fatigue research into a single text and that the focus was on some of the most prevalent fatigue hypotheses that have produced significant research interest and/or entered public consciousness, and some contemporary issues in fatigue research. It is important that readers remember this and do not see the book as the final word on all possible causes of sport and exercise fatigue. The book is a good place to start, but further study and exploration is encouraged (see Section 10.3).

The book has also focussed almost exclusively on physiological causes of fatigue or causes that at least have a physiological component in their hypothesis/model. Doubtless there are potential contributions to fatigue in sport and exercise from psychological, nutritional (beyond energy availability), and biomechanical variables, in addition to the interesting perspective on sport and exercise, fatigue brought by aspects of pathophysiology and other pathologies. Hopefully, this book may act as a stimulus for other authors to address such factors in a similar way.

10.3   Staying informed

Our understanding of fatigue in sport and exercise has expanded and deepened exponentially in the last few decades, due in part to the development of new technologies and research methodologies as mentioned in Section 10.1. There is no reason to believe that this rate of knowledge development will stop; in fact, it is more likely to increase. The rapidly evolving landscape of fatigue research reinforces the need to keep your knowledge up to date. Doing so will allow you to share the correct knowledge with colleagues/clients/students/athletes and will help to prevent the perpetuation of outdated concepts.

It is easy to say that knowledge should remain up to date but it is another thing to achieve it (particularly in the wide-ranging and conflicting world of sport and exercise fatigue research). This section will provide some hints and tips for maintaining a contemporary knowledge base in sport and exercise fatigue, as well as some things to be aware of to ensure that knowledge is being gained from the most appropriate and trusted sources. The following is not an exhaustive list; it is more a core strategy that can be employed to assist you in staying informed. Use the advice as you see fit and explore other ways of keeping informed that work for you.

10.3.1   *Ways to stay informed*

10.3.1.1   *Access the primary literature*

While this strategy may be the most obvious one, it is also the most important. Simply put, "access the primary literature" means "read the research"! More specifically, it means read original research designed to address a focussed research question related to fatigue in sport and exercise. This is not only a useful strategy but it is also deceptively difficult, particularly in a topic that covers as many bases as fatigue research. Accessing the primary literature will likely throw up some tricky questions and scenarios, for example:

- Do I need to look back at the historical research in order to better understand the contemporary studies?
- If I should look at the historical work, how far back should I go?
- What are the "seminal" studies in each particular field of fatigue research?
- There is so much potentially relevant original work in each field of fatigue research; I feel lost before I even begin.

Some of the potential stumbling blocks that may be encountered when trying to develop and maintain a knowledge base of fatigue in sport and exercise may be alleviated by initially accessing a recent review of research on the topic. A literature review can come in at least two forms. A narrative review is where the author collates a comprehensive number of studies related to the topic of the review and describes the studies with a particular focus on methodological approach, key results, and the interpretation of those results by the original authors. Narrative reviews are therefore overviews of a topic, with the collation of the studies not driven by a regimented protocol of selection (thereby precluding replication) and potentially open to author bias. Systematic reviews try to overcome these limitations. Systematic reviews attempt to review a body of evidence with the aim of addressing a particular question. For example, a systematic review could address the question: *does attainment of a critical core temperature cause fatigue during exercise in the heat in highly trained marathon runners?* The authors of the review would then set about searching for all available literature related to this question using multiple methods of study retrieval (online databases, searching of study reference lists, etc.). Importantly, the authors would need to access all literature on the topic regardless of the study findings, as a systematic review must be unbiased in its presentation of knowledge. Each study is then assessed for eligibility against pre-defined criteria and included or excluded from the review. Included studies are then evaluated in terms of their methodological approach, and key findings are summarised and combined to provide an "answer" to the original question and to provide evidence-based recommendations for further study that may be needed. Sometimes a systematic review will include statistical analysis, such as in meta-analyses where a standardised effect size is calculated for the effect of the intervention in each individual study, and these effect sizes can be compared and/or combined to gain a clearer view of the magnitude of effect of an intervention. Importantly, the authors of a systematic review will publish their study retrieval and assessment protocol in full detail so that it could be replicated (much in the same way as authors of original studies publish their methodology). If the systematic review procedure was sufficiently rigorous and unbiased, then replication of the process should lead to the same conclusions.

While review articles are a useful tool for gaining an overarching insight into a topic, they are still a summary of the topic and are not a substitute for reading the primary literature. Therefore, reviews should be used as a starting point in understanding a topic, and as a way of identifying key early and more contemporary primary literature.

10.3.1.2   *Identify the "key players"*

Keeping your knowledge of fatigue in sport and exercise up to date may prove challenging due to the large amount of existing research, the rate of new publications, and the breadth of the field. It may help to streamline your literature searches by identifying the names of key authors or research groups that have a track-record of publications in a particular area(s) of sport and exercise fatigue. Online research databases incorporate an advanced search facility where keyword-based searches can be focussed by the addition of among other selections, publication date ranges, and the names of author(s). Using these tools may enable you to track down relevant historical and contemporary papers in a more efficient way.

While it is critical to the development and maintenance of your knowledge to search databases of peer-reviewed research publications, other avenues of information should not be discounted. For example, many academics and researchers produce expert statements, guest articles, and other contributions for popular sport, health, fitness, and medical publications such as magazines, websites, and lay-books. One of the main reasons many academics/researchers do this is to improve communication between producers of science and potential consumers of that science and thereby demonstrate real-world impact of their research findings. This is particularly important for academics as sometimes it is difficult to implement research findings in a real-world setting. If key players involved in researching fatigue in sport and exercise are making the effort to achieve greater real-world impact, then students of sport and exercise fatigue should make the most of such opportunities.

10.3.1.3   Social media

Other ways in which academics/researchers may engage is via social media. In recent years, many researchers have developed a presence on social media and professional networking sites such as ResearchGate, Twitter, and Linkedin, among others. These sites are freely available to the public, only requiring registration to create a user profile. Once registered, users can "follow" other users and gain access to the information they share.

Sites such as ResearchGate encourage users to post research publication lists and conference presentations, allowing followers to see the track-record, as well as the latest work, of authors who's work they are interested in. These sites often have the facility to post questions on topics, which other users who have interest/expertise in the question can answer. Sites such as Linkedin also allow users to post research publications, as well as such information as employment history and research interests. Such sites may also allow users to "advertise" their skills and services, thereby encouraging professional networking. Finally, sites such as Twitter allow users to post short comments/observations about any topic they wish, links to other websites/articles/publications, and allow users to enter conversation with one another.

It is increasingly common for academics/researchers to use social media to increase awareness of their research. This is often done by simply discussing ongoing research, seeking advice/collaborations on a proposed research study, or providing "sneak-peeks" of new research data pre-publication. Many researchers also provide links to contemporary research of others that they find interesting or relevant, thereby providing another avenue for discovering new research. Academics may also enter discussions and debates with one another, which sometimes provides a unique opportunity to gain access to the combined knowledge and perspectives of a researcher and his/her professional network.

Social media can be a powerful tool in gaining a greater understanding of current knowledge in a particular area of research, the key people who are developing this knowledge, emerging developments in the field, and providing communication access to the key players in ways that may not otherwise be possible. However, it is important to carefully cultivate a social media presence. Things to consider include which individuals/groups to follow, what information you may wish to share with users, and that any communication with fellow users should be carried out in a professional manner. Finally, even though you may be engaging on social media with professional academics and researchers, it should be remembered that much of the comments and information shared may be based on opinion and will not necessarily have gone through any formal vetting/review process. Therefore, be wary of taking all social media communications at face value and consider doing additional research or asking further questions as required.

10.3.1.4 Professional memberships

Several large sport and exercise science governing bodies/organisations exist who's purpose includes acting as professional registers and support structures for those working in various aspects of the sport and exercise science industry and working to raise and maintain the professional standards of sport and exercise science. Examples of such bodies (there are many others) include the British Association of Sport and Exercise Sciences (BASES), the European Congress of Sports Science (ECSS), and the American College of Sports Medicine (ACSM). Many of these organisations offer membership to those working in different roles within sport and exercise science, and to students of the discipline.

Some governing bodies, particularly BASES and the ACSM, periodically publish position statements written by experts in the field. These position statements represent the most up to date viewpoint on a particular topic and may also include recommendations and guidelines as appropriate. For example, a periodic position statement regarding fluid intake in sport and exercise is published by the ACSM. This position statement provides a review of the literature related to dehydration, rehydration, and fluid intake strategies in sport and exercise, makes inferences regarding the strength of existing evidence within each of these aspects, and provides recommendations for fluid intake practices. Governing bodies and organisations also organise special working groups comprised academics from specific fields that work to develop research strategies and foster collaborative research opportunities. An annual student conference is held by BASES and is open to all undergraduate and postgraduate sport and exercise science students, who can submit to present their research at the conference. The conference also features talks and other presentations by established academics and researchers, as well as networking opportunities and career advice. Most governing bodies/organisations also regularly publish their own members' magazine containing news from across the sport and exercise sciences, expert letters and articles, and opportunities to write in with questions about various aspects of sport and exercise science. Finally, many governing bodies/organisations hold short workshops on a variety of topics and issues in sport and exercise science, where attendees can address the issues and debate the latest findings.

Becoming a member of one or more of these governing bodies/associations can provide access to the above facilities. Such access provides another way of keeping up to date with the goings on in sport and exercise science in general, and possibly with research into fatigue in sport and exercise.

10.3.2   Potential problems when trying to stay informed

10.3.2.1   The mainstream media

It is important to be able to address the mainstream media (newspapers, online news websites, television/radio) reporting of scientific findings from a critical perspective. This is because reporting in the mainstream media can be subject to misinterpretation (of study findings, researcher interviews/comments etc.), misunderstanding (for example, by the reporter or editor), reporter/publisher bias (a particular "spin" placed on a study finding to reflect the agenda of the publication), and sensationalism (dramatically overstating or overreaching the study findings to make the implications significantly more positive, negative, or impactful). Such reporting can contribute to inaccurate perceptions of scientific concepts by the lay-person, and to the persistent belief in incorrect information that has been alluded to at various points throughout this book. As a student of the sciences, it is important that you can identify such reporting issues (perhaps using some of the strategies discussed in Section 10.3.1 and others you develop yourself) and pass this on to others who may not have the same background knowledge to do this for themselves (see Section 10.4). By doing this, you will contribute to the more accurate viewing of science as a gradual development in knowledge over many small steps, rather than large leaps and sweeping generalisations. You may also help to prevent the development of "incorrect truths" arising from misrepresented scientific research.

10.3.2.2   Who is making the claims?

Section 10.3.1.3 discussed how social media can be a very useful tool for accessing the latest news, views, and research findings. However, the section also cautioned that even though social media interactions may be with key players in the field (see Section 10.3.1.2), many of the views shared might be based on personal perspectives and may not have been formally vetted/reviewed for accuracy or substantiation. The same applies to individuals making claims/statements about scientific findings via all forms of media. It is important to consider who is making the statements/claims to evaluate their veracity. Key questions that may help you to do this include:

- What is the professional background of the individual?
- Is the individual involved in the research on which the claims are based, or is the research being used "second hand"?

- What companies/organisations does the individual work for?
- Does the individual have any financial/commercial/professional affiliations that could present a conflict of interest or potentially bias the statements they are making?

A healthy dose of scepticism is a good thing as it motivates you to look a little deeper and not passively accept all that you see or hear.

10.4 A final word

Writing this book has at times been quite challenging. One of the reasons for this is because it can be daunting (and sometimes disheartening) to delve into the huge body of literature into fatigue in sport and exercise to answer questions, challenge misconceptions, or simply provide more insight into any of the myriad topics in this area. My role as an academic and researcher has afforded me experience of sifting through research studies and collating findings to reach a consensus about current knowledge in a topic. Nevertheless, it was at times exasperating to go through this process with the fatigue literature due to the volume of disparate and contradictory research findings that have been published over the years and continue to be published today. Going through this process has given me a clearer appreciation (and sympathy!) for students of the sport and exercise sciences, and any other interested individuals, who try to do the same thing to further their knowledge. My experiences have also reinforced the importance of one of the key aims of the book: to collate current thinking on some key hypotheses/theories in sport and exercise fatigue in a clear, easy-to-understand way.

I hope that this aim has been achieved. I hope that you feel able to use this book as a starting point or a guide for your studies into fatigue in sport and exercise. I also hope that you have been provided with an informative and thought-provoking insight into some of the current thinking in this field. Finally, I hope that you feel motivated and inspired to use the knowledge and insights gained from reading the book in whatever ways are appropriate to you both personally and professionally, and to spread this new knowledge and insight to friends and colleagues. In the preface, I mentioned that the reader should not expect that at the end of the book, they would know precisely what causes fatigue in sport and exercise as many of the answers to this question have not yet been found. You probably now understand the accuracy of this statement! However, even if you are motivated simply to spread the word on all that we *don't* yet know regarding fatigue in sport and exercise, this would be useful as well as accurate. In the process of communicating the complexity of fatigue and the limitations to our knowledge, you will also communicate that many of the long-held beliefs regarding what causes fatigue are limited in their ability to explain fatigue or have even been disregarded as causes of fatigue in sport and exercise. The message is that in whatever way is relevant to you, it is beneficial to talk about fatigue in sport and exercise.

Index

Note: **Bold** page numbers refer to tables and *italic* page numbers refer to figures.

Printed in the United States
by Baker & Taylor Publisher Services